THE Blue Zones Kitchen

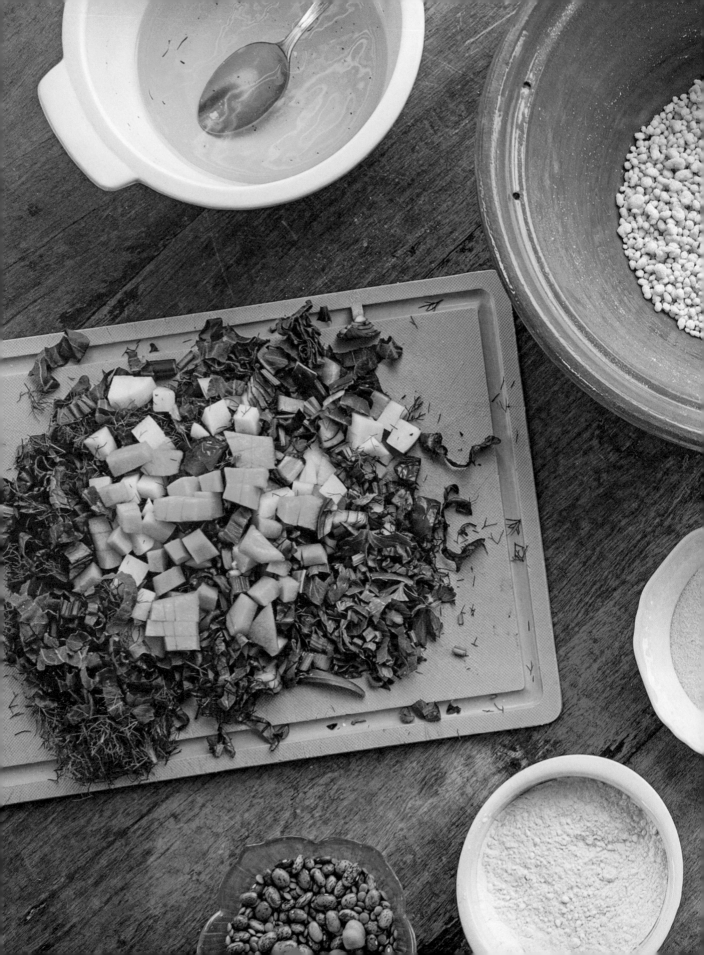

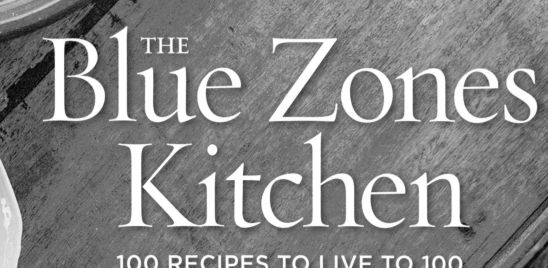

THE
Blue Zones
Kitchen

100 RECIPES TO LIVE TO 100

DAN BUETTNER

WITH PHOTOGRAPHS BY DAVID McLAIN

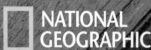

NATIONAL GEOGRAPHIC

WASHINGTON, D.C.

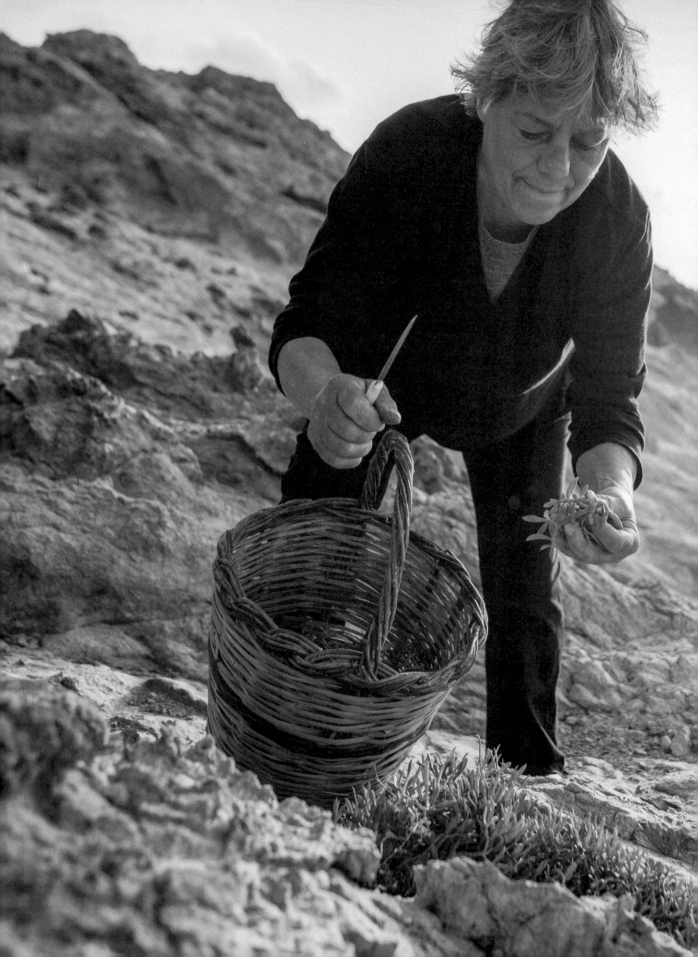

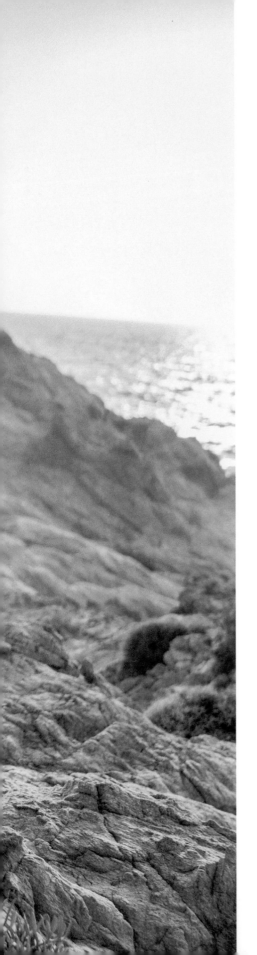

CONTENTS

In Ikaria, locals forage for wild greens on the rocky seaside. Many dishes use these greens, which may contribute to the blue zone's lower rates of dementia.

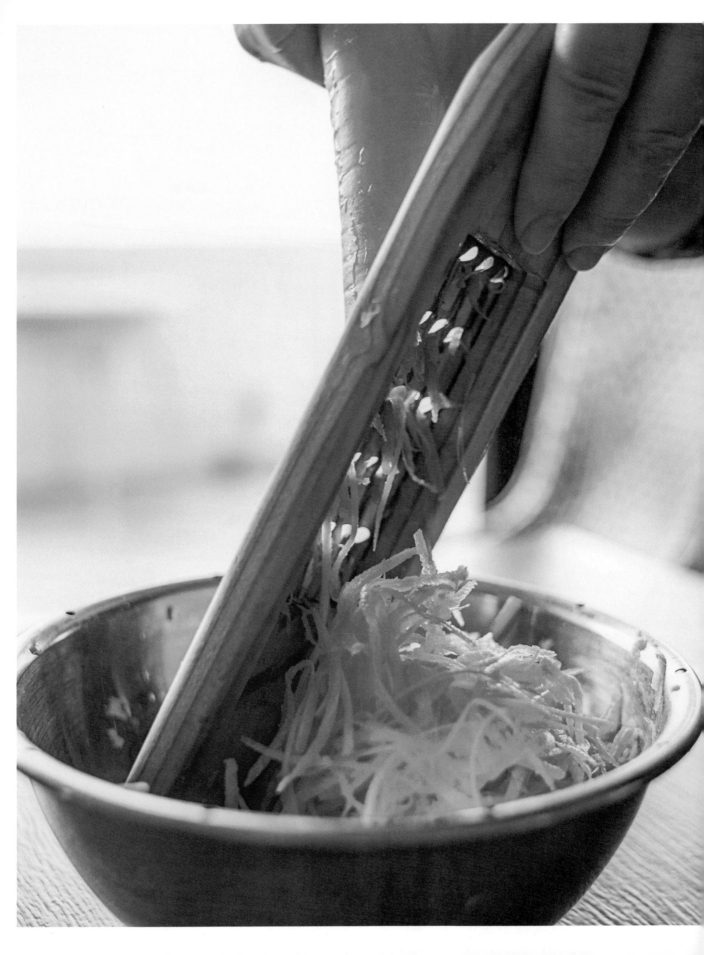

RECIPES

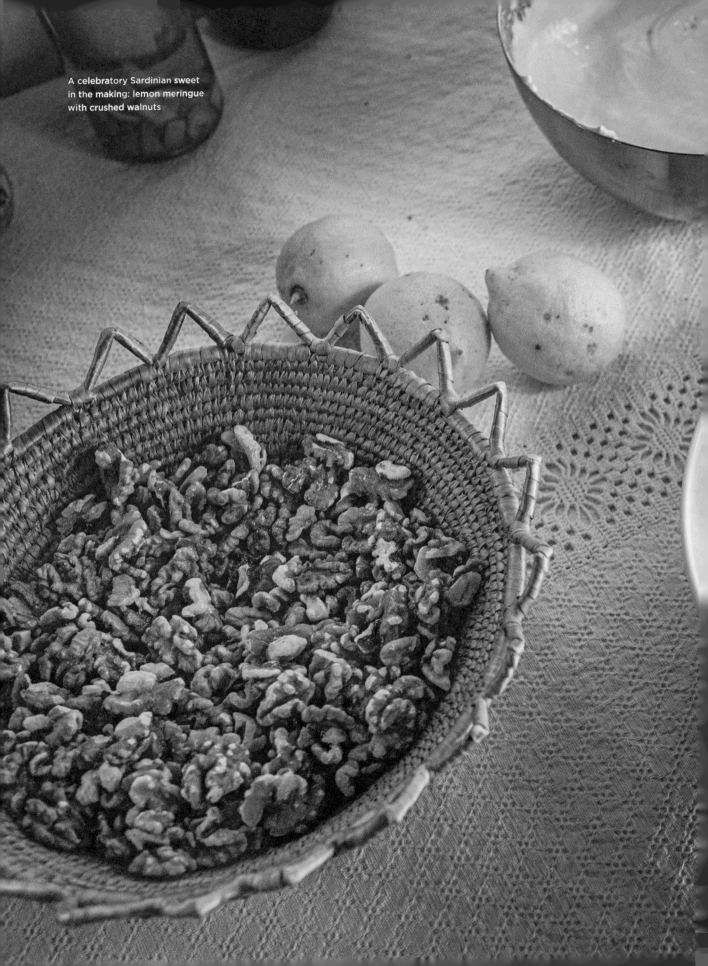

A celebratory Sardinian sweet in the making: lemon meringue with crushed walnuts

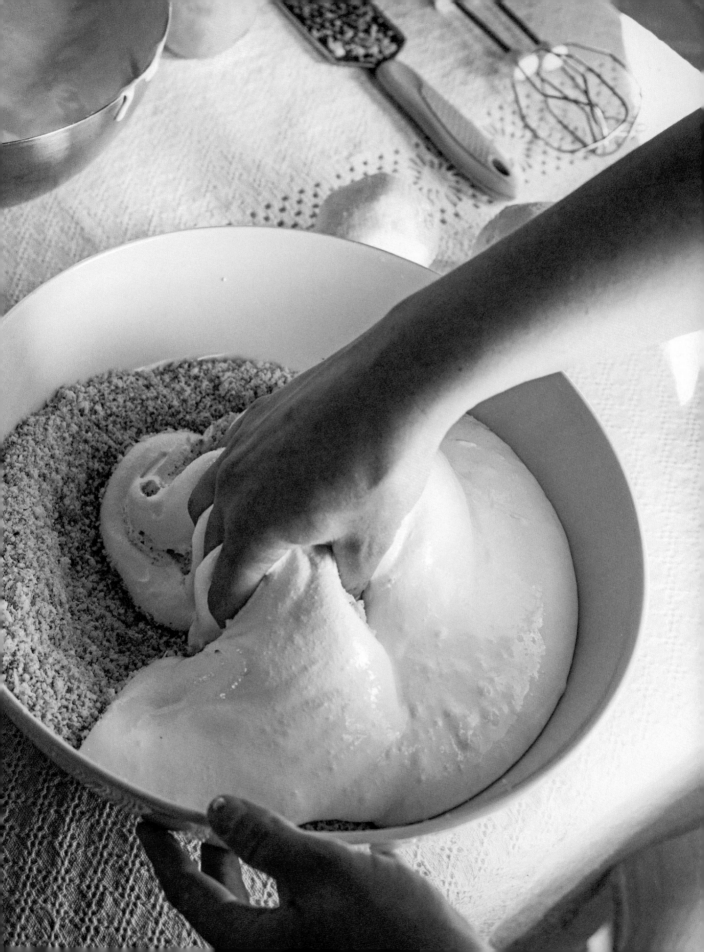

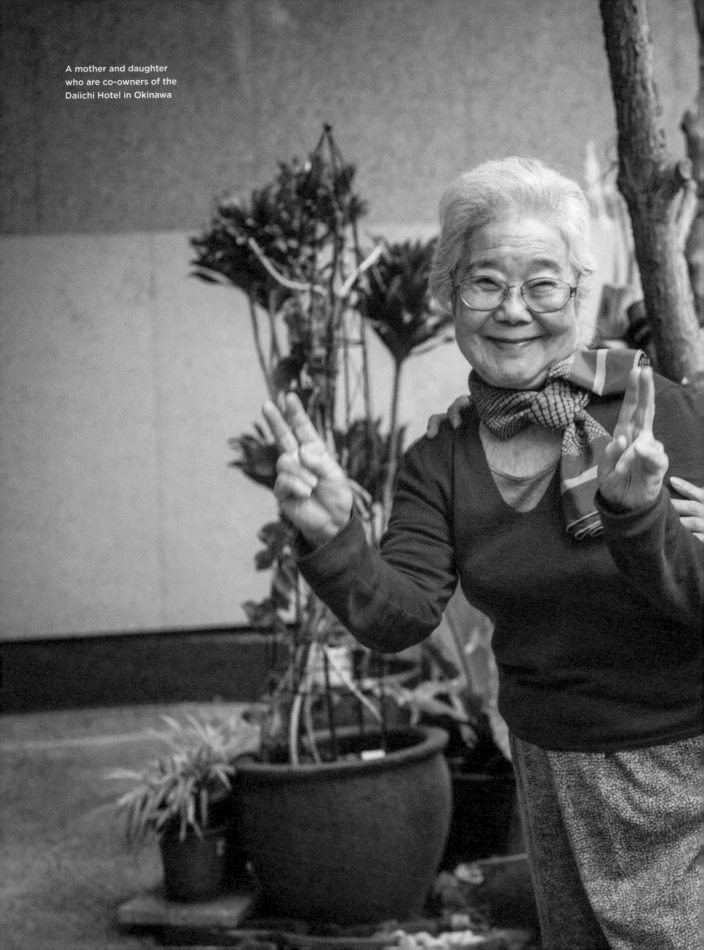
A mother and daughter
who are co-owners of the
Daiichi Hotel in Okinawa

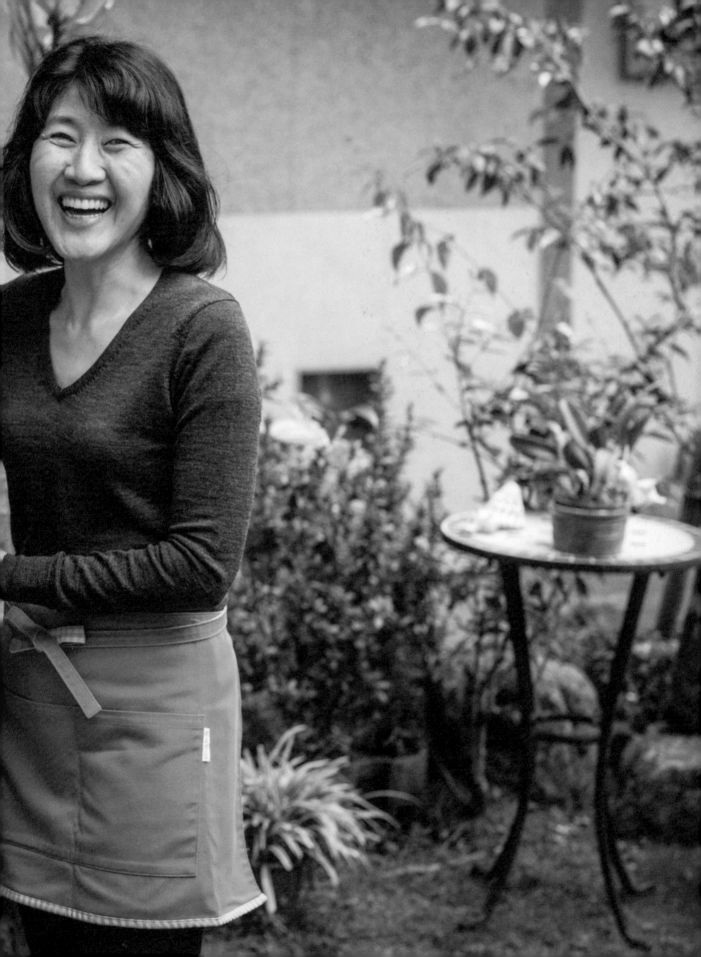

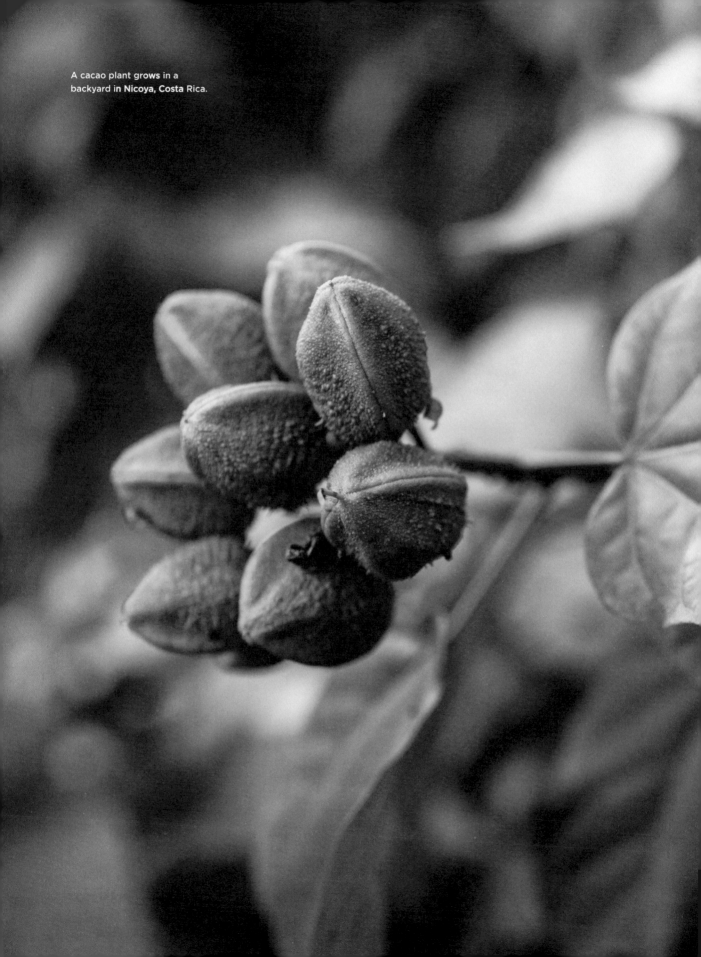
A cacao plant grows in a backyard in Nicoya, Costa Rica.

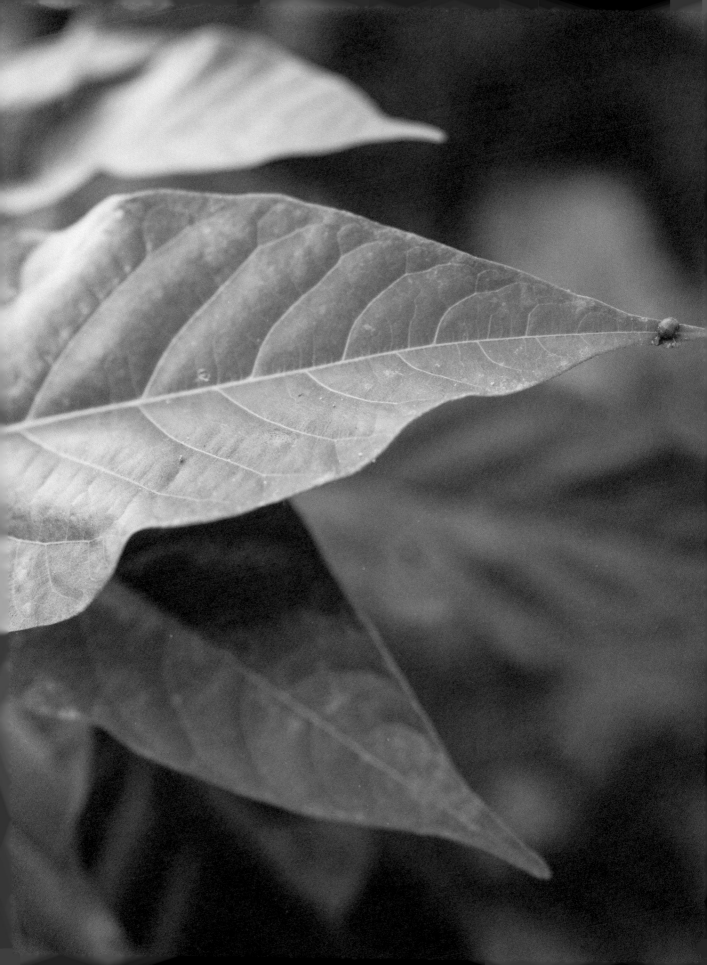

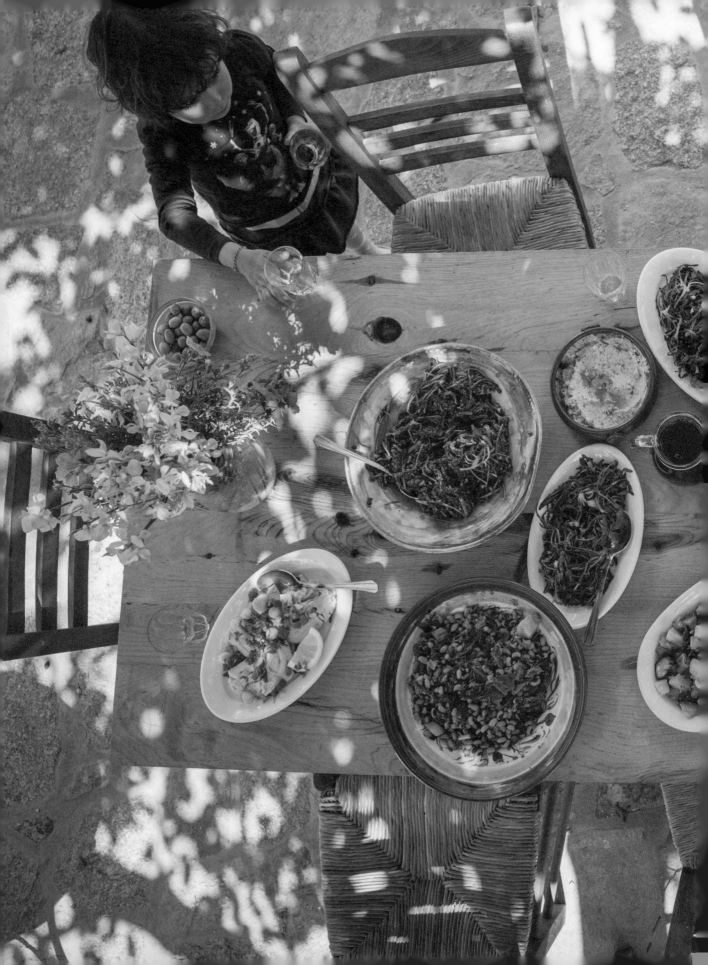

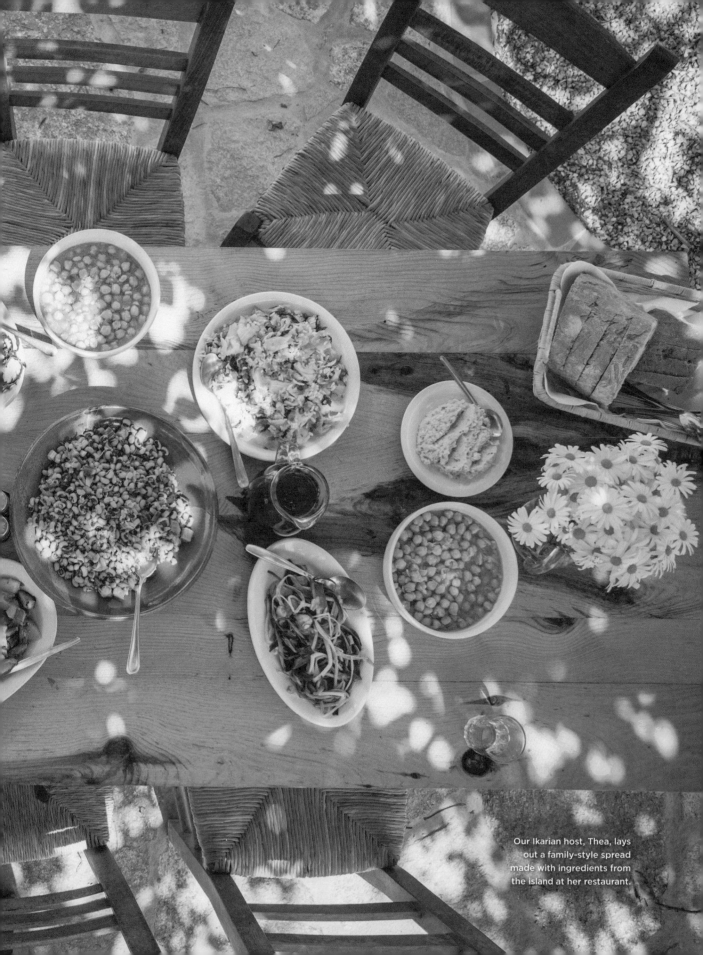

Our Ikarian host, Thea, lays out a family-style spread made with ingredients from the island at her restaurant.

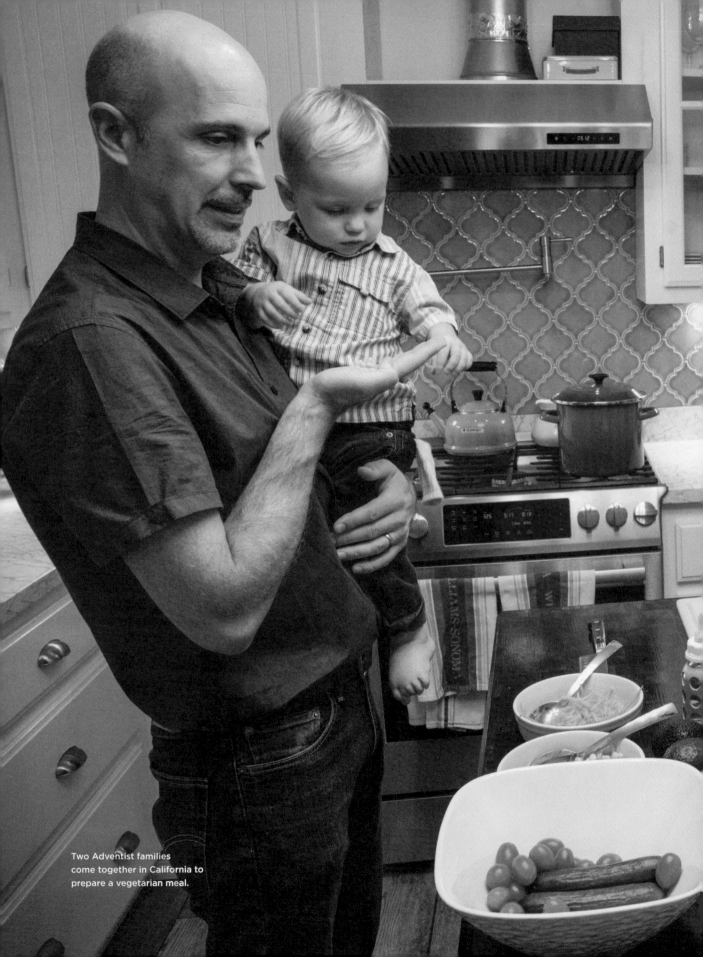

Two Adventist families come together in California to prepare a vegetarian meal.

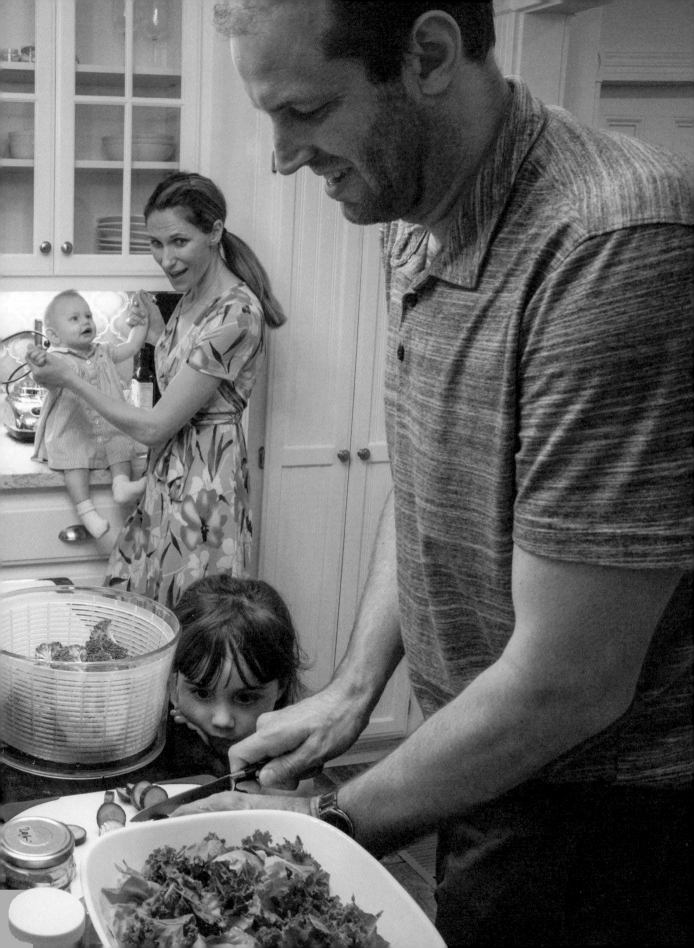

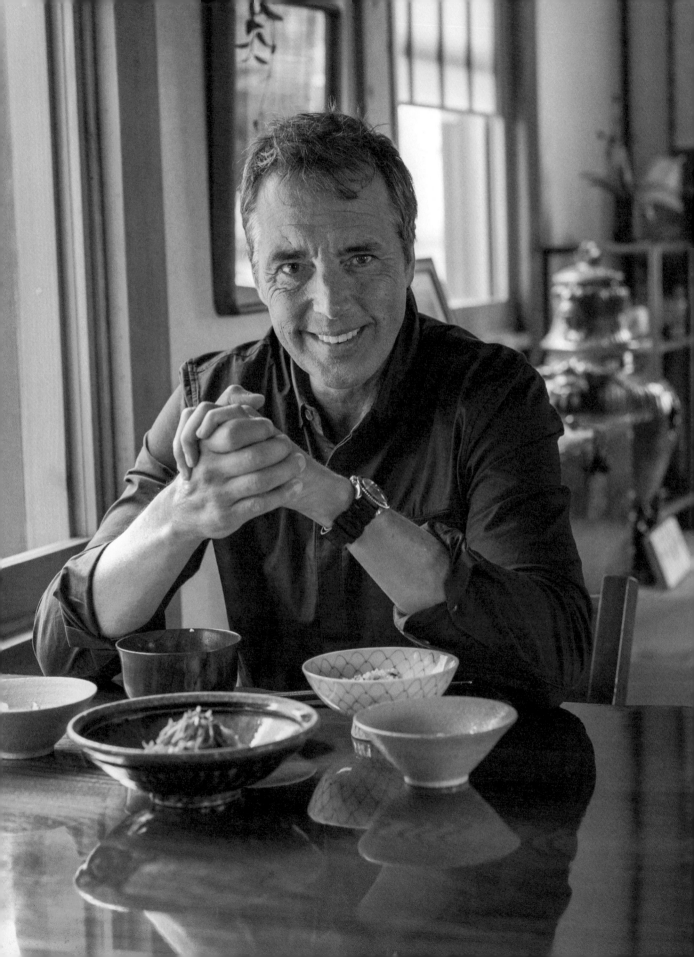

INTRODUCTION

I f you want to live to a healthy 100, eat like healthy people who've lived to 100. • About 15 years ago, in conjunction with National Geographic, I set out to reverse-engineer a formula for longevity. Working with renowned doctors and experts Gianni Pes and Michel Poulain, I identified the places around the world where people live the longest, drawing a line around each area in blue ink. Together, we created the

concept of Blues Zones: the set of characteristics that have produced the world's longest lived people. Their secrets can help you live a longer, better life.

In Sardinia we found the world's longest lived men in a string of mountainous villages. On the South Pacific islands of Okinawa, we found villages that produced the world's highest percentage of centenarians—mostly women. In Ikaria, Greece, we found the "Island Where People Forget to Die"—10,000 or so residents who not only live long lives but also suffer the world's lowest rates of dementia. On Costa Rica's Nicoya Peninsula, we found an entire population likely to reach a healthy age of 90. And in and around Loma Linda, California, we discovered a group of Seventh-day Adventists who live up to a decade longer than other Americans.

These people don't live longer because of supplements, pills, or hocus-pocus antiaging serums. They do so because their surroundings nudge them into the right behaviors.

What does work? We found that those who live in the blue zones move naturally every 20 minutes or so. Their streets are built for humans, not cars; going to a friend's house, out to eat, or to work is an opportunity for a walk.

Dan enjoying a traditional breakfast at the Daiichi Hotel

Their houses aren't full of mechanical conveniences: They still do work by hand, grinding corn or kneading bread. They grow a garden.

People aren't lonely, because it simply isn't an option. If after a few days people don't show up to the town festival, church, or even the village café, someone will generally check in on them. Electronic gadgets haven't yet taken over: People talk face-to-face instead of on Facebook.

Moreover, blue zones residents have a sense of purpose (the Okinawans call it *ikigai,* and the Nicoyans call it *plan de vida*). Their lives are imbued with meaning from age 10 to age 100, and their brand of purpose is not just hobbies or golf. It also includes a sense of responsibility: for their community, family, or the next generation.

And of course, blue zones inhabitants live longer because they've eaten the right foods—and avoided the wrong ones—for most of their lives. Ninety to 100 percent of their diet consists of whole, plant-based fare. They eat this way not because they possess heroic discipline, but because fruits, vegetables, tubers, nuts, beans, and whole grains are cheap and accessible. Their kitchens are set up so it's easy to make those foods; they spend time with people who eat the same way; and they possess time-honored recipes to make healthy food taste good. Taste is the most important ingredient in any longevity recipe.

People in blue zones areas also lead healthy, energetic lives. Before the 1970s, fewer than 2 percent of people in Okinawa and Sardinia were overweight and obese. Then something terrible happened. Beginning in the 1970s, paved roads and electrification arrived in blue zones areas, bringing pizzas, burgers, chips, and sodas. The Standard American Diet overwhelmed taste buds, pushing out the nuanced flavors and textures of traditional diets, and the diseases of affluence quickly followed. In Sardinia, the diabetes rate has soared to 10 percent. And Okinawa, once home to the world's longest lived population, is now home to the unhealthiest people in Japan. The villages are still there, the centenarians are still living, but life expectancy in younger generations is plummeting.

The longevity phenomenon is disappearing in blue zones, but its secrets survive—mostly in the kitchens of older people. People who've grown up eating the foods of their ancestors aren't looking to trade them in for packaged junk. Older people who possess the skills, recipes, and culinary wisdom of previous generations carry forth a tradition that is centuries—or millennia—old.

For this book, I went back to each of the five blue zones areas. I persuaded older people to allow me to watch them cook everyday foods. In most cases, I spent the better part of a day perched on a stool, observing exactly how to make the food that has produced the world's longest lived people.

In blue zones areas, people ate meat and sweets, but mostly as celebratory foods. Everyday meals were composed of simple peasant fare, made with fresh, plant-based ingredients. Some of the recipes require time to prepare, but the vast majority take less than a half hour. Another plus: Most of the ingredients are cheap—beans, whole grains, herbs. This completely destroys the myth that you need to be rich to be healthy; in fact, the reverse is true.

Along the way, I met experts who could help me explain why the foods people ate led to longer lives: Dr. Makoto Suzuki and Drs. Craig and Bradley Willcox in Okinawa; geneticist Dr. David Rehkopf in Costa Rica; Dr. Gary Fraser in Loma Linda; Dr. Christina Chrysohoou in Ikaria; and the great Gianni Pes in Sardinia. Here are a few cooking tips for eating to 100:

• **USE FEWER INGREDIENTS:** Blue zones diets tend to use the same 20 or so ingredients over and over. Less variety may help keep people from overeating and keep the immune system strong.

• **ADD CRUCIFEROUS VEGETABLES:** Cruciferous vegetables like broccoli, cabbage, and cauliflower have been known to help protect the heart, stave off cancer, and lower oxidative stress. In Sardinia, we discovered that because people add cruciferous vegetables to their daily minestrone, the thyroid functions differently and may help slow down the metabolism and help you live longer. (Think of turning down the flame of a lighter.)

MAPPING THE BLUE ZONES

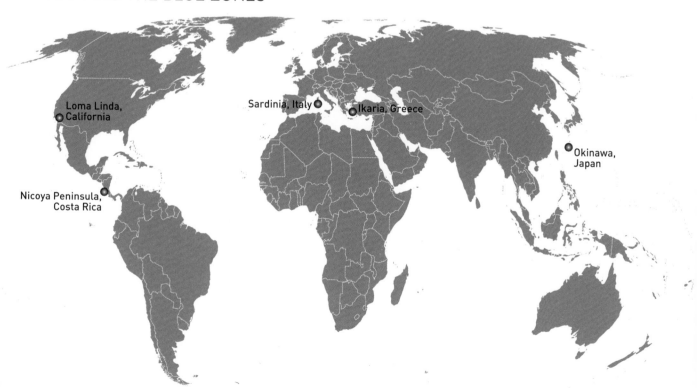

• **MAKE BEANS TASTY:** In America, cooks tend to make meat the focus of their ingenuity; in the blue zones, beans are the main story. They're cooked into soups and stews, enhanced with spices, and complemented by grains and vegetables. Moreover, nuts, beans, and grains are a much healthier source of protein than meat or eggs; they're also high in fiber and complex carbohydrates. And finally, they're cheap, they're versatile, and they allow subtle flavors to shine through.

• **FINISH DISHES WITH OLIVE OIL:** Olive oil's monounsaturated fatty acids break down quickly when oils are heated beyond the smoking point of about 375 degrees Fahrenheit. In blue zones, room temperature olive oil is added to breads, drizzled over vegetables, and added to soups and stews.

• **SUPPLEMENT WITH FRESH HERBS AND SPICES:** Rosemary, oregano, sage, mint, garlic, turmeric, and mugwort all possess well-documented medicinal values; they also add flavor while imparting healing properties. Since most bioactive properties in herbs degrade as soon as you pick them, it's best to use them fresh. People in blue zones often get their herbs from a kitchen garden, which doubles as a live medicine chest.

• **FIBER IS MORE IMPORTANT THAN WE THOUGHT:** Grains, greens, nuts, and beans not only contain the protein, complex carbohydrates, vitamins, and minerals that keep our heart healthy and our mind sharp, and prevent cancers, they also feed the eight pounds of bacteria living in our gut. Some of that bacteria produces toxins like choline; others produce compounds that reduce inflammation, regulate our metabolism, and fuel our immune system. The toxin-producing bacteria tend to feed off meat and eggs, while the healthy bacteria favor fiber.

• **ENJOY YOUR MEALS WITH RED WINE:** We've all heard plenty about polyphenols and antioxidants, which occur more often in red than white wine. But it turns out that red wine, along with a blue zones (plant-based) diet, almost triples the absorption of antioxidants. Additionally, 90 to 95 percent of wine polyphenols are metabolized in the gut, where good bacteria convert them to powerful compounds that lower inflammation and decrease leaky gut syndrome.

Finally, it's important to remember that eating for longevity is not just about what you eat, but how you eat. Blue zones teach us that dining with family, pausing before a meal to express gratitude, fasting occasionally, eating

Freshly picked lemons and a cat in slow-paced Ikaria

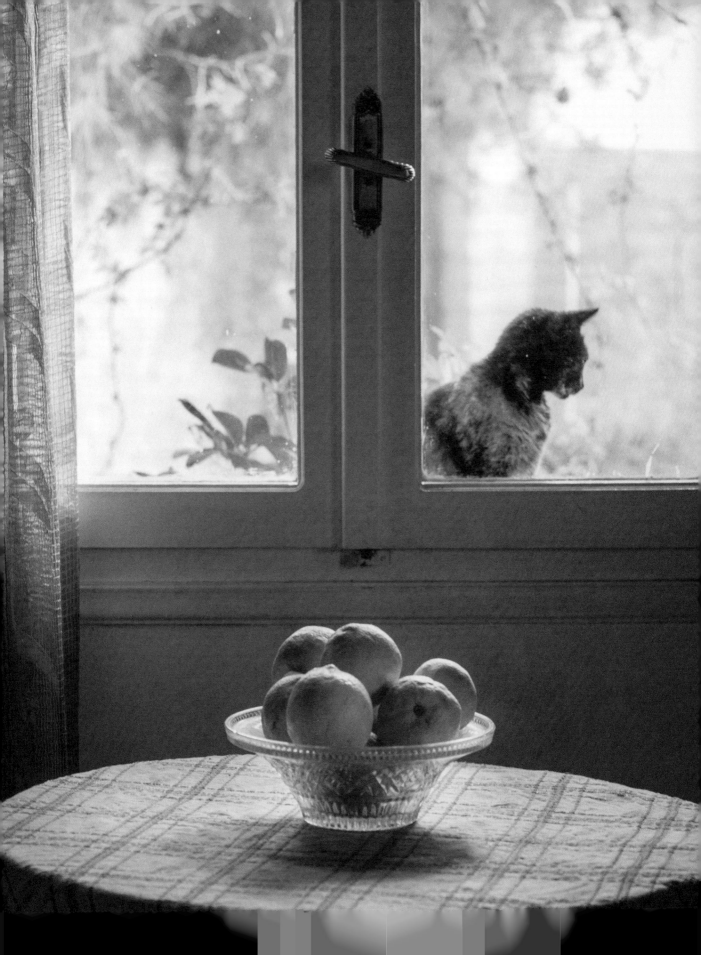

a big breakfast, and trying to eat all of your calories in an eight-hour window helps you stay healthier, live longer, and feel better.

In Sardinia, people pass each other on the street and greet each other by saying, *Akentannos*—May you live to 100! So here's to making it to your 100th birthday—and may the people sitting around your table be there to count every year!

THE BLUE ZONES FOOD GUIDELINES

In these pages, we've distilled more than 150 dietary surveys of the world's longest-lived people to reveal the secrets of a strong longevity regimen. These 11 simple guidelines reflect how the world's longest lived people ate for most of their lives.

1. ENSURE THAT YOUR DIET IS 90 TO 100 PERCENT PLANT BASED

While people in four of the five blue zones consume meat, they do so sparingly, using it as a celebratory food, a small side, or as a way to flavor dishes. People in the blue zones eat an impressive variety of garden vegetables and leafy greens (especially spinach, kale, beet and turnip tops, chard, and collards) when they are in season; they pickle or dry the surplus to enjoy during the off-season. Beans, greens, sweet potatoes, whole grains, fruits, nuts, and

A steaming walnut "meat" loaf (see page 268 for recipe) is sliced for serving in Loma Linda.

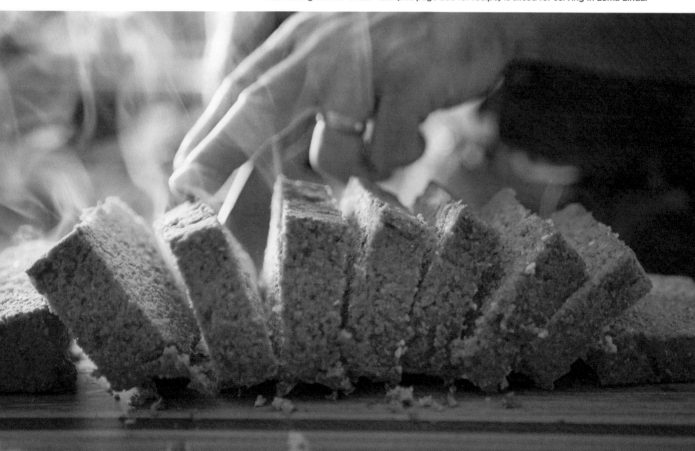

seeds dominate blue zones meals all year long. Olive oil is also a staple in the blue zones. Evidence shows that olive oil consumption increases good cholesterol and lowers bad cholesterol. In Ikaria, for example, we found that for middle-aged people, about six tablespoons of olive oil daily seemed to cut the risk of premature mortality in half.

2. RETREAT FROM MEAT

Averaging out consumption across the blue zones, we found that people ate about two ounces or less of meat about five times per month.

The Adventist Health Study 2, which has been following 96,000 Americans since 2002, has determined that the people who lived the longest were vegans or pesco-vegetarians who ate a small amount of fish. Vegetarian Adventists will likely outlive their meat-eating counterparts by as many as eight years.

While you may want to celebrate from time to time with meat, we don't recommend it as part of a blue zones diet. Okinawans probably offer the best meat substitute: extra-firm tofu, which is high in protein and cancer-fighting phytoestrogens.

3. GO EASY ON FISH

If you must eat fish, consume fewer than three ounces up to three times weekly. In most blue zones, people ate small amounts of fish, up to three small servings a week. Usually, the fish being eaten are small, relatively inexpensive varieties like sardines, anchovies, and cod—middle-of-the-food-chain species that are not exposed to the high levels of mercury or other chemicals that pollute our gourmet fish supply today.

Again, fish is not a necessary part of a longevity diet, but if you must eat it, elect varieties that are common and not threatened by overfishing.

4. REDUCE DAIRY

Cow's milk doesn't figure significantly in any blue zones diet (except that of some Adventists). Goat and sheep milk products figure prominently into the Ikarian and Sardinian blue zones. We don't know if it's the goat's milk or sheep's milk that makes people healthier, or if it's the fact that they climb up and down the same hilly terrain as the goats. Interestingly, though, most goat's milk is consumed not as liquid, but as yogurt, sour milk, or cheese.

5. CUT DOWN ON EGGS

People in all the blue zones eat eggs about two to four times per week. Usually they eat just one as a side: Nicoyans fold an egg and beans into corn tortillas; Okinawans boil an egg in soup; those in Mediterranean blue zones—Sardinia and Ikaria—fry an egg to eat with bread, almonds, and olives for breakfast.

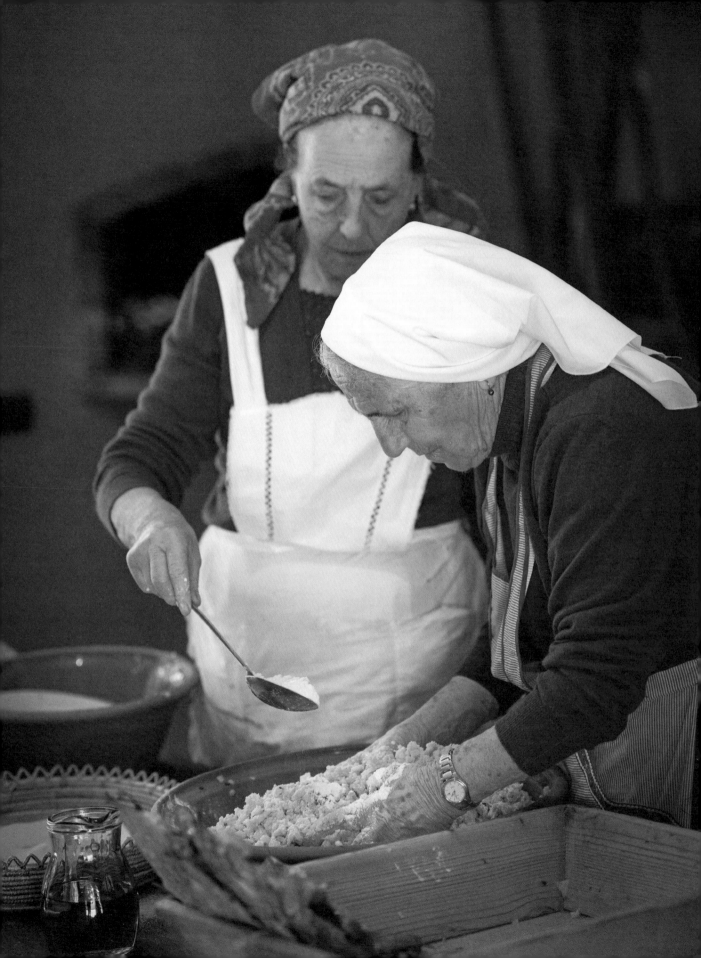

Blue zones eggs come from chickens that range freely and don't receive hormones or antibiotics.

People with diabetes and heart disease often limit their egg consumption for health reasons. Eggs aren't a key component for living a long life so we don't recommend them—but if you must eat them, try to eat no more than three per week.

6. EAT A DAILY DOSE OF BEANS

Beans reign supreme in the blue zones and are the cornerstone of every longevity diet in the world: black beans in Nicoya; lentils, garbanzo, and white beans in the Mediterranean; and soybeans in Okinawa. People in the blue zones eat at least four times as many beans as Americans do on average—at least a half cup per day—and so should you.

Why? Beans are packed with more nutrients per gram than any other food on Earth. On average, they are made up of 21 percent protein, 77 percent complex carbohydrates, and only a few percent fat. Because they are fiber-rich and satisfying, they'll likely help to push less-healthy foods out of your diet.

7. SLASH SUGAR

Consume only 28 grams (7 teaspoons) of added sugar daily. People in the blue zones eat sugar intentionally, not by habit or accident. They consume about the same amount of naturally occurring sugars as North Americans do, but only about a fifth as much added sugar—no more than seven teaspoons a day. Between 1970 and 2000, the amount of added sugar in the American food supply rose by 25 percent (about 22 teaspoons of added sugar per day)—generally, the result of the insidious, hidden sugars mixed into soda, yogurt, and sauces.

If you must eat sweets, save cookies, candy, and bakery items for special occasions—ideally as part of a meal. Limit sugar added to coffee, tea, or other foods to no more than four teaspoons per day. Skip any product that lists sugar among its first five ingredients.

8. SNACK ON NUTS

Eat two handfuls of nuts per day. A handful weighs about two ounces, the average amount that blue zones centenarians consume: almonds in Ikaria and Sardinia, pistachios in Nicoya, and all varieties of nuts with the Adventists. The Adventist Health Study 2 found that nut eaters outlive non-nut eaters by an average of two to three years. So try to snack on a couple handfuls of almonds, Brazil nuts, cashews, walnuts, and/or peanuts every day.

Two Sardinian women prepare squash pancakes to be cooked in a wood-fired oven.

9. SOUR ON BREAD

If you can, strive to eat only sourdough or 100 percent whole wheat bread. Most commercially available breads start with bleached white flour, which metabolizes quickly into sugar and spikes insulin levels. But blue zones bread is either whole grain or sourdough; in Ikaria and Sardinia, breads are made from a variety of whole grains such as wheat, rye, or barley, each of which offers a wide spectrum of nutrients.

Whole grains have higher levels of fiber than most commonly used bleached flours. Some traditional blue zones breads are made with naturally occurring bacteria called lactobacilli, which "digest" the starches and glutens while making the bread rise. The process also creates an acid—the "sour" in sourdough. The result is bread with less gluten than breads labeled "gluten free," with a longer shelf life and a pleasantly sour taste that most people like. Traditional sourdough breads actually lower the glycemic load of meals, making your entire meal healthier, slower burning, easier on your pancreas, and more likely to make calories available as energy than stored as fat.

10. GO WHOLE

Strive to eat foods that are recognizable. People in the blue zones traditionally eat whole foods, which are made from a single ingredient—raw, cooked, ground, or fermented—and are not highly processed. Residents eat raw fruits and vegetables; they grind whole grains themselves and then cook them slowly. They use fermentation—an ancient way to make nutrients bioavailable—in the tofu, sourdough bread, wine, and pickled vegetables they eat. And they rarely ingest artificial preservatives. Blue zones dishes typically contain a half dozen or so ingredients, simply blended together.

11. DRINK MOSTLY WATER

If possible, strive to avoid soft drinks (including diet soda). With very few exceptions, people in blue zones drink only coffee, tea, water, and wine. (Soft drinks, which account for about half of Americans' sugar intake, were unknown to most blue zones centenarians until recently.) Here's why:

Water: Adventists recommend seven glasses of water daily. They point to studies showing that being hydrated facilitates blood flow and lessens the chance of a blood clot.

Coffee: Sardinians, Ikarians, and Nicoyans all drink coffee. Research associates coffee drinking with lower rates of dementia and Parkinson's disease.

Tea: People in every blue zone drink tea. Okinawans prefer green varieties, which have been shown to lower the risk of heart disease and several cancers. Ikarians drink brews of rosemary, wild sage, and dandelion—all herbs known to have anti-inflammatory properties.

Red Wine: People who drink—in moderation—tend to outlive those who don't. (This doesn't mean you should start drinking if you don't drink now.) People in most blue zones drink one to three small glasses of red wine per day, often with a meal and with friends.

AUTHOR'S NOTE

As you'll see, I've chosen only plant-based recipes for this book. First and foremost, because the daily meals in blue zones were overwhelmingly vegetarian. Second, because if you're eating healthy, plant-based food, you're much more likely to live to 100 than if you're eating like an average American. In a typical year, Americans eat 208 pounds of meat and get 130 percent of their daily sugar and 70 percent of their calories from processed foods. We can't escape meat: Open a menu at the vast majority of restaurants and every appetizer and entrée will be animal based. This book will provide a refuge. Whether you're cooking for yourself, your family, or your friends, the recipes here will be delicious and will put you on a path to live to 100. Enjoy!

After church, Loma Linda Adventists gather together to share food at a community potluck.

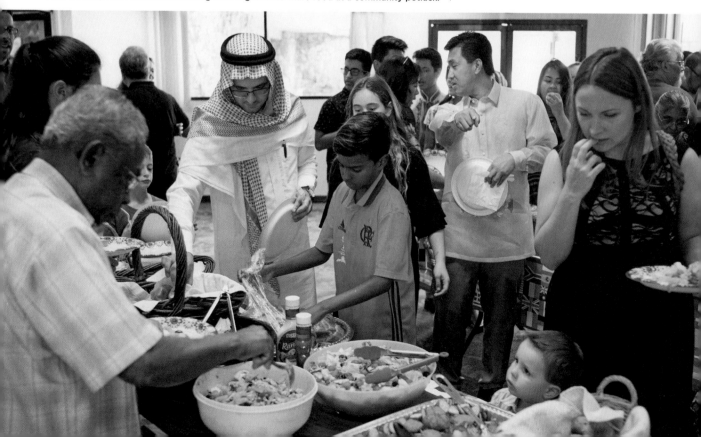

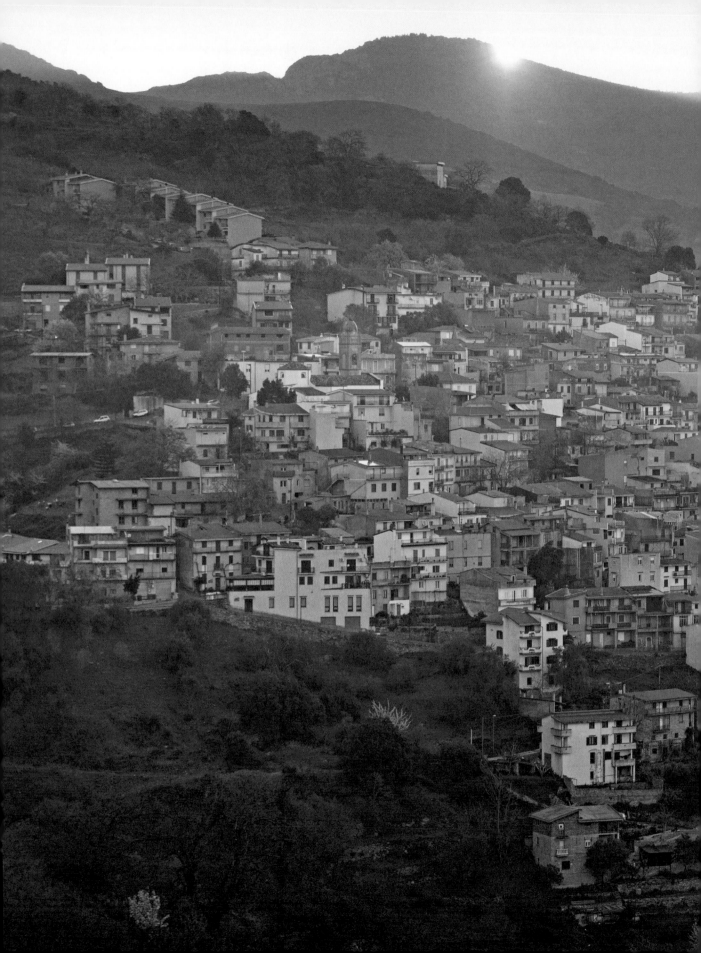

The sun rises over a tight-knit
but isolated village tucked away
in the hills of Sardinia.

CHAPTER ONE

Sardinia

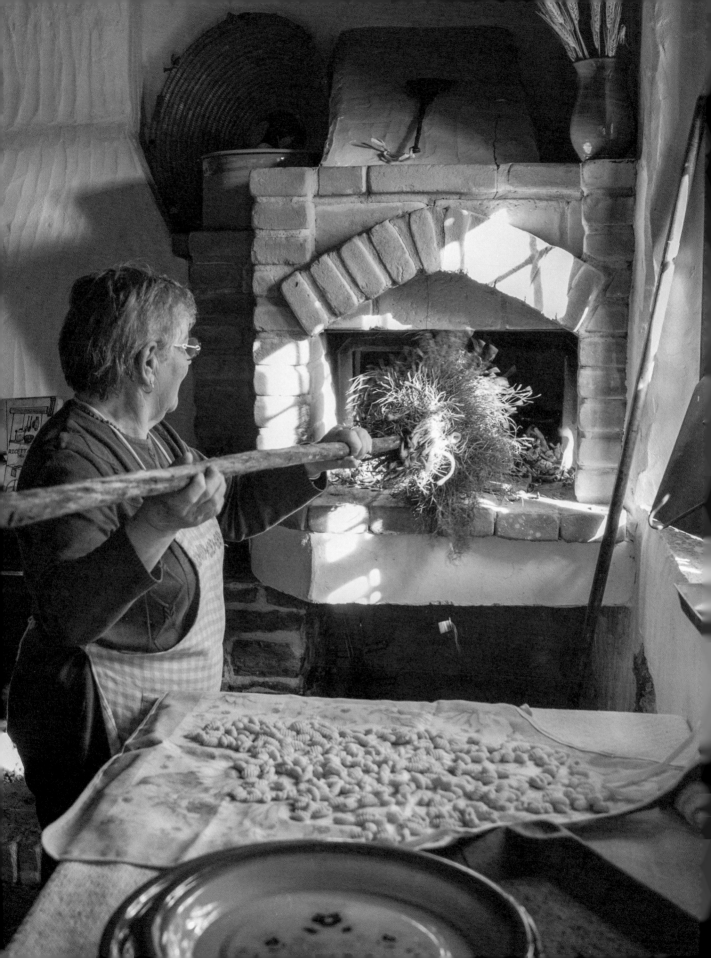

Sardinia, Italy

I t's a spring afternoon at a small farm outside of Urzulei, ground zero of Sardinia's blue zones hot spot, home to the world's longest lived men. We're on an island 200 miles off the western coast of Italy, in the central highlands that were originally settled by Bronze Age people. Today sunbeams angle through blossoming cherry trees, pooling warmly on terraced gardens of herbs and spring vegetables. Across a leafy valley, a granite-tipped mountain peak looms large.

Inside a small plaster-and-stone farmhouse, a slight woman with a shock of wild hair and a floral apron stirs an earthen pot. "Minestrone," she explains with a smile as we peer into the simmering mélange of beans, freshly picked zucchini, onions, tomatoes, garlic, and thyme (page 47). The soup smells savory and homey, redolent of a roast, but with none of the gaminess.

Nearby, a table spread with *carta de musica* flatbread (page 65), a fresh dill-and-cucumber salad, and a thick carafe of garnet-red Cannonau wine awaits us. "Sit," Pina Lorrai commands, deploying the region's generous albeit predatory hospitality. She wipes her hands on her apron, pours us wine in stout glasses, and serves the steaming dishes. Their delicate flavor helps explain much of Sardinia's extraordinary longevity.

As it happens, minestrone possesses all the characteristics of world-class longevity food. The Sardinian version—a pot of healthy amino acids—delivers all the protein necessary for human sustenance. The beans and vegetables also provide a huge dose of fiber, which feeds healthy gut bacteria, complex (or slow-burning) carbohydrates, and compounds that may regulate metabolism.

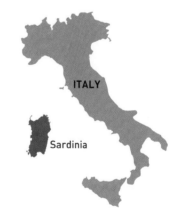

ITALY

Sardinia

Handmade *Iaddedos* (Sardinian gnocchi, see page 60) dry on an apron as a woman cleans and flavors a wood-burning oven with wild fennel.

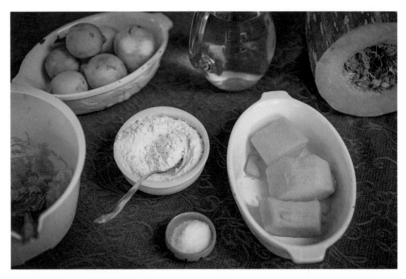

Ingredients are readied for making a traditional Sardinian supper.

And, since its ingredients morph with the seasons, so too does the flavor.

Each of the blue zones' Sardinian villages—Artzana, Baunei, Villagrande, Seulo, Urzulei, and Talana—champions its own recipe. All versions are a peasant's delight: sublimely flavored, cheap, and full of variations of the same longevity-promoting ingredients—beans, barley, seasonal vegetables, potatoes, and Mediterranean herbs. One pot captures a millennia of culinary expertise, as well as dependable produce (of which Sardinians never tire). Indeed, a typical lunch consists of minestrone, bread, and a small glass of Cannonau. Dinner is often made of leftovers, which tastes even better because the flavors have had time to harmonize. The nine siblings of the record-setting Melis family (collective age 852 years) claimed they ate minestrone (page 48) every day of their lives.

Repetitive as this may sound, dietary monotony may be an important component of longevity. "Too many ingredients create molecular stress in your body," says Sassari University professor Gianni Pes, one of the world's foremost longevity experts. He's been studying Sardinia's diet for more than 30 years, surveying centenarians from around the world. "When you eat too many types of food, you're asking your immune system to work harder and undertake stress," he told me. "When our immune systems are confronted with foreign invaders—whether it's a bacteria, virus, or new molecule—they turn on genes to mount a defense. We only have so many genes to 'turn on' before our immune systems begin to wear out. Eating the same food every day may preserve them."

Wine is another factor that may contribute to Sardinia's longevity—specifically, the very high antioxidant content of Cannonau wine, which accompanies most meals and social gatherings. Made from juice pressed from local Grenache grapes, it ferments for 15 days with flavonoid-rich seeds and skins. The result is a wine with arguably the world's highest antioxidant content.

Cruciferous vegetables—onions, cabbage, and especially kohlrabi—also play a longevity role because they modulate thyroid function. Dr. Pes explains, "A low-functioning thyroid may help you live longer in the way that a Cricket lighter with the flame turned down lasts longer. Cruciferous vegetables turn down your thyroid function."

Sardinia's diet has undergone three major shifts over the life span of the centenarians here. Before 1940, people mostly ate a high-carb diet of bread, sheep's milk cheese (mostly rich Parmesan-like pecorino), and garden vegetables. After World War II, soldiers returning from the mainland brought pastas. During this time, Sardinians developed their version of gnocchi (page 60) and spaghetti. Meat consumption—mostly pork and lamb—increased but only during times of celebration and rarely more than five times monthly. The prosperity of the 1970s brought paved roads and American influences to Sardinia. Many shepherds abandoned their pastures and

A young girl, raised on a working farm, very much enjoys eating her vegetables (wild greens, see page 214).

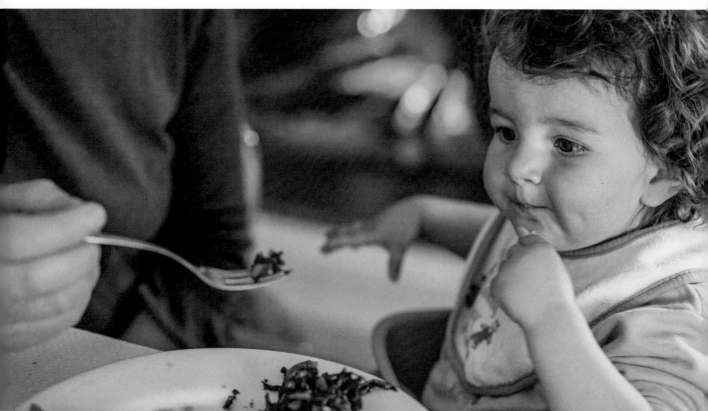

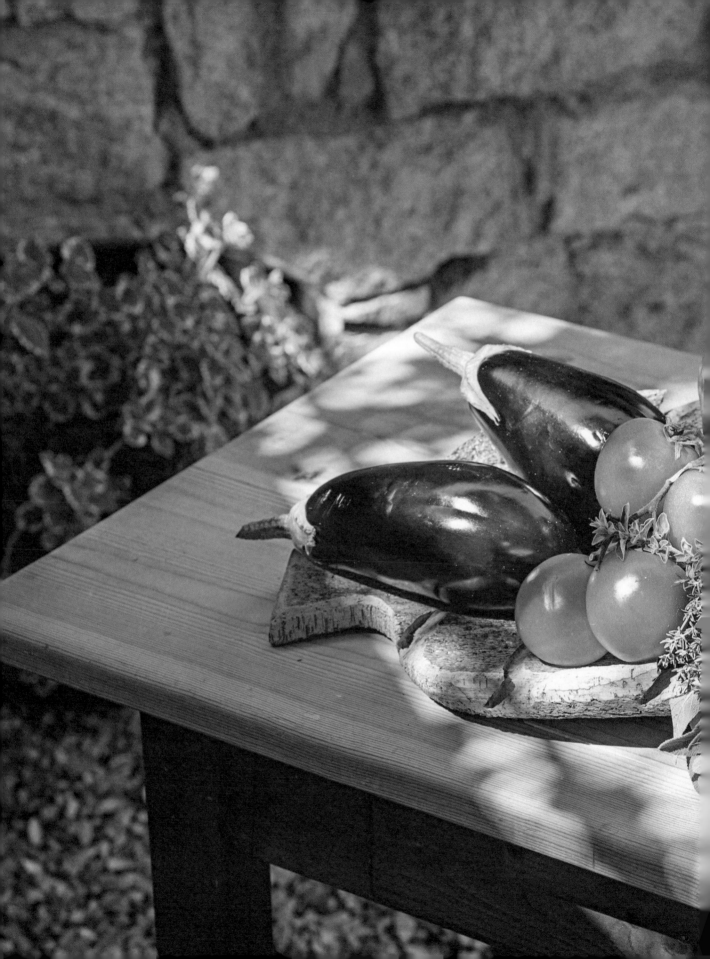

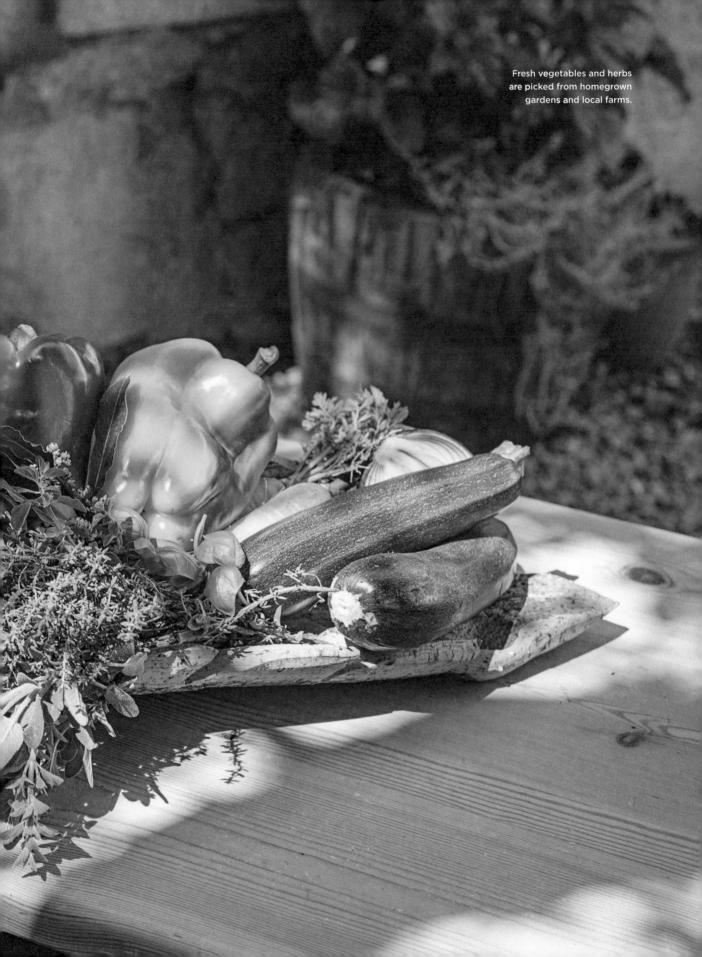

Fresh vegetables and herbs are picked from homegrown gardens and local farms.

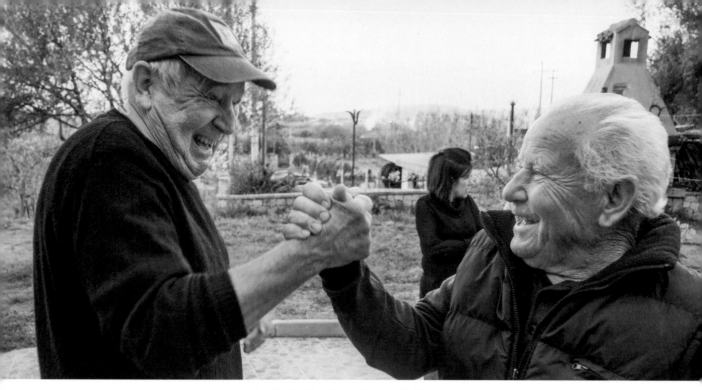

Dan's father, Roger Buettner (left), engages in a game of strength with an older Sardinian we met on our travels through the blue zone.

moved into towns. The predictable processed and Western foods—chips, sodas, sugary yogurts, pizza, burgers—began to nudge out fresh vegetables. As in all blue zones hot spots, life expectancy has begun to ebb.

But not all traditions have been lost. In the 15 years that photographer David McLain and I have been traveling to Sardinia, we've marveled at how its residents put family first and celebrate their elders. Unlike America, where about 50 percent of seniors will spend time in a retirement community, aging parents here live at home and are seen as repositories of wisdom. They tend the garden, help raise children, and pass down Sardinia's unique longevity diet. Some data suggests that older Sardinians living in the family home gain 15 years of life expectancy over those living in retirement homes.

AT THE COMMUNITY bakery in Seulo, we had a chance to observe elder wisdom at work. Reina Boi, the senior baker, oversaw operations and provided the starter dough for the bread (a prized ingredient that her family has cultivated for generations). The starter's live cultures leaven dough, and in the process, break down the simple sugars and proteins to yield a bread that has 1 percent of the gluten of normal white bread and slows down sugar absorption by as much as 25 percent.

When the loaves came out of the oven, Reina skewered a piece with a knife and presented it to me. Still warm, it tasted chewy and tart and rich in a way that didn't call for butter. It occurred to me that this culinary heirloom has been making every meal marginally healthier for generations.

"This is the highlight of my week," said 36-year-old Francesca Ghiani, the youngest member of the group. In tight jeans, a Gore-Tex jacket, and apron, she's a visual icon of shifting traditions. "Every week, I learn something new from the older ladies—and not just about cooking. We ridicule men, support each other, and pass down traditions. When I have a problem, someone here has been through it before, and they help me through. Plus, I take fresh bread back to my family every week."

In Artzana, a village whose name means "pure air," we met three friends who call themselves "The Women of San Antonio"—Anna Stochino, Iole Demurtas, and Franca Piras. Each year, they bring feuding factions of the village together to resolve disputes over platters of gnocchi, pasta, and *anguli 'e cibudda* (Sardinian pizza).

At Nuraghe Murtarba, a bed-and-breakfast located on a working farm outside of Talana, I witness four generations of the Fracas-Perroni family debate the best way to make sourdough bread. The older generations favor semolina, wheat germ, and apple cider vinegar with long fermentation times; the younger generation favors a simpler recipe that uses honey.

In our exploration, we found that food was never just fuel, but a ritual to cement family ties, to consolidate friendships, or to share hospitality. The meals begin with a hoisted glass of Cannonau, and the timeless Sardinian blessing that could not be more fitting:

"*Akentannos!*—May you live to 100!" bellows the host. "And may you be here to count the years!" reply the guests. *

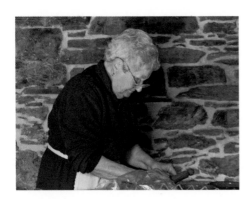

Reina Boi, 80 YEARS OLD

At a century-old community bakery in Seulo we met with a dozen village women whose ages spanned six decades as they gathered to make bread. The senior baker, a short, vigorous woman of 80 named Reina Boi, commanded the process. She dispensed advice and signaled when the dough was ready and the oven hot enough. She had also provided the sourdough starter from a small jar that contained what looked like frothy curdled milk—a secret ingredient her family has cultivated for generations. It contained live cultures of lactobacillus, a probiotic.

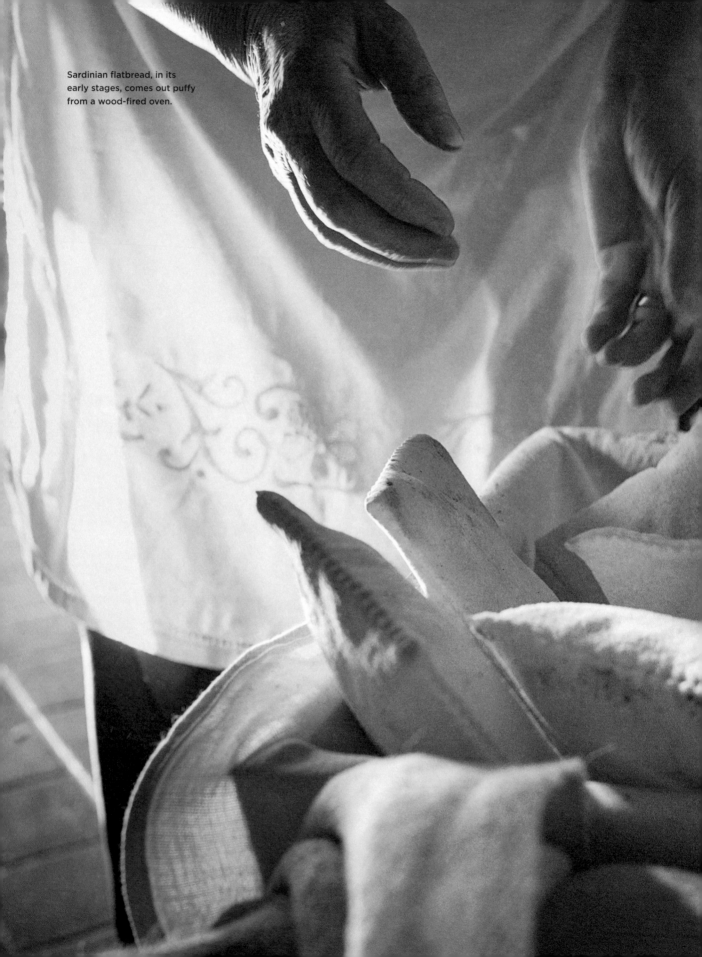

Sardinian flatbread, in its
early stages, comes out puffy
from a wood-fired oven.

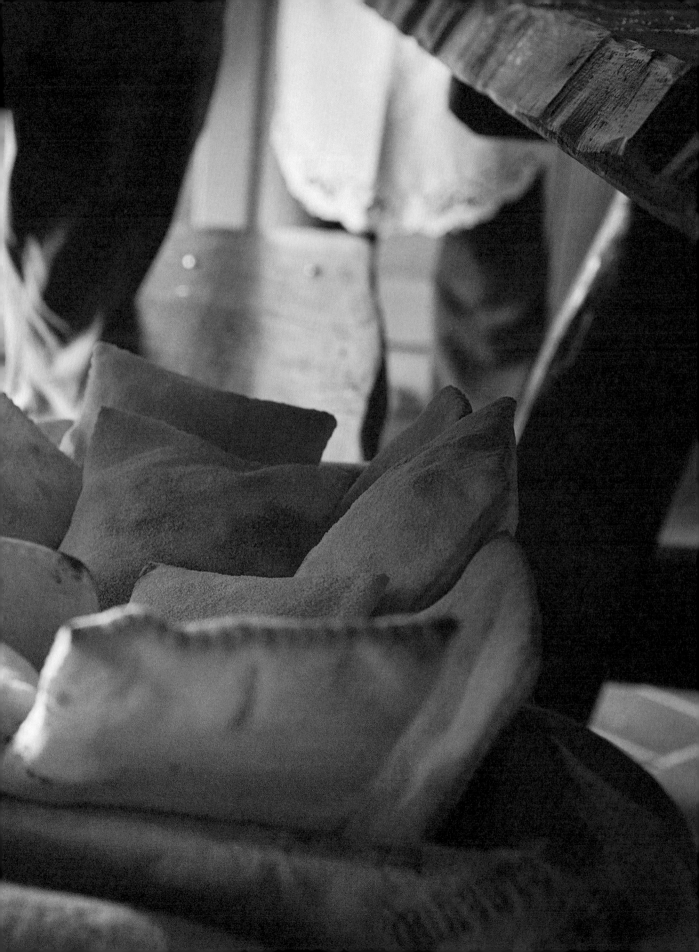

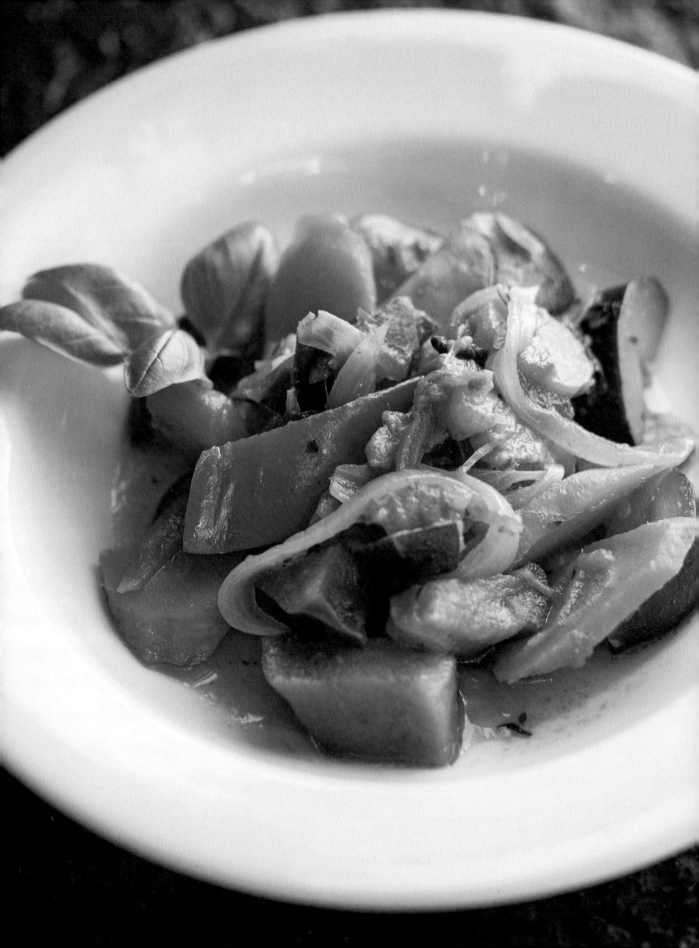

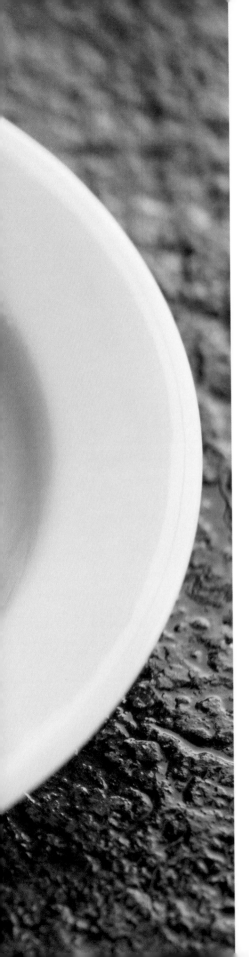

Veggie Cassola

TOTAL COOK TIME: 70 MINUTES | MAKES 4 SERVINGS

Talana, like the other villages in the Sardinian blue zones area, is located a day's journey from the sea (and until 1960, a two-day round-trip trek was required to reach the coast). To avoid the travel, villagers produced their food in the highlands around their homes instead of relying on seafood. During the summer, when their gardens offer a bounty of fresh vegetables, this hearty dish appears on the dinner table of Sardinian shepherds most nights of the week.

1 zucchini, cut into ½-inch dice

1 large onion, chopped

2 large red or yellow bell peppers, chopped

2 carrots, peeled and coarsely chopped

1 Italian eggplant, cut into ½-inch dice

½ cup extra-virgin olive oil

Salt and pepper (optional)

1 bunch parsley, washed and chopped

5 leaves basil

1 sprig thyme, stemmed and minced

1 sprig oregano, stemmed and minced

3 bay leaves

Preheat oven to 300 degrees.

In a large bowl, toss all vegetables with olive oil. Add salt and pepper to taste.

Toss with herbs, then spread out evenly on a large roasting pan.

Roast for 1 hour.

Remove bay leaves, then serve with crusty bread or Sardinian flatbread (page 65).

Quick Greens and Onions

TOTAL COOK TIME: 15 MINUTES | MAKES 4 SERVINGS

Consuming cooked greens is one of the greatest predictors of longevity; we surveyed 670 people over the age of 60 and found that those most likely to survive the next 10 years were eating at least a quarter of a cup every day. Cooking greens, incidentally, breaks down cell walls in the plants to release nutrients. This simple recipe offers a flavorful way for you to incorporate this powerful longevity food into your daily diet.

1 sweet onion (like Vidalia), thinly sliced

1 to 2 tablespoons extra-virgin olive oil

3 pounds greens (spinach, Swiss chard, or beet greens), washed

Salt and pepper (optional)

In a large pan, sauté the onion in olive oil for 5 minutes, or until translucent.

Add all the greens; cover and cook over low heat for 5 minutes or until cooked and brightly colored. Add a couple tablespoons of water, as needed, to steam.

Remove from heat and chop.

Season with salt and pepper to taste. Serve hot or cold.

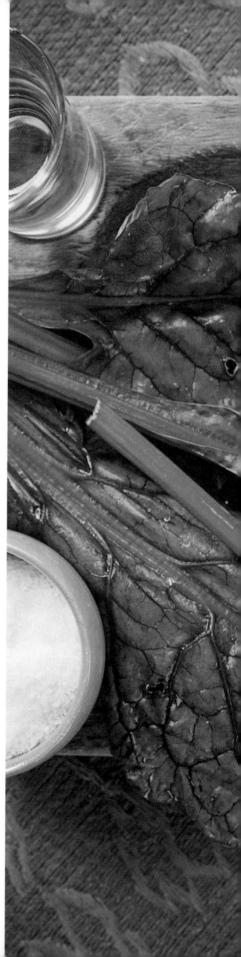

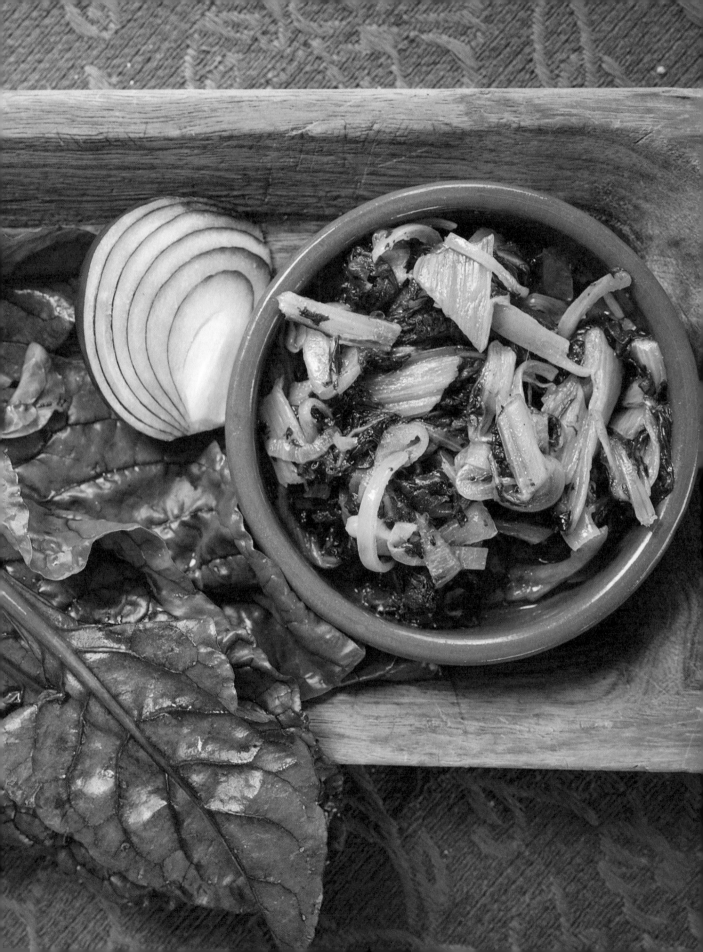

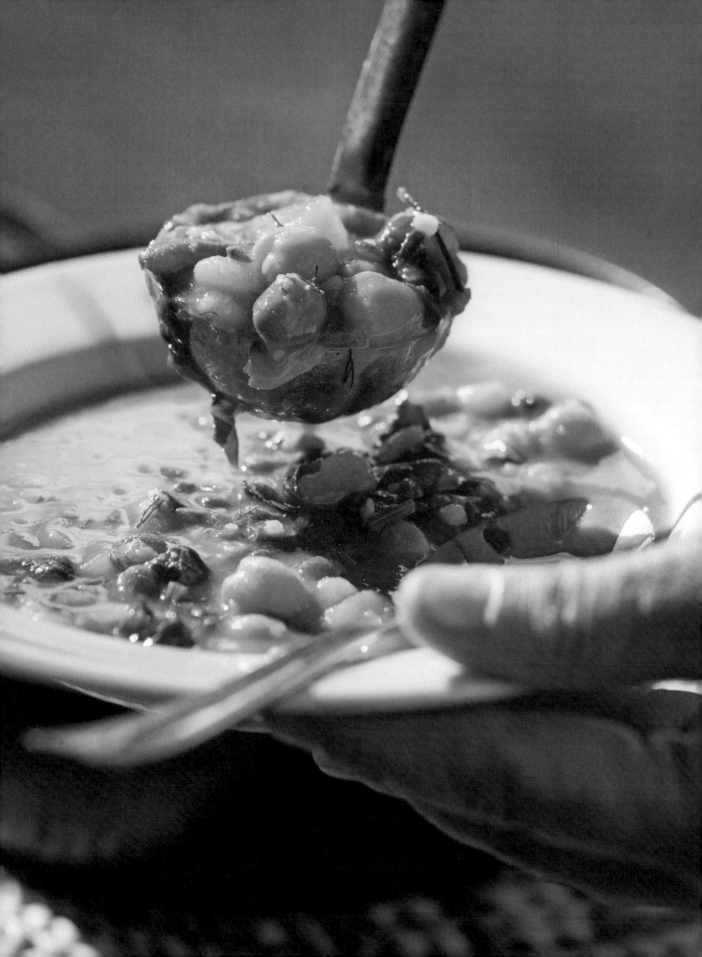

Minestrone Three Ways

Each of the six villages in Sardinia's blue zones area prides itself on recipes for both summer and winter minestrones; these chunky and hearty fresh vegetable soups are made and enjoyed year-round with in-season vegetables. Not only do these fragrant soups provide several helpings of vegetables, but they also deliver a full daily dose of beans, my favorite longevity supplement. This bountiful dish is eaten for lunch every day by the world's longest lived family, the Melises (see their version on the next page).

In America, we tend to eat only fennel bulbs, but Sardinians take full use of the aromatic fronds, which are also rich in antioxidants. The fresh herbs and fennel give these hearty soups a fresh and sprightly lift. You can make any of these with canned beans, but using dried beans will result in a deeper flavor. And, as longevity scientist Gianni Pes points out, a longer cooking time enhances the bioavailability of more nutrients, such as the lycopene in tomatoes, as well as carotenoids and other antioxidants.

MINESTRONE WITH FENNEL AND WILD GARLIC

TOTAL COOK TIME: 8 HOURS IF USING DRIED BEANS; 90 MINUTES IF USING CANNED BEANS | MAKES 8 SERVINGS

¼ cup red beans, dried or canned (see preparation note)

¼ cup chickpeas, dried or canned (see preparation note)

¼ cup dried fava beans

¼ cup lentils

2 large potatoes, peeled and cut into 1-inch cubes

1 onion, chopped

1 bunch beet or Swiss chard leaves

2 fennel bulbs and stalks, washed and chopped

1 fresh tomato

2 garlic cloves

1 stalk celery, chopped

2 cups cubed pumpkin or other squash (zucchini, yellow, butternut, acorn)

4 to 5 stalks wild garlic, garlic scapes, or garlic chives

¼ cup *fregula* pasta

3 quarts water

If using dried beans:
Soak beans at least 6 hours, or overnight; drain and rinse.

Peel the fava beans by squeezing each one between your thumb and other fingers. The skins should slip off pretty easily.

In a soup pot, simmer beans in water to cover for 45 minutes to 1 hour, adding lentils after 30 minutes.

Drain beans and lentils.

If using canned beans:
Rinse and simmer beans and lentils in water to cover for 30 minutes, then drain.

For the minestrone:
In large soup pot, combine beans with all vegetables in water and bring to a boil.

Lower heat to medium-low and simmer for 15 minutes.

Add *fregula* and simmer for another 15 minutes.

Serve with crusty bread and a drizzle of olive oil.

(Minestrone Three Ways continued)

HERBED LENTIL MINESTRONE WITH WILD FENNEL (right)

TOTAL COOK TIME: 40 MINUTES | MAKES 5 SERVINGS

¾ cup dried chickpeas, soaked overnight (or one 15-ounce can, drained)

¼ cup lentils

1 white onion, chopped

1 tablespoon extra-virgin olive oil

4 sun-dried tomatoes, coarsely chopped

Small bunch of mint, finely chopped

Sprig of rosemary, stem removed

1 bay leaf

1 wild fennel bulb with fronds, coarsely chopped

¼ pound peeled potatoes, cubed

1½ cups barley

Salt and pepper (optional)

In a soup pot, combine all ingredients. Cover with water to an inch above the top of the other ingredients.

Bring to a boil and reduce to a simmer.

Cook for about 30 minutes.

Add salt and pepper to taste.

Remove bay leaf before serving.

MELIS FAMILY MINESTRONE

TOTAL COOK TIME: 8 HOURS IF USING DRIED BEANS; 30 MINUTES IF USING CANNED BEANS | MAKES 8 SERVINGS

7 tablespoons extra-virgin olive oil, divided

1 medium yellow or white onion, chopped (about 1 cup)

2 medium carrots, peeled and chopped (about ⅔ cup)

2 medium celery stalks, chopped (about ½ cup)

2 teaspoons minced garlic

One 28-ounce can crushed tomatoes

3 medium yellow potatoes, peeled and diced (about 1½ cups)

1½ cups chopped fennel (bulbs, stalks, and fronds)

¼ cup loosely packed fresh Italian flat-leaf parsley leaves, chopped

2 tablespoons chopped fresh basil leaves

½ cup dried and peeled fava beans, soaked overnight (or one 15-ounce can, drained)

½ cup dried cranberry beans, soaked overnight (or one 15-ounce can, drained)

⅓ cup dried chickpeas, soaked overnight (or ½ 15-ounce can, drained)

6 to 8 cups water

⅔ cup Sardinian *fregula,* Israeli couscous, or *acini di pepe* pasta

½ teaspoon salt

½ teaspoon freshly ground black pepper

Warm 3 tablespoons of olive oil in a large soup pot or Dutch oven set over medium-high heat.

Add the onion, carrots, and celery; cook, stirring often, until soft but not browned, about 5 minutes. Add the garlic and cook until fragrant, about 20 seconds.

Stir in the tomatoes, potatoes, fennel, parsley, and basil, as well as the drained beans and chickpeas. Add enough water (about 6 to 8 cups) so that everything is submerged by 1 inch.

Raise the heat to high and bring pot to a full boil. Reduce the heat to low and simmer slowly, uncovered, until the beans are tender, adding more water as necessary, about 1½ hours. If using canned beans, simmer for only 10 minutes.

Stir in the pasta, salt, and pepper. Add up to 2 cups of water if the soup seems too dry. Continue simmering, uncovered, until the pasta is tender, about 10 minutes.

Pour 1 tablespoon of olive oil into bowl before serving.

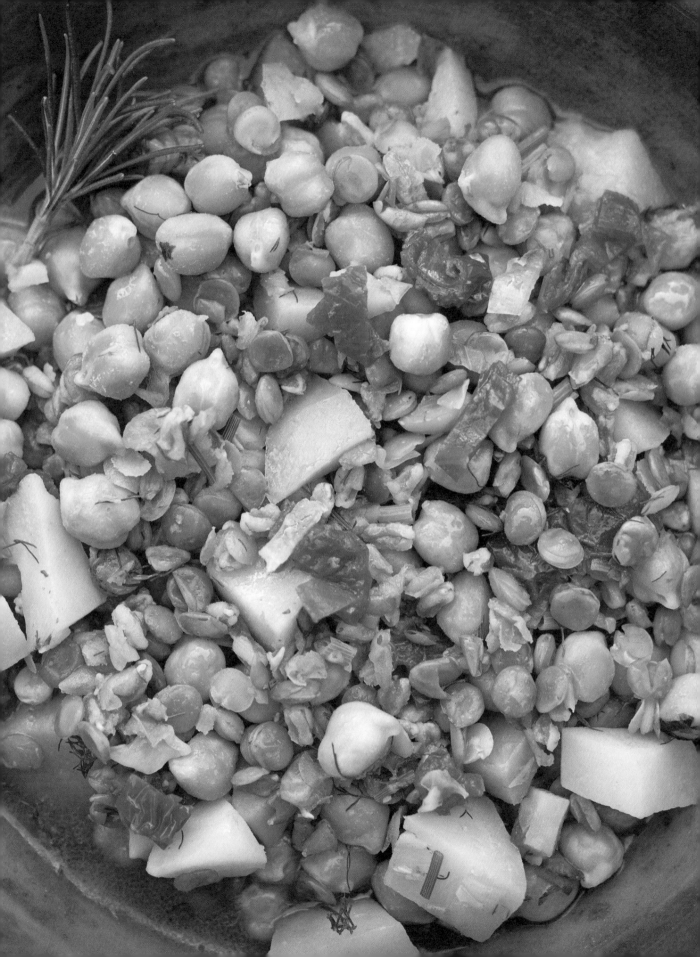

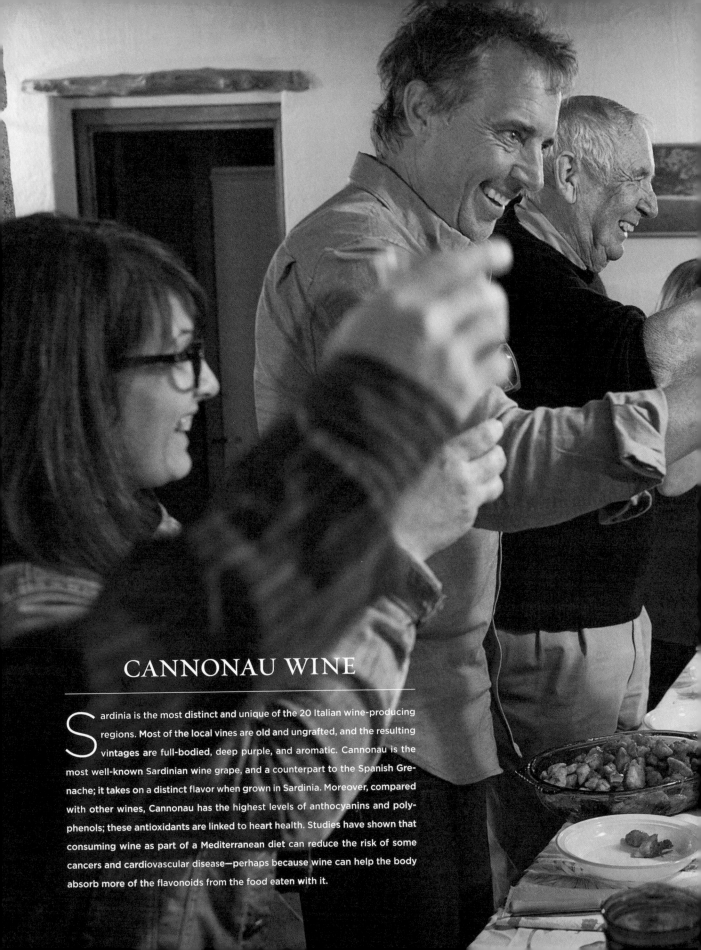

CANNONAU WINE

Sardinia is the most distinct and unique of the 20 Italian wine-producing regions. Most of the local vines are old and ungrafted, and the resulting vintages are full-bodied, deep purple, and aromatic. Cannonau is the most well-known Sardinian wine grape, and a counterpart to the Spanish Grenache; it takes on a distinct flavor when grown in Sardinia. Moreover, compared with other wines, Cannonau has the highest levels of anthocyanins and polyphenols; these antioxidants are linked to heart health. Studies have shown that consuming wine as part of a Mediterranean diet can reduce the risk of some cancers and cardiovascular disease—perhaps because wine can help the body absorb more of the flavonoids from the food eaten with it.

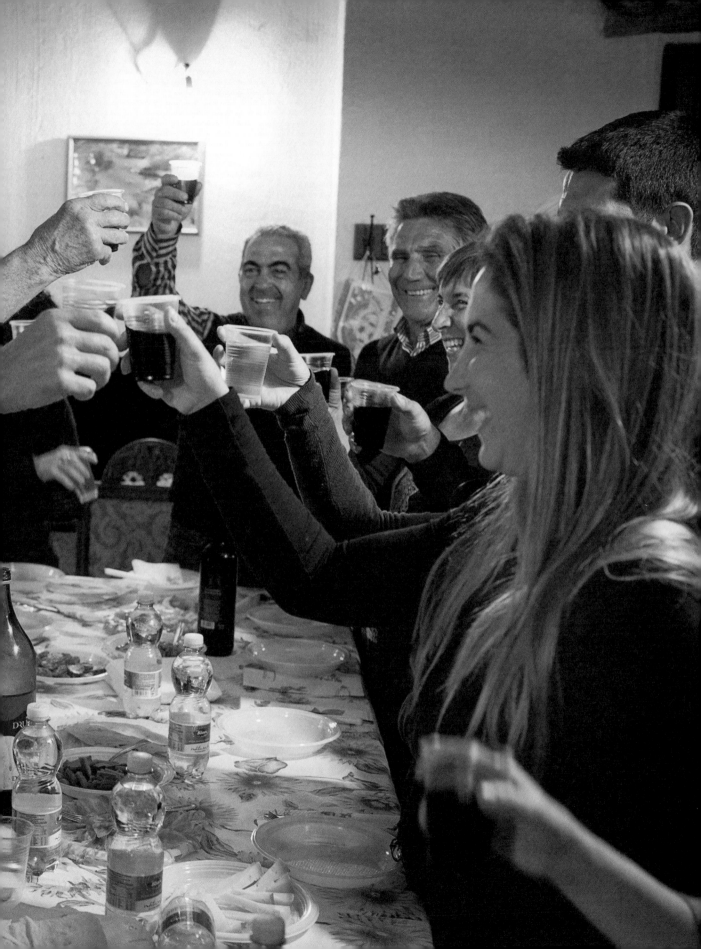

Fresh Fava Beans With Mint and Scallions

TOTAL COOK TIME: 25 MINUTES | MAKES 4 SERVINGS

Aromatic wild herbs grow everywhere in Sardinia's highlands, inland from the flashy coast. In the company of fava beans, which are central to the Sardinian diet, these herbs deliver protein, fiber, and deliciousness.

Fava beans, sometimes called broad beans, are one of the earliest vegetables to become available each spring. Sardinians eagerly await the appearance of the first fava and enjoy them in a number of ways, including raw and cooked. This simple dish brings out the best in seasonal eating—a sacred spring rite in Sardinia. It also tastes great with chickpeas for a variation that you can enjoy year-round.

4 tablespoons extra-virgin olive oil, divided

Small bunch wild garlic or scallions

2 cups fresh fava beans,* shelled

1 cup water

½ cup chopped fresh mint

Salt and pepper (optional)

In a large pot, sauté scallions in 2 tablespoons of oil for 1 minute, until wilted.

Add fava beans and water; stir to combine.

Simmer for about 10 minutes, or until the fava beans are soft.

Drain the fava beans and scallions and return to pot.

Immediately add mint and remaining olive oil to the warm beans and toss.

Add salt and pepper to taste before serving.

*You can also make this dish with frozen or canned fava beans. If using frozen, defrost and rinse beans; if using canned, drain and rinse. Next, warm drained beans for 2 to 3 minutes in a sauté pan with scallions in 2 tablespoons of extra-virgin olive oil. Remove from heat and immediately add mint and olive oil to warm beans and toss. Add salt and pepper to taste.

Fennel and Potato Cassola

TOTAL COOK TIME: 35 MINUTES | MAKES 4 SERVINGS

Wildly aromatic fennel grows all over Sardinia like a weed, especially in the spring and early summer. It gives a unique and sweet aroma to all types of traditional dishes. This stew is a delightful balance of flavors and textures: The potato provides heartiness, the onion provides depth and sweetness, and the fennel provides a slight licorice flavor.

3 baby fennel bulbs, stemmed, cored, and sliced into thin pieces

1 sweet onion (like Vidalia), roughly chopped

2 to 3 potatoes, washed, peeled, and cut into 1-inch cubes

3 tablespoons extra-virgin olive oil

2 cups water, divided

3 bay leaves

Salt and pepper (optional)

In a large sauté pan, sauté fennel, onion, and potatoes in olive oil over medium-high heat until they are mostly cooked through—about 10 minutes.

Add 1 cup of water and bay leaves.

Cook over medium heat until water boils off, about 6-7 minutes.

Add another cup of water and continue to cook until vegetables are cooked through, about 6-7 minutes.

Remove from heat, discard bay leaves, and add salt and pepper to taste.

Cabbage and Sun-Dried Tomato Sauté

TOTAL COOK TIME: 20 MINUTES | MAKES 4 SERVINGS

Though cabbage is arguably one of the healthiest and least expensive vegetables, Americans don't do a very good job of including it in their diet, other than in coleslaw that's been weighed down with heavy mayo and sugar. This Sardinian specialty uniquely deploys the sweet, savory quality of sun-dried tomatoes to what could otherwise be a bland dish.

4 sun-dried tomatoes, rinsed and chopped

2 small heads cabbage, thinly sliced

1 cup green onions, sliced

1 sweet onion (like Vidalia), thinly sliced

3 tablespoons extra-virgin olive oil

Salt and pepper (optional)

Set a large sauté pan over medium-high heat, cook all vegetables in olive oil for 10 to 12 minutes, or until cooked through but not too brown.

Stir and toss frequently and turn down heat to medium (if needed) to avoid burning.

Add salt and pepper to taste before serving.

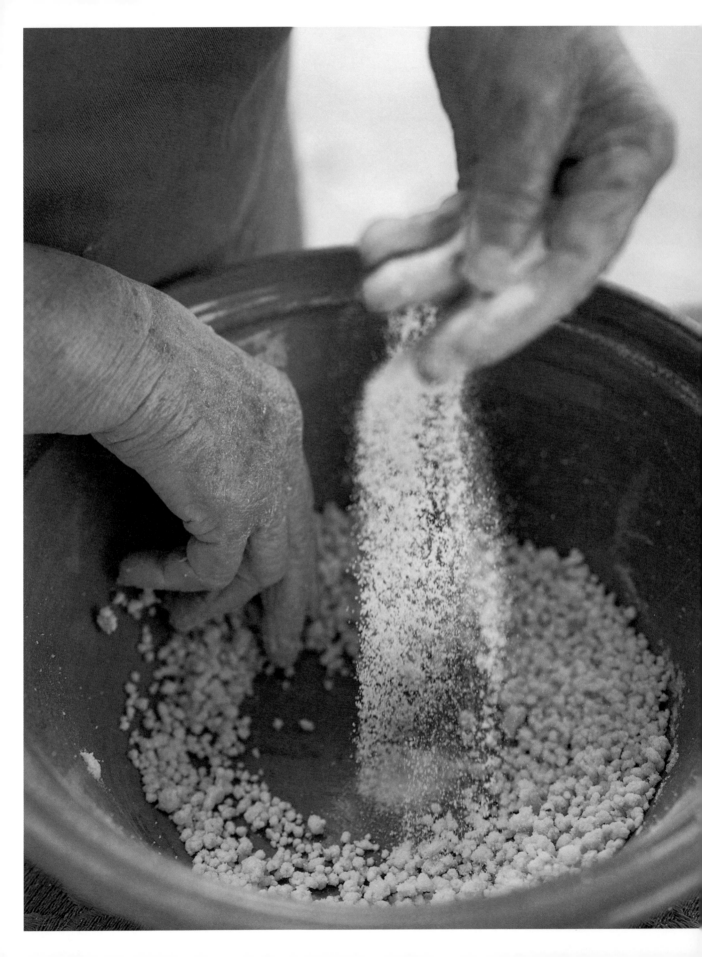

Toasted Fregula With Asparagus

TOTAL COOK TIME: 50 MINUTES | MAKES 4 SERVINGS

Inspired by North Africa's couscous, Sardinians created *fregula*, their own version of semolina pasta. To make *fregula*, they rub semolina flour and water together in a circular motion to form a round shape. Traditionally they then sun dry and toast it, giving it a rich, nutty flavor. While spaghetti and other types of pasta are used in Sardinia, *fregula* is more widely used on the island.

½ sweet onion, minced

1 pound asparagus, stems cut off, washed and cut into ¼-inch pieces

2 tablespoons extra-virgin olive oil, plus more for garnish

½ pound *fregula* pasta

4 cups vegetable broth

Salt and pepper (optional)

In a soup pot, sauté onion and asparagus in olive oil until onion is wilted, about 5 minutes. Add *fregula* and sauté for about 5 minutes—or until lightly browned—over medium heat.

Slowly add the broth, letting it absorb fully, about 10 minutes. Remove from heat.

Lightly toss pasta and veggies, and let sit, covered, for about 30 minutes.

Add salt and pepper to taste and drizzle with olive oil to serve.

Spaghetti With Walnut Pesto

TOTAL COOK TIME: 40 MINUTES | MAKES 6 SERVINGS

While basil and pine nut versions may be the most familiar variations to Americans, Italy boasts dozens of different types of pestos, often featuring parsley, mint, and other herbs. These sauces predate the introduction of tomatoes in Italian cuisine, which according to food historians didn't happen until the 18th century, as tomatoes were assumed to be poisonous. This uniquely Sardinian dish boasts a rich and bright flavor from the nuts and the parsley.

¾ cup walnuts

1 pound spaghetti or linguine

6 quarts water

2 large cloves garlic, finely chopped

2 tablespoons chopped fresh Italian parsley

½ cup extra-virgin olive oil

2 tablespoons salt

1 cup (¼ pound) freshly grated pecorino cheese (optional)

Grind the walnuts in a food processor until chopped but not overprocessed (avoid mincing or forming a paste).

Cook pasta in a large pot until almost al dente; drain and reserve one cup of cooking water.

In a very large sauté pan, cook the nuts, garlic, and parsley in the olive oil over low heat until the garlic is soft, about 8-9 minutes.

Add pasta and gently mix to combine with sauce.

Add as much of the reserved cooking water as you need to get the sauce consistency you like—probably ¼ to ½ cup.

If using cheese, add pecorino to pasta and serve immediately.

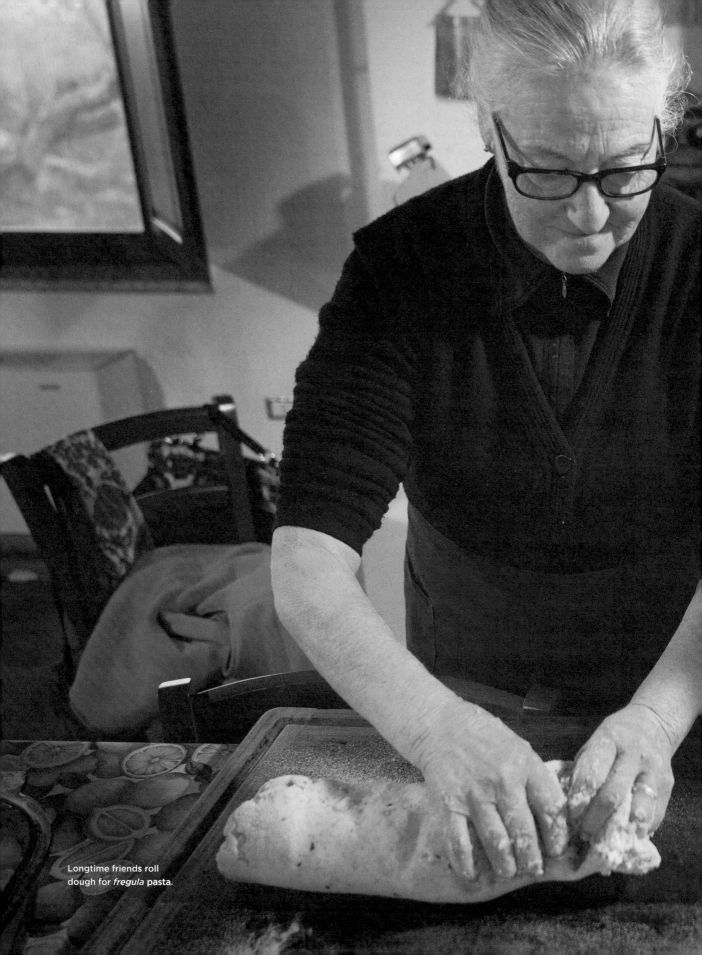

Longtime friends roll dough for *fregula* pasta.

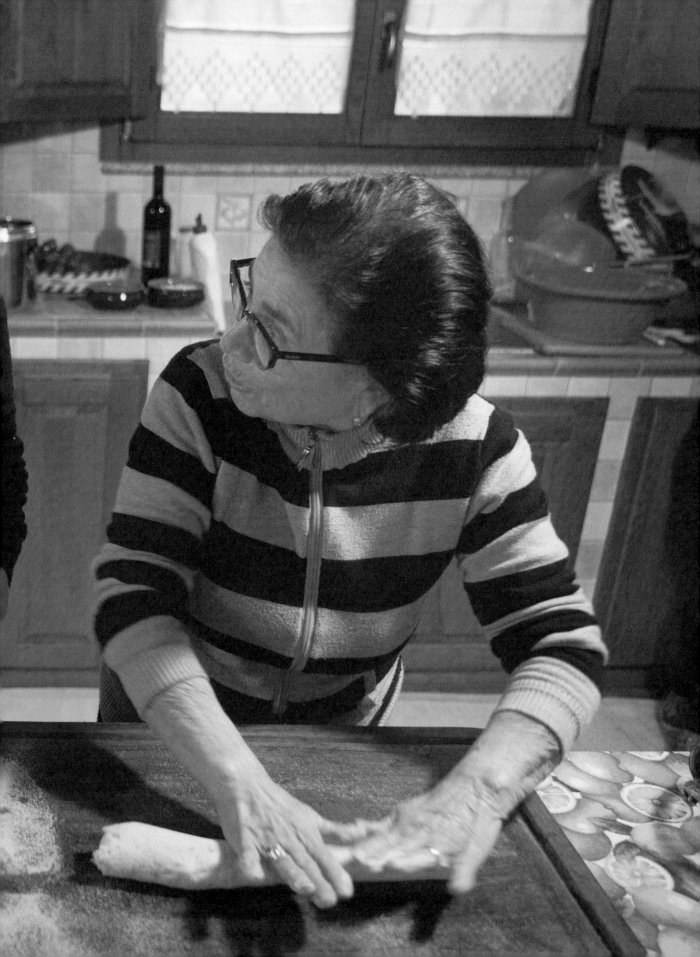

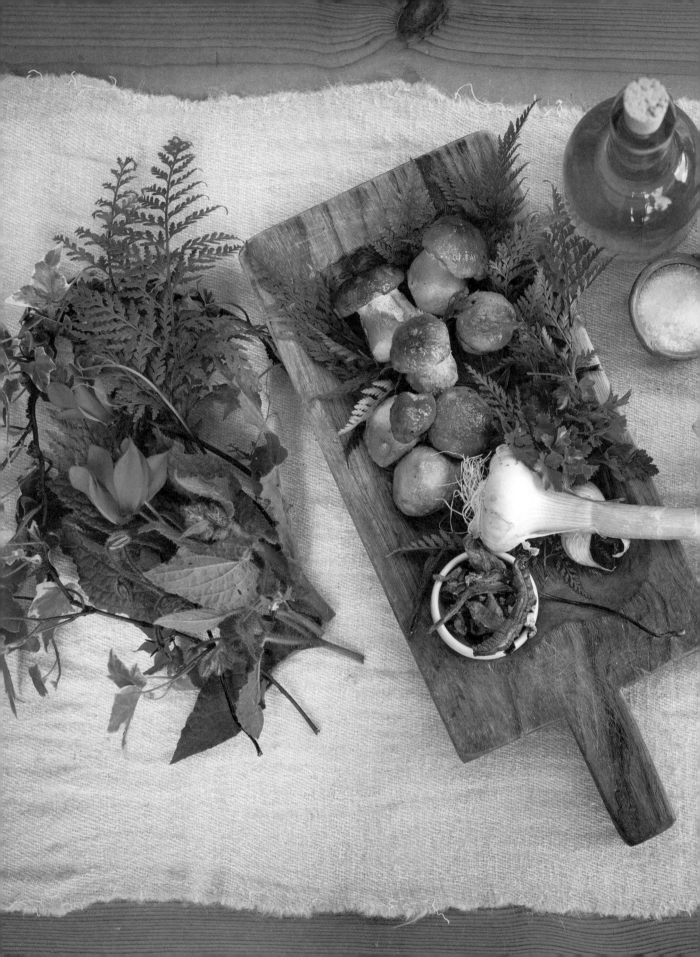

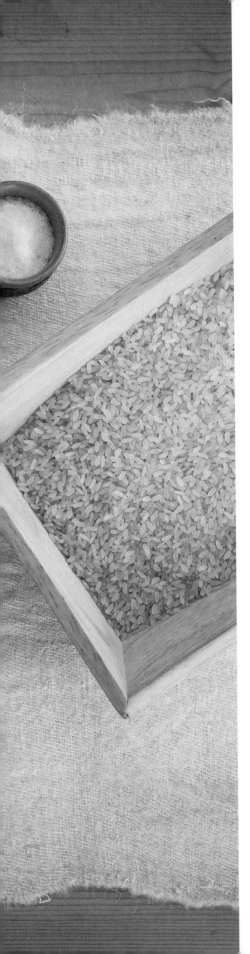

Porcini Mushroom Risotto

TOTAL COOK TIME: 1 HOUR | MAKES 4 SERVINGS

This plant-forward risotto offers all the flavor and none of the saturated fat of its Northern Italian cousin. In many ways, this dish is more similar to Spanish paella (Spain ruled Sardinia for centuries) than it is to the more widely known Italian risotto. The meatlike texture and hearty flavor of porcini mushrooms is unrivaled, since they don't lose their flavor and fragrance during cooking. This low-maintenance version of the traditional risotto is very forgiving—just make sure to remember to stir it while it's simmering on the stove.

½ white onion, minced

5 dried porcini mushrooms (or other dried wild mushroom), soaked in warm water for 30 minutes

2 cloves garlic, minced

6 cups water

Bunch parsley, minced

2¼ cups arborio rice

2 cups fresh porcini mushrooms (or a variety of other mushrooms like chanterelles, stemmed shiitakes, or cremini)

Salt and pepper (optional)

¼ cup extra-virgin olive oil (optional)

Grated pecorino cheese (optional)

In a soup pot, add onion, dried mushrooms, garlic, and water.

Bring to a boil and simmer over medium-low heat for about 20 minutes.

Add parsley, rice, and fresh mushrooms and simmer for another 25 minutes, or until rice is done. Be sure to stir the rice every few minutes so that it doesn't burn.

Season with salt and pepper to taste before serving and add cheese, if using. Drizzle with olive oil to finish.

Ladeddos With Tomato Sauce

TOTAL COOK TIME: 35 MINUTES | MAKES 4 SERVINGS

Pasta lovers will love this one—here the Sardinian version of gnocchi, called *ladeddos,* is accented with a touch of mint. This Sardinian custom is not something American chefs have fully adopted but should; mint adds a unique, fresh element to savory dishes. The traditional gnocchi is made with flour, potatoes, eggs, and some cheese, but *ladeddos* are more simply prepared with potatoes, semolina, and salt.

2 pounds potatoes, peeled (Yukon gold work well, but any will do)

4 cups whole wheat flour

4 cups semolina flour

1¼ teaspoons salt

5 teaspoons chopped mint

2 tablespoons extra-virgin olive oil

Quick and Chunky Tomato Sauce (page 66)

Bring a salted pot of water to a boil.

Boil potatoes until half tender, about 15 minutes. Drain and let cool.

Rice the potatoes with a potato ricer or masher in a medium bowl.

Add flour, semolina, and salt and knead to combine thoroughly into a smooth, firm dough that should not be too sticky.

Roll the dough into snakes, about 1 inch thick, and cut into 1-inch pieces.

Bring another pot of water to a boil; drop pasta into boiling water and cook until the pieces float to the top, about 4 minutes.

Drain, toss with mint and olive oil, and serve with tomato sauce.

Pro tip: Simmer sauce in a separate pan while the gnocchi cooks. After you drain the gnocchi, immediately add it to the simmering sauce for about 30 seconds; this melds the sauce to the gnocchi.

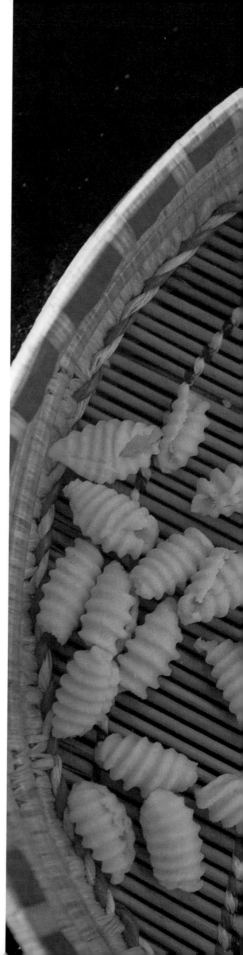

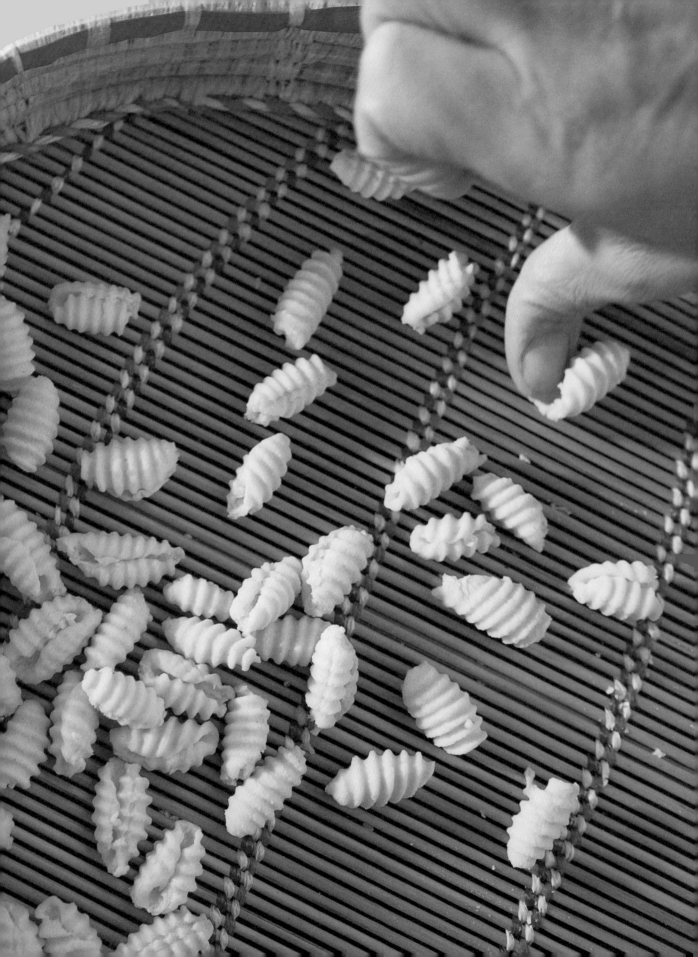

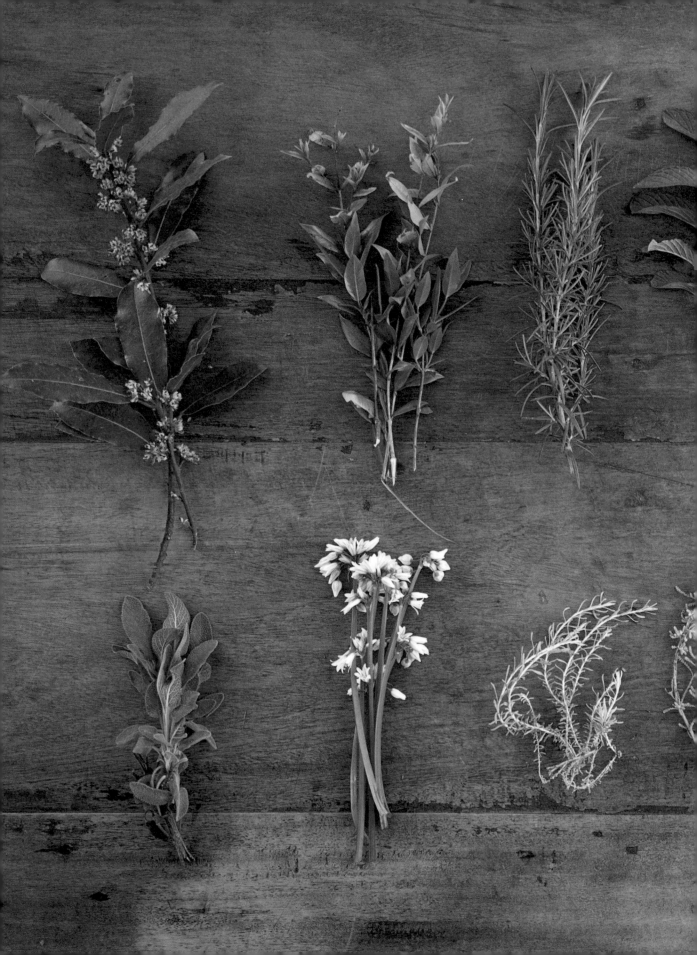

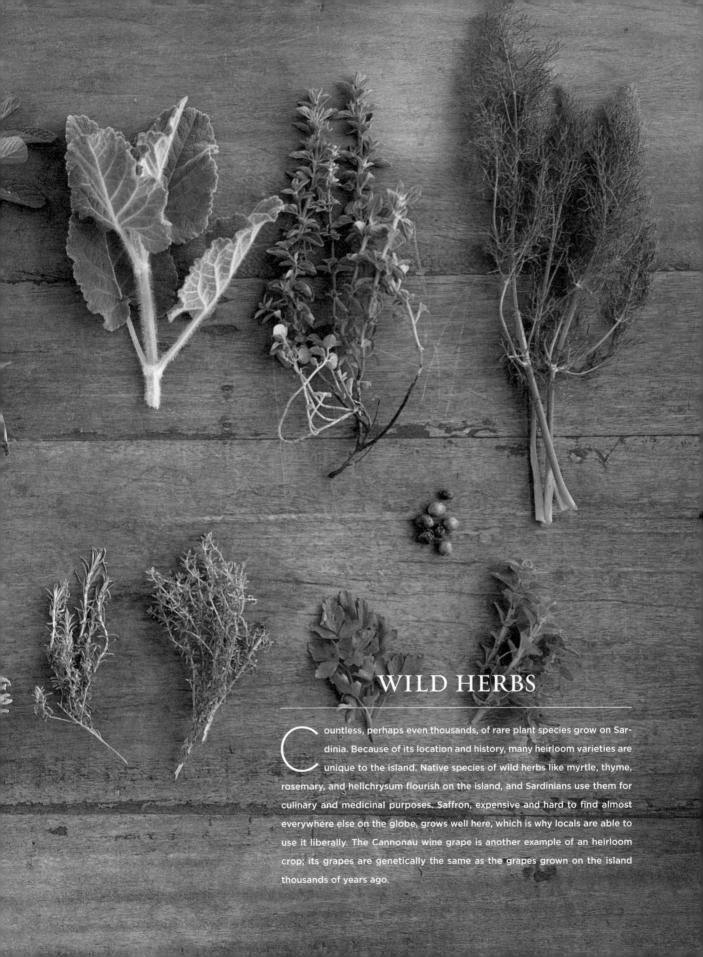

WILD HERBS

Countless, perhaps even thousands, of rare plant species grow on Sardinia. Because of its location and history, many heirloom varieties are unique to the island. Native species of wild herbs like myrtle, thyme, rosemary, and helichrysum flourish on the island, and Sardinians use them for culinary and medicinal purposes. Saffron, expensive and hard to find almost everywhere else on the globe, grows well here, which is why locals are able to use it liberally. The Cannonau wine grape is another example of an heirloom crop; its grapes are genetically the same as the grapes grown on the island thousands of years ago.

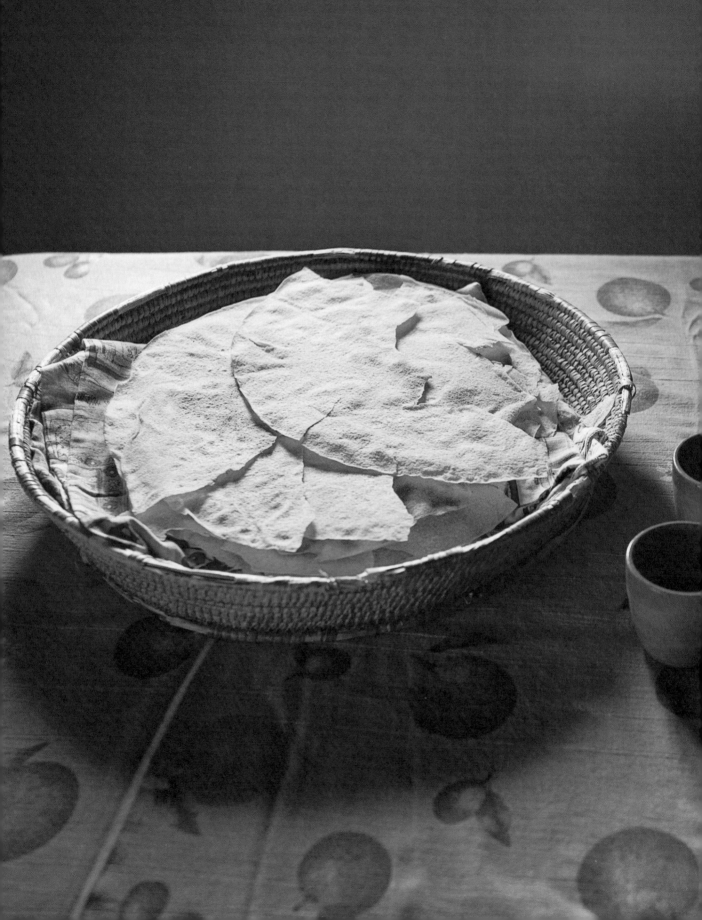

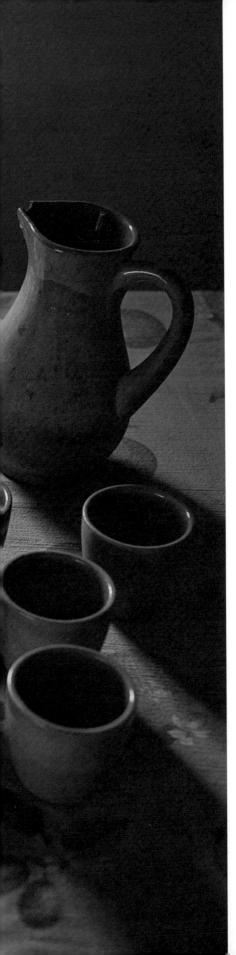

Sardinian Flatbread

TOTAL COOK TIME: 70 MINUTES | MAKES 4 SERVINGS

One of the most distinctive Sardinian foods, *pane carasau* is a crisp, thin bread that is shaped in rounds. Owing to its appearance and crackling sound, it is also called sheet music bread (*carta de musica*) in other parts of Italy. This bread dates back to ancient times, when shepherds herding their flocks needed a food that would not go bad while they were away from home for long stretches—and *pane carasau* can keep without refrigeration for a year or so.

Made from durum wheat, yeast, water, and salt, this flatbread is first baked so that it inflates into a balloon shape, then cut along the circumference of the bread into two thin sides, flipped so that the porous sides are on the outside, and then baked again to achieve its characteristic crispness and color. Traditionally, village women make the bread once a month in a group effort.

In Sardinia, *pane carasau* graces the table at almost every meal, and it also forms the base of many other dishes, such as a layered lasagna-type dish (page 69), in a pizza-like dish called *pane frattau* (page 66), and in the ever popular *pane guttiau*. *Pane guttiau* is *pane carasau* drizzled with olive oil, sprinkled with salt, and toasted or grilled quickly until golden brown. Pair it with sweet green olives and a glass of wine for a lovely Sardinian antipasto.

You can also buy *pane carasau* at gourmet grocers and online.

1½ cups all-purpose flour

1½ cups semolina flour

1½ cups warm water, plus more if needed

1 packet (¼ ounce) active dry yeast

Pinch of salt

Extra-virgin olive oil and coarse sea salt, for serving

In a large mixing bowl, combine flours, water, yeast, and a pinch of salt; mix thoroughly to form a soft but firm dough.

Divide the dough into quarters; cover and let rest for an hour.

Preheat oven to 375 degrees.

Using a rolling pin and lightly floured surface, roll each quarter of dough into paper-thin rounds.

Bake on a lightly oiled baking pan for 2 minutes.

Flip and bake for another 2-3 minutes, or until bread is crispy and brown.

To serve, brush or drizzle lightly with olive oil and sprinkle with coarse sea salt.

Quick and Chunky Tomato Sauce

TOTAL COOK TIME: 15 MINUTES | MAKES 6 SERVINGS

Sardinians use this sauce on pasta, *fregula*, or crisp flatbread (page 65) or as a dipping sauce for fresh baked bread. Studies show that people who consume a lot of tomatoes reduce their risk of ovarian or prostate cancer. The Sardinian tomato, *pomodoro sardo*, is larger than a cherry tomato but smaller than the garden variety American tomato. For this recipe, you can substitute with Roma tomatoes or grape tomatoes.

10 medium Roma tomatoes or 25 to 35 grape tomatoes, coarsely chopped

1 onion, roughly chopped

1 clove garlic, minced

3 to 4 leaves basil, chopped

2 tablespoons extra-virgin olive oil

Salt and pepper (optional)

In a sauté pan, sauté all ingredients in olive oil until onion is not quite transparent, about 8-10 minutes.

Sauce will be chunky but not broken down all the way.

Remove from heat and stir in salt and pepper to taste.

Sardinian-Style Pizza

TOTAL COOK TIME: 30 MINUTES | MAKES 4 SERVINGS

This easy-to-whip-up dish—our version of *pane frattau*—is similar to pizza with tomato sauce, but the crust is Sardinian flatbread. Alternatively, you can cut a whole-wheat pita in half to make a round base and toast it until warm and crisp.

1 clove garlic, minced

3 tablespoons extra-virgin olive oil, divided

One 28-ounce can roasted San Marzano tomatoes

5 to 6 fresh basil leaves, sliced

Sea salt and pepper (optional)

2 cups low-sodium vegetable broth

8 rounds *pane carasau* (page 65)

¼ cup grated pecorino cheese (optional)

In a sauté pan, cook the garlic in 1 tablespoon of olive oil over medium heat until it begins to sizzle, about 2-3 minutes.

Add tomatoes, basil, and a pinch of sea salt. Bring to a simmer and cook for 15 minutes.

Season to taste with salt and pepper and remove sauce from heat.

In a large pan, warm vegetable broth over medium-high heat for 5 minutes.

Drop the bread rounds, one at a time, into the pan and let soak for about 30 seconds.

Remove from the pan and transfer bread onto individual plates.

Spoon tomato sauce over each bread round, spreading evenly. Garnish with pecorino, if using.

Summer Pasta With Fresh Tomato and Basil

TOTAL COOK TIME: 30 MINUTES | MAKES 4 SERVINGS

Inspired by the fresh ingredients from Sardinia—often grown and picked in the gardens found in local back-yards—the simple, delicious balance of tomatoes and seasonings in this recipe is my own creation. I love to whip it up in late summer, when the basil and tomatoes in my own garden are perfectly ripe.

3 to 4 cups water

4 tomatoes (Roma will work well here)

1 clove garlic

¼ red onion, minced

¼ cup extra-virgin olive oil

½ cup finely chopped fresh basil

1 pound angel hair or capellini pasta

Red pepper flakes (optional)

Salt and pepper (optional)

Bring water to a boil in a medium soup pot.

Add tomatoes to water to parboil. Remove after 1 minute.

When cool enough to handle, remove skins from the tomatoes and coarsely chop.

In a large mixing bowl, combine the tomatoes, garlic, onion, olive oil, and basil; let sit for 10-20 minutes so the flavors combine.

While the fresh tomato sauce is marinating, cook pasta according to package directions.

Drain pasta, then immediately toss with fresh tomato sauce.

Season with red pepper flakes, salt, and pepper to taste before serving.

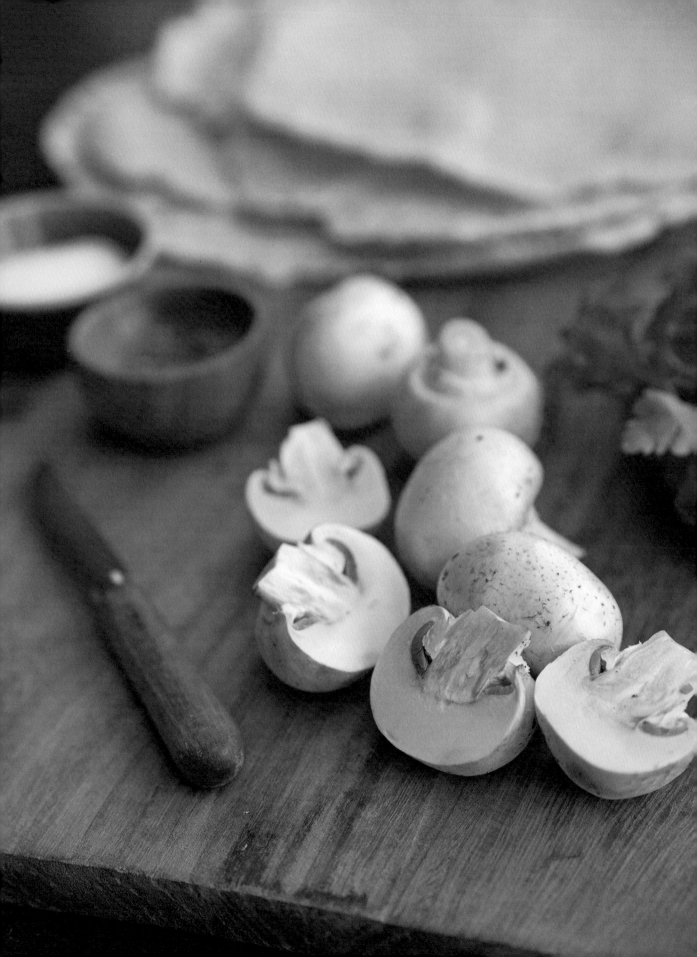

Sardinian Lasagna

TOTAL COOK TIME: 50 MINUTES | MAKES 4 SERVINGS

In Sardinia, this layered dish—a cross between lasagna and a casserole—is both everyday comfort food and a special occasion dish. You can make this to use up some leftover *pane carasau* (page 65), the Sardinian flatbread, or as a dish worthy of dinner guests. If you're not making your own flatbread, you can buy it at specialty gourmet grocers or at online retailers.

1 pound white button mushrooms, stalks and tops separated and finely chopped

Extra-virgin olive oil

Splash of dry white wine

Salt and pepper (optional)

¼ cup minced parsley

3 cups unsweetened soy milk

¾ tablespoon all-purpose flour

Pinch of ground nutmeg

6 rounds *pane carasau* (page 65)

1 clove garlic, minced

¼ cup grated pecorino cheese (optional)

In a pan over medium-high heat, sauté mushroom tops in a little olive oil for 2-3 minutes.

Add chopped stalks and cook for another 2 minutes.

Add a splash of white wine and continue cooking for another 3-4 minutes. Season with a dash of salt and pepper, to taste, and add parsley.

Remove from heat and set aside.

Pour half the soy milk into a cold saucepan. Add flour and mix well with a whisk, until it starts to thicken.

Add the rest of the milk, a pinch of salt, a pinch of nutmeg, and a couple drops of olive oil; whisk together. Heat mixture on the stove over medium-high heat until the béchamel becomes creamy and thick.

Remove from heat and set aside.

Preheat oven to 350 degrees as you build the lasagna.

Spread a thin layer of béchamel on the bottom of an oiled, deep baking pan.

Quickly dip each *pane carasau* in a bowl of warm water, then place in the dish and cover with a layer of béchamel and mushrooms.

Continue to layer *pane carasau*, béchamel, and mushrooms until you run out. Top with a final layer of béchamel and grated cheese, if using.

Bake for about 15 minutes, or until lightly toasted on top.

Let rest for 5 minutes before slicing and serving.

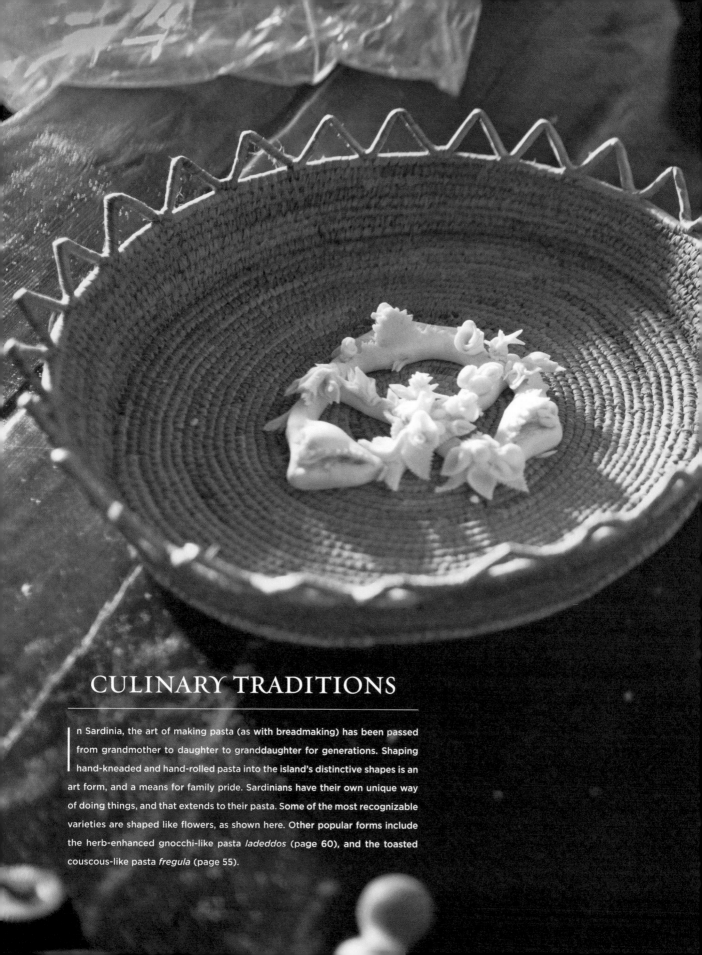

CULINARY TRADITIONS

n Sardinia, the art of making pasta (as with breadmaking) has been passed from grandmother to daughter to granddaughter for generations. Shaping hand-kneaded and hand-rolled pasta into the island's distinctive shapes is an art form, and a means for family pride. Sardinians have their own unique way of doing things, and that extends to their pasta. Some of the most recognizable varieties are shaped like flowers, as shown here. Other popular forms include the herb-enhanced gnocchi-like pasta *ladeddos* (page 60), and the toasted couscous-like pasta *fregula* (page 55).

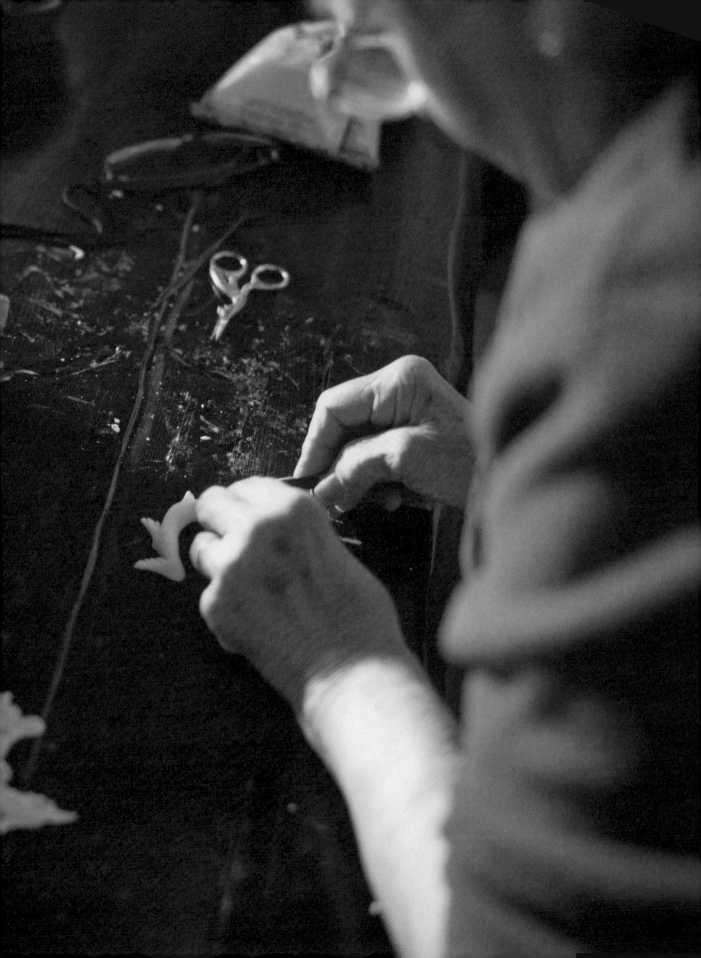

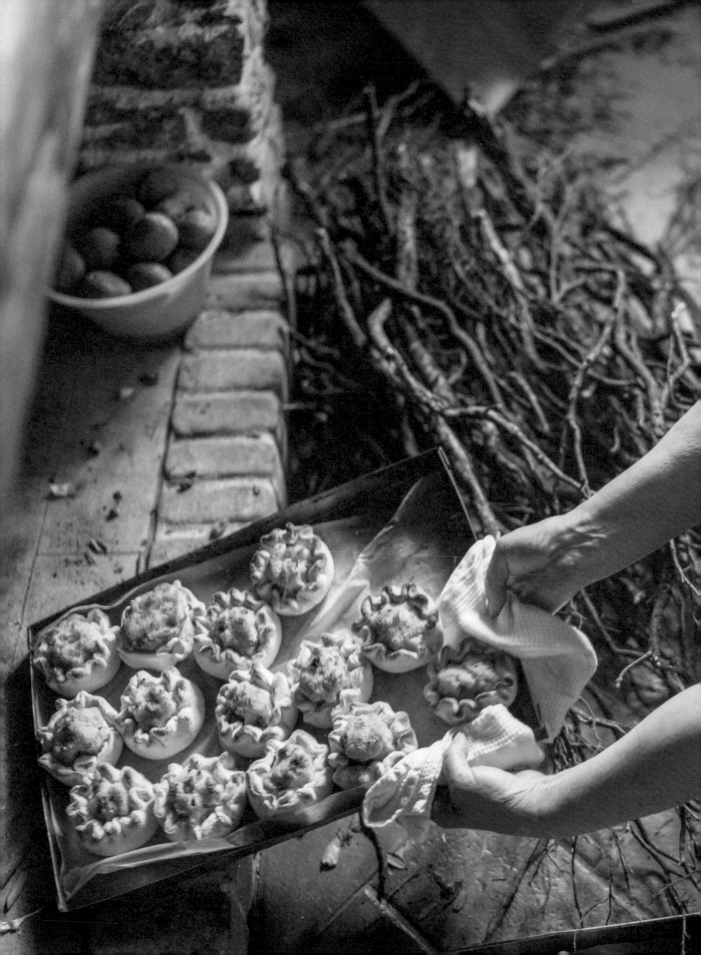

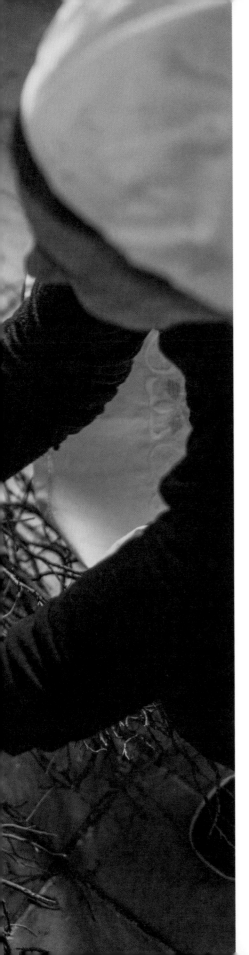

Mini Sweet Potato Tarts

TOTAL COOK TIME: 75 MINUTES | MAKES 6 SERVINGS

These mini pies are inspired by Sardinia's sweet and savory baked creations but are made easier with ready-made pie crust or phyllo dough shells. There are a few traditional Sardinian dishes that use sweet potato as the filling—from baked tarts to ravioli-like stuffed pasta. Roasted sweet potatoes become very sweet and sticky as they cook, so you don't need much additional sweetener to create these easy treats.

4 large sweet potatoes (red, white, yellow, or orange work)

1 large ready-made pie crust or 12 mini phyllo shells

2 tablespoons oatmeal

2 tablespoons pecans, crushed

2 tablespoons maple sugar or brown sugar

Preheat the oven to 375 degrees.

Bake potatoes with skin on for 45 minutes. You can do this in advance.

When done and cool enough to handle, slip potatoes out of skins. Potatoes will be soft; mash in a bowl.

Cut pie crust into six 3- to 4-inch rounds. Press rounds into a muffin tin and freeze for at least 10 minutes.

Bake the crusts for 12 minutes at 375 degrees.

Meanwhile, combine oats, crushed pecans, and maple sugar together in a small bowl.

Remove crusts from oven and fill with mashed sweet potatoes. Bake for 10 more minutes.

Remove from oven and top with nut and oat crumble.

Bake mini pies for another 10 minutes, or until the crust is golden brown.

Sweet Pumpkin Fritters

TOTAL COOK TIME: 20 MINUTES | MAKES 4 SERVINGS

Squash and sweet potatoes are cornerstones of longevity diets in all blue zones areas, so I was pleasantly surprised to see pumpkins growing in the highlands of Sardinia. And the very first recipe we discovered there was this tasty confection called *thippulas:* soft and smooth on the inside and sweet and crisp on the outside.

With its delicate flavor, saffron—more readily available and affordable in Sardinia than in the United States—is a wonderful addition to this dish. If your budget affords it, then we recommend including it in your fritters, but this recipe is perfectly delicious without it as well. Besides being a prized culinary spice around the world, saffron, recent research shows, is made up of chemical compounds that support respiratory, digestive, and heart health.

One 15-ounce can pumpkin
  puree*

Pinch of salt

1 cup flour (more if needed)

1 tablespoon baking powder

1 cup water

½ teaspoon saffron (optional)

Zest from ½ lemon

½ cup applesauce

Olive or vegetable oil, for frying

¼ cup confectioners' sugar

In a medium bowl mix together all ingredients, except oil and sugar, to make the dough.

In a large skillet, heat 1 inch of oil to 350 degrees. If you don't have a candy thermometer, dip the handle of a wooden spoon into the oil. If the oil bubbles around the handle, it's ready for frying.

Spoon tablespoons of dough into hot oil to make fritters, making sure to leave space between them, and cook them in batches.

Fry both sides for 2-3 minutes or until golden, and then transfer to a paper towel–lined plate.

Roll lightly in sugar and serve warm.

*The flesh of a Sardinian pumpkin differs from the jack-o-lantern pumpkins in America, which are too fibrous and watery. That's why we've subbed in canned pumpkin puree. But you can also substitute pureed acorn or butternut squash.

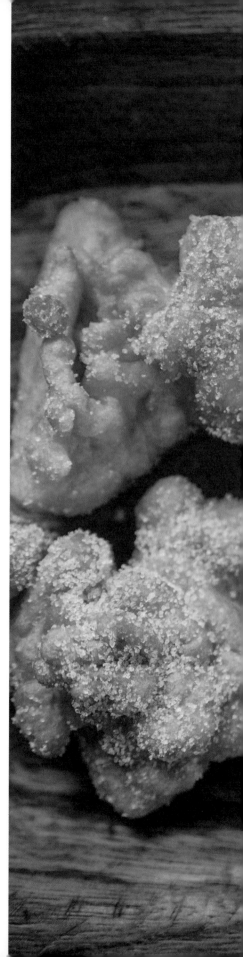

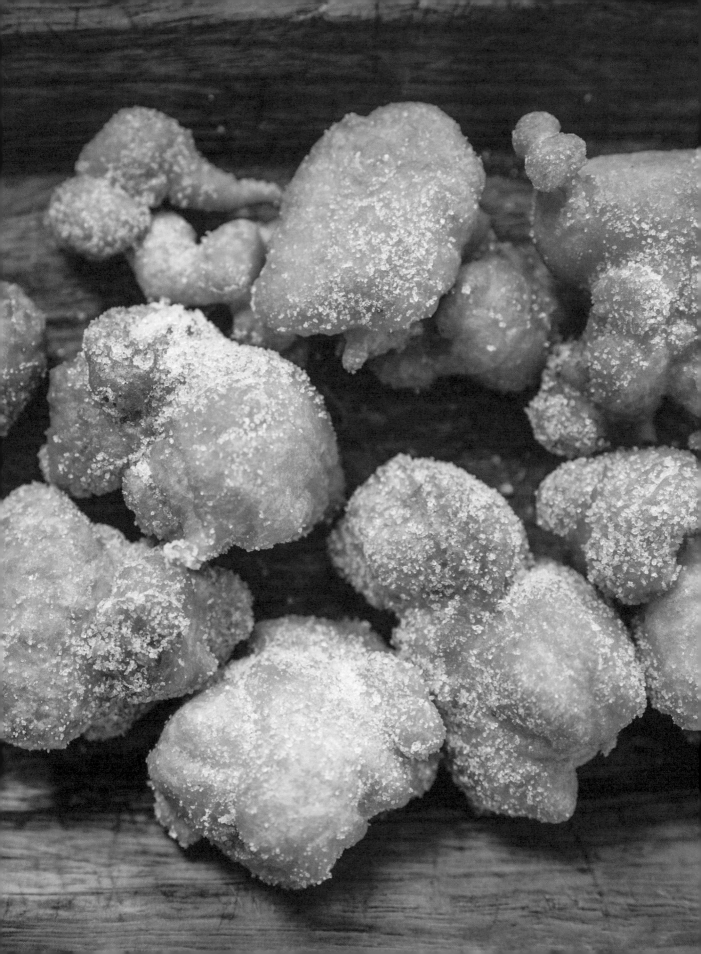

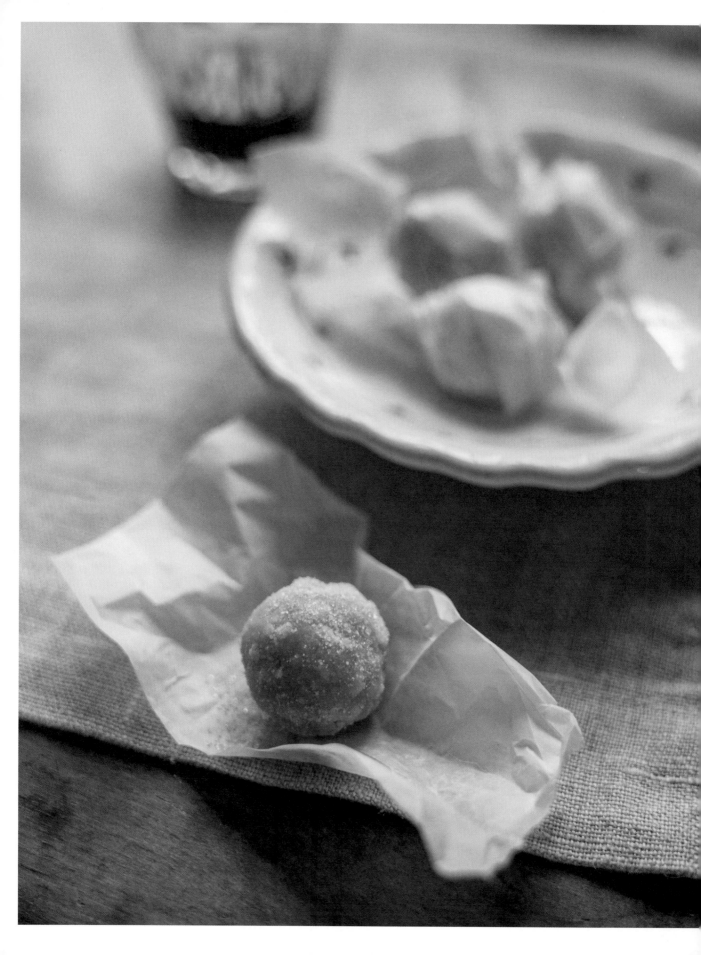

Almond Cookies

TOTAL COOK TIME: 30 MINUTES | **MAKES 16 SERVINGS**

Almonds appear regularly in Sardinian cooking. Nuts are a staple in all blue zones regions, and almonds are associated with losing weight, increasing good cholesterol, and lowering blood pressure. These traditional almond cookies—*goeffus,* as they are called in Ogliastra, one of the villages in the Sardinian blue zones region—are simple to make and taste delicious flavored with fresh lemon zest.

6 cups almonds, blanched and peeled

⅔ cup sugar, divided

3 tablespoons orange flower water

Zest of 1 whole lemon

In a 300-degree oven, toast almonds for 10 minutes.

In a food processor or high-powered blender, process almonds until they reach the consistency of coarse almond flour.

In a sauce pot, combine ½ cup sugar and orange flower water. Heat over very low heat until the syrup becomes thick.

Add the almond flour into the syrup, mixing to combine over heat for a couple minutes.

Turn off heat and add lemon zest, mixing to combine.

When cool enough to handle, roll dough into walnut-size balls with hands.

Roll the balls in remaining sugar.

Let almond balls dry completely and wrap in tissue paper, twirling the sides like candy wrappers.

Keep in glass jars or another covered container.

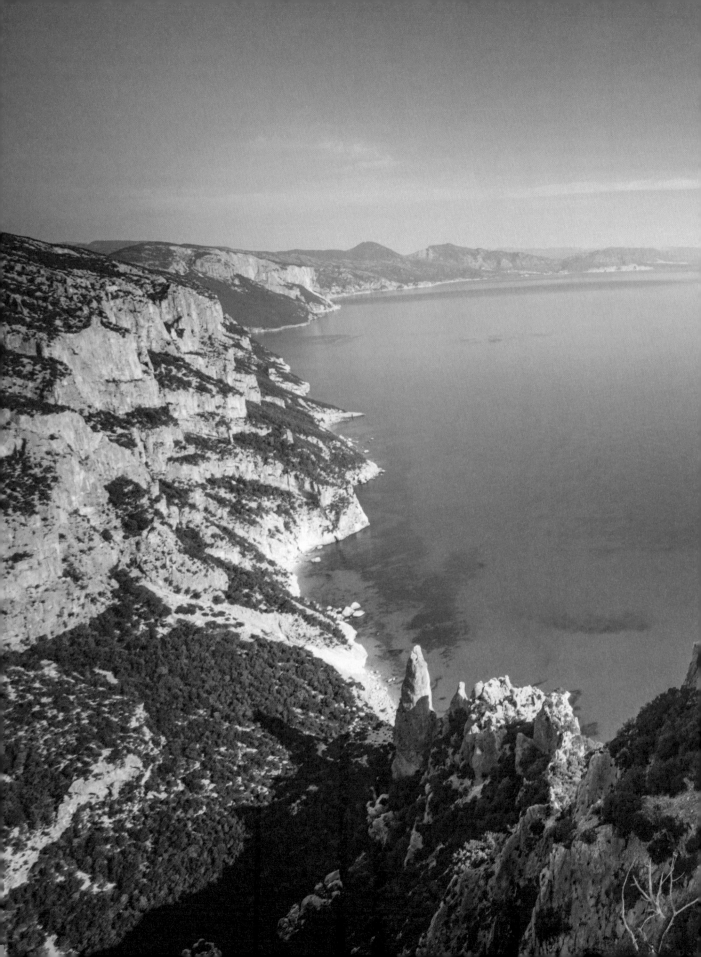

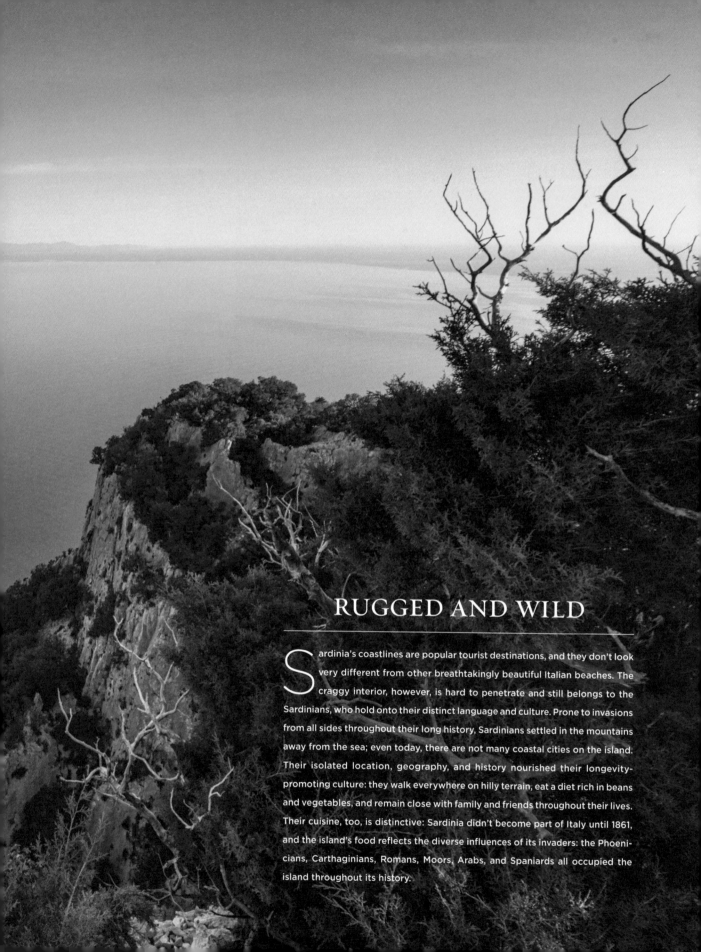

RUGGED AND WILD

Sardinia's coastlines are popular tourist destinations, and they don't look very different from other breathtakingly beautiful Italian beaches. The craggy interior, however, is hard to penetrate and still belongs to the Sardinians, who hold onto their distinct language and culture. Prone to invasions from all sides throughout their long history, Sardinians settled in the mountains away from the sea; even today, there are not many coastal cities on the island. Their isolated location, geography, and history nourished their longevity-promoting culture: they walk everywhere on hilly terrain, eat a diet rich in beans and vegetables, and remain close with family and friends throughout their lives. Their cuisine, too, is distinctive: Sardinia didn't become part of Italy until 1861, and the island's food reflects the diverse influences of its invaders: the Phoenicians, Carthaginians, Romans, Moors, Arabs, and Spaniards all occupied the island throughout its history.

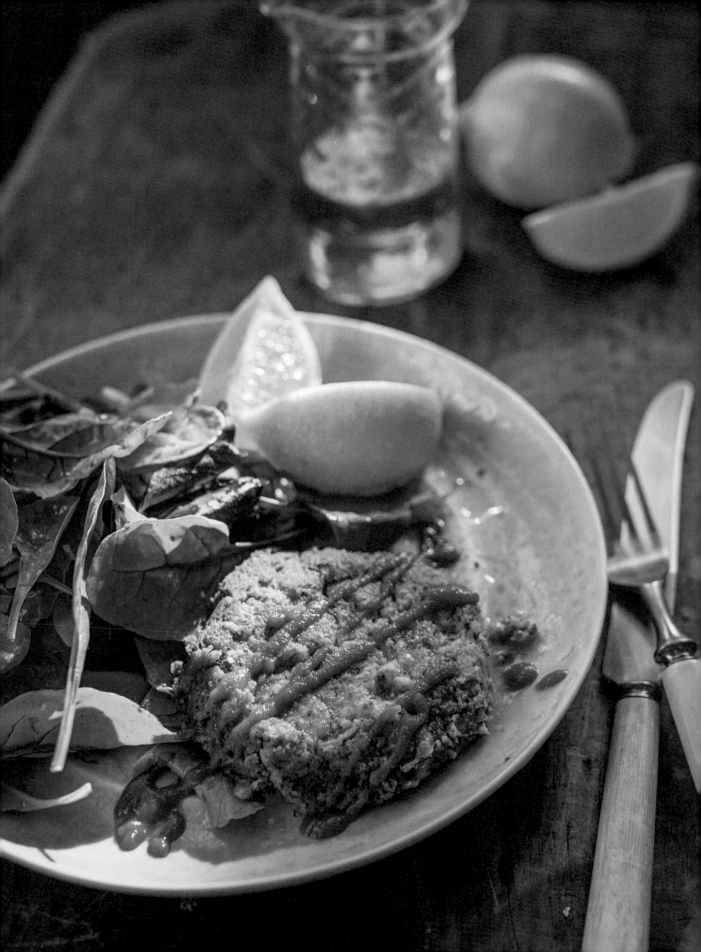

Chickpea (Falafel) Patties

TOTAL COOK TIME: 25 MINUTES | **MAKES 6 SERVINGS**

These falafel-inspired patties are full of flavor and spice but are lighter and easier to make as they aren't deep fried.

The largest certified blue zones community in the United States, Fort Worth started on its Blue Zones Project journey in 2014. More than 300 businesses and organizations have signed on to improve the health of their employees and customers, and nearly 90,000 residents are involved in the movement.

Since 2014, Fort Worth has seen dramatic improvements: a 31 percent decrease in smoking, a 17 percent increase in people exercising three times a week, and important gains in overall well-being and life satisfaction. In the past five years, Fort Worth has moved from 185th to 31st healthiest city in the nation.

2 cups dried chickpeas (or four 15-ounce cans, drained)

5 garlic cloves

½ sweet onion, sliced

1 cup cilantro

1 cup parsley

3 teaspoons ground cumin

2 teaspoons ground coriander

1 teaspoon salt

½ teaspoon black pepper

⅛ teaspoon ground cardamom

1 tablespoon baking powder

Extra-virgin olive oil, as needed

Lemon wedges, for serving

If using dried chickpeas, place them in a large bowl. Cover with at least 6 cups of water. Allow to soak for 18-24 hours. Drain well. If using canned, skip this step.

Place the chickpeas and the remaining falafel ingredients (except olive oil and lemon) into a food processor. Grind until the mixture begins to hold together, scraping down the sides of the bowl occasionally.

Take a handful of the mixture and form a ball. If the mixture holds together, it's ready to be formed. If it doesn't hold together, grind it further. Don't add water, as this will make the dough too wet and it won't hold together.

Form the falafel into ¼-inch-thick patties.

Heat a medium skillet over high heat. When the skillet is hot, add enough oil to generously coat the pan and create a thin layer.

When the oil is hot, gently add the falafel patties to the skillet. Cook for a total of around 4 minutes, 2 minutes on each side or until browned. Remove to a paper towel–lined plate to cool.

Serve in a sandwich or on top of a sturdy salad with a squeeze of lemon.

❋ By Chef Sandra Lewis, Life at the Table, Blue Zones Project Fort Worth, Texas

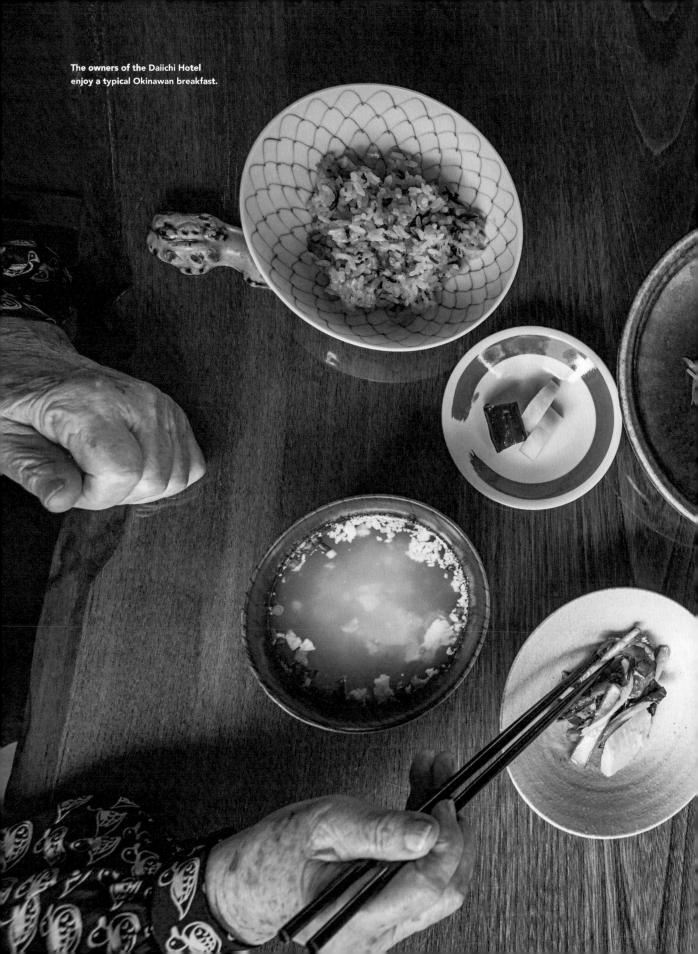

The owners of the Daiichi Hotel enjoy a typical Okinawan breakfast.

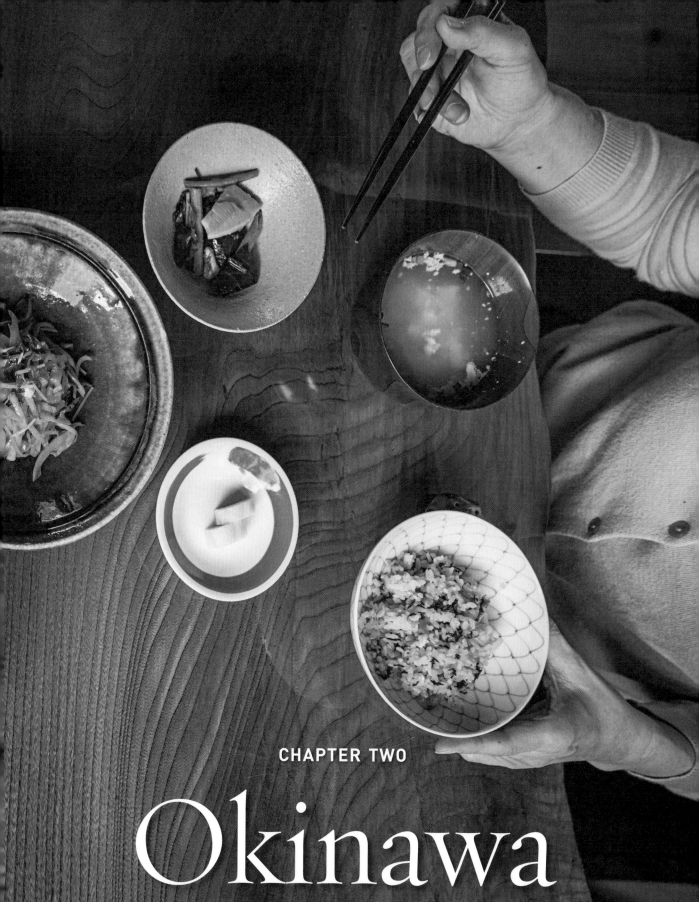

CHAPTER TWO

Okinawa

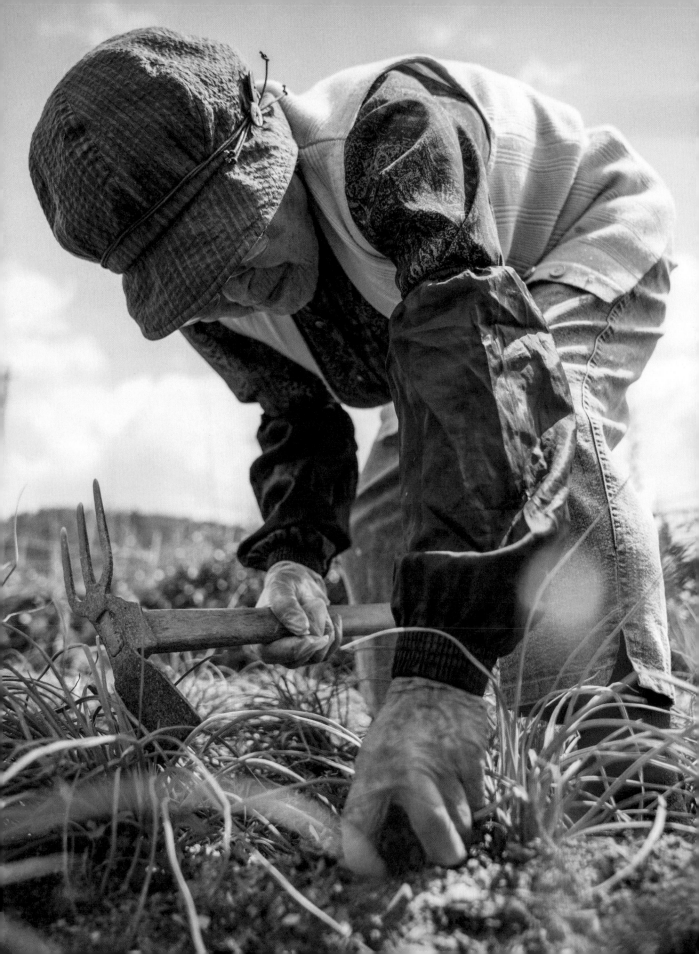

Okinawa, Japan

Combining subtle flavors from Southeast Asia, East Asia, and some of the world's most powerful longevity ingredients, the Okinawan diet has produced not only the world's longest lived population but also some of Asia's most delicious food. • Okinawa is a Pacific archipelago that was once known as the Ryukyu Kingdom. Its location—south of most of the Japanese islands, roughly 800 miles south of Tokyo, 400 miles east of the coast of China, and 300 miles

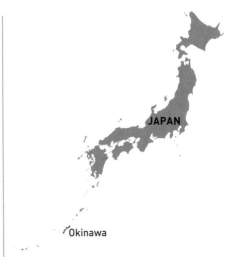

north of Taiwan—has meant that it has served as a trading post for centuries. For hundreds of years, China exerted most of the culinary influence, along with the traditional Chinese medicine practice of categorizing foods as cooling or warming foods. When Japan annexed Okinawa in 1879, the Japanese culinary influence grew stronger. Today Okinawan cuisine is a delicious blend of Chinese, Southeast Asian, and Japanese cooking styles, along with its native tropical vegetables and fruits. You won't find many of these regional dishes and delicacies anywhere else.

Through the mid-20th century, when the current crop of Okinawan centenarians were developing as young adults and establishing lifelong eating habits, the quotidian diet consisted mainly of tubers, garden-grown greens and vegetables, tofu, and a little seafood. About 60 percent of all calories came from just one source: a purple variety of sweet potato known locally as *beni imo*. Why? Mostly because typhoons blew through the islands several times a year, wiping out most other crops but sparing these underground tubers. The Okinawan sweet potatoes were abundant, easy to

Fuji Kinoshita, well into her 90s, carefully tends to her vegetable garden as she has for her entire life.

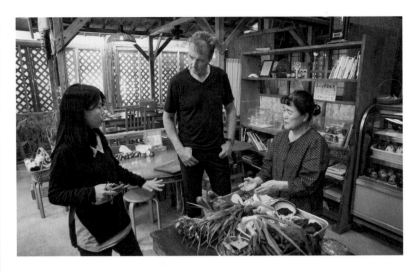

Dan and his translator talk with a shop owner about the benefits of local ingredients.

prepare, and—dressed up with garlic chives or sesame oil—could be made to taste delicious.

Over the centuries, Okinawan cooking assimilated white rice, sugarcane, and many of the other wild vegetables you might see in an Asian market. Okinawans' use of bitter melon, as well as herbs and spices like turmeric, is evidence of the southern and southeastern Asian influence. In the 16th century, a semisavage strain of black swine arrived on the island and proliferated slowly; by the late 19th century, most households kept a family pig, and pork found its way into Okinawan cuisine (though mostly as a celebratory food).

Okinawans readily adopted the Japanese trick of using pungent flavors to enhance the taste of healthy vegetables. Most of the 24 recipes I've captured in these pages rely on a cup or so of dashi (see page 105), a rich broth commonly made from bonito flakes (flakes of dried, smoked bonito fish) and sea kelp. This "sea forward" broth brings the prized umami character to their food. A few ladles of dashi in your vegetable stir-fry can convert a plate resembling a compost pile to a tsunami of deliciousness. The resulting dish has fewer calories than a hamburger, with five times the nutrients.

MOST OF WHAT WE KNOW about Okinawa's longevity diet comes from Blue Zones collaborators Bradley Willcox and his brother Craig, along with their mentor, Dr. Makoto Suzuki. For more than a half century and in their best-selling book, *The Okinawa Program,* they've chronicled what Okinawans have eaten traditionally and how the ingredients may explain longevity. They reveal that Okinawan tofu is firmer and more packed with protein and phytonutrients; turmeric, used in teas and soups, is a powerful antioxidant and anticancer agent; and *goya,* the main ingredient in *champuru* stir-fries, has powerful compounds that control blood sugar. Plus, the ubiquitous purple sweet potato is high in B vitamins and potassium, and it has a higher concentration of the antioxidant anthocyanin (from purple pigment) than blueberries.

Lately, the brothers have been investigating FOXO3, what they call a "genius gene." It helps our cells clean up waste and reduces inflammation in the body. (Chronic inflammation is at the root of every major age-related disease.) FOXO3 also helps cells detect a malfunction and signals the cell to destroy itself, lowering the chances of cancer. And what activates FOXO3? Turmeric, kelp, green tea, and tofu—all four pillars of the traditional Okinawa diet.

Like all other blue zones regions, several nondietary factors explain longevity on Okinawa. First, the word "retirement" doesn't exist in the native dialect. Instead *ikigai,* or "a reason for being," imbues every adult life. Having a strong sense of purpose is associated with about eight extra years.

Other longevity advantages include the Okinawan propensity to support each other by forming *moais* (pronounced moe-eye), or committed social circles, and by practicing *yuimaru,* the spirit of mutual aid. Traditionally, Okinawan peasants didn't have access to bank loans, so they'd form groups of five to eight

At a cooking school, the teacher shows students how to make tofu and veggie champuru (page 97).

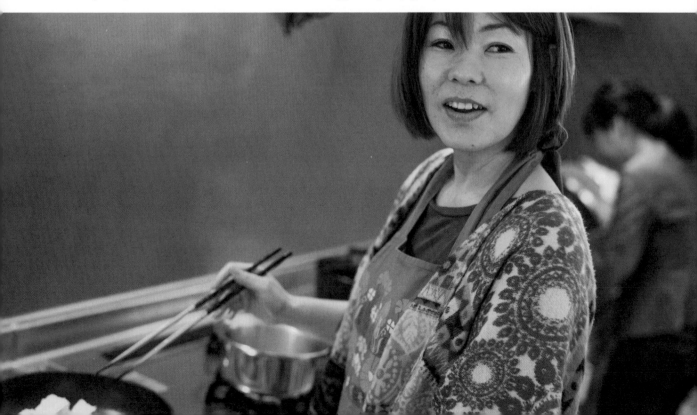

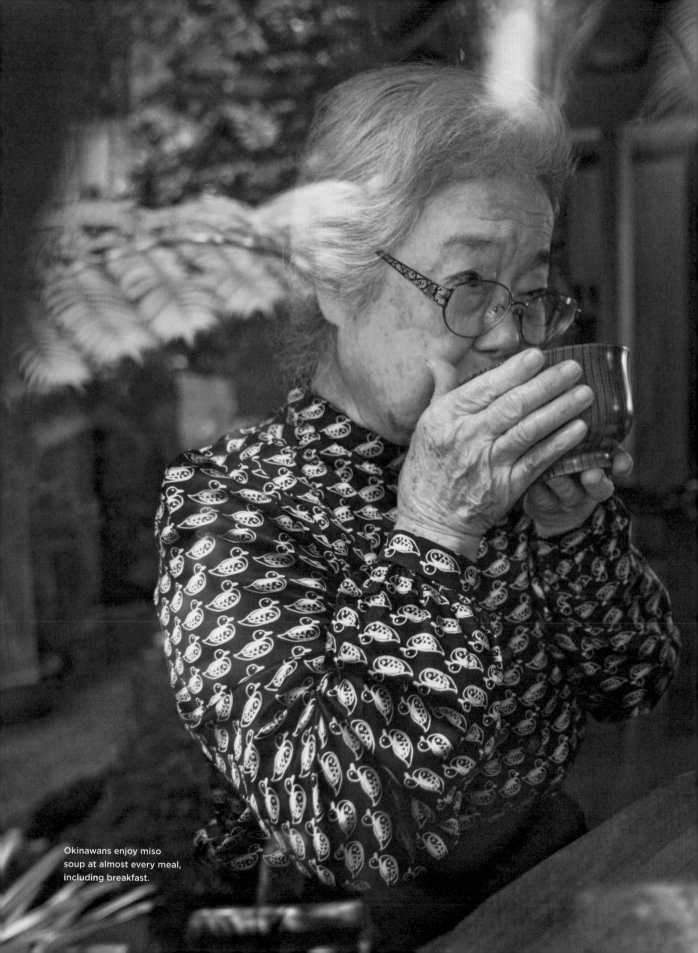

Okinawans enjoy miso soup at almost every meal, including breakfast.

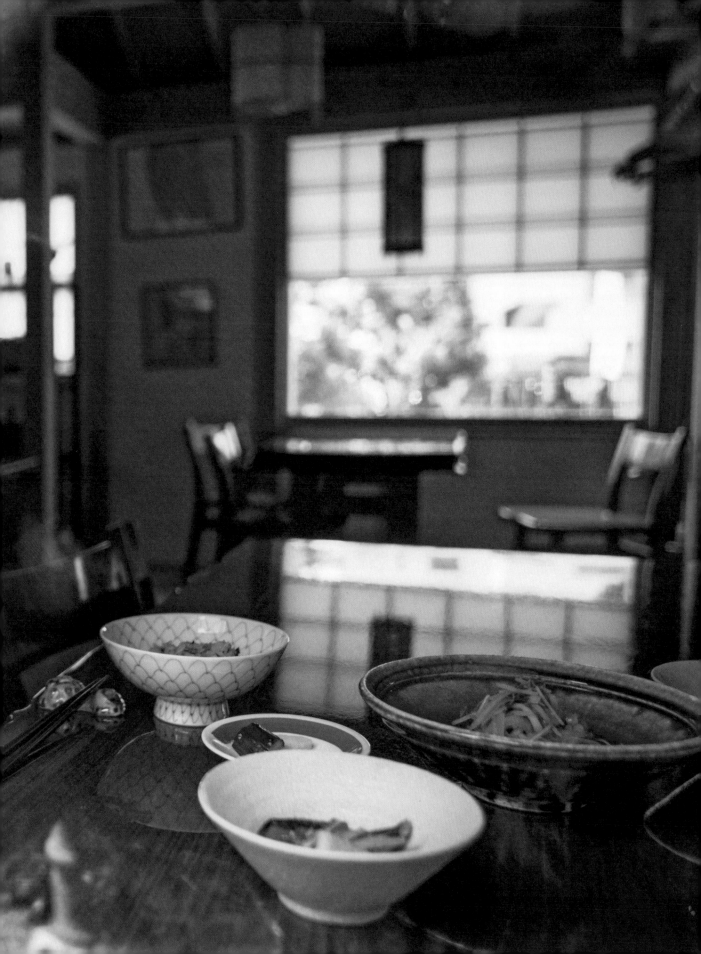

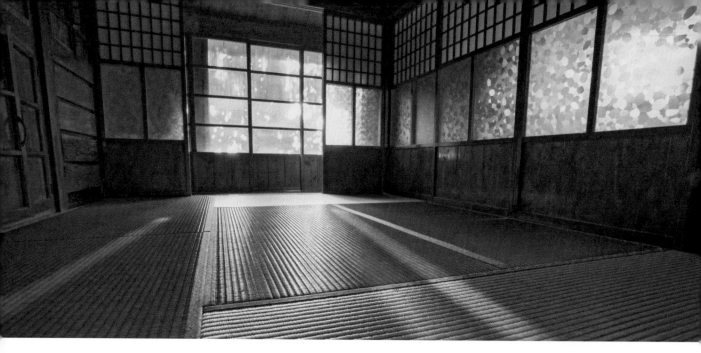

This traditional home is emblematic of the spaces Okinawans grow up in.

people and agree to meet regularly. At each meeting, *moai* members would chip in a sum of money to be given to the member with the greatest need. Through the middle of the 20th century, *moais* helped the community, providing aid to farmers needing to buy seed or covering the medical costs of a sick child. While *moais* are still popular in Okinawa, they're now mostly a social affair, and an excuse to gather around a meal. Nevertheless, the bond is authentic, and *moai* members tend to support each other, literally and figuratively. This ancient practice helps prevent loneliness, an increasingly prevalent ailment in the modern world that can be as bad for your health as a smoking habit.

SADLY, OKINAWA'S PROPENSITY toward longevity is slipping away. American GIs introduced canned Spam to the island, which found ready customers among the war-ragged, calorie-starved population. Today Okinawa is one of the world's largest consumers of this canned pork product, which the World Health Organization classifies in the same category as smoking when it comes to promoting cancers. By the 1970s, white rice had largely replaced the much more nutritious sweet potato as the staple food. The U.S. military base, a forest of fast-food restaurants (including the world's biggest A&W Root Beer stand) and a snarl of highways has paved over much of Okinawa's culture of longevity. Although this place once produced the world's longest lived people, they're now the most obese of Japan's 47 prefectures. And, though the jury is still out, in all likelihood Nagano is poised to overtake Okinawa as Japan's blue zones area. Why? Because Nagano is making efforts to limit junk food availability: a proven strategy that hasn't yet been implemented by Okinawa's leaders.

In an attempt to capture a style of cooking that is dying away, I traveled to Okinawa and visited cooks and kitchens that were still preparing food the old-fashioned way. To hunt down the recipes that follow, David McLain and I traveled with my 83-year-old dad, Roger, Fulbright scholar Jordan Kondo, and our translator, Naomi, to the villages of Ogimi and Motobu, on the northernmost tip of Okinawa, where vestiges of longevity cuisine still endure.

Cordon Bleu–trained chef Yoshiki Toyokawa took us four stories deep into a cave that was once used as a bomb shelter to show us how to make *tofuyo* or "royal" tofu. What starts as a plain tofu undergoes a regal transformation when marinated in a rice mold in Okinawan sake (*awamori*); it's then stored in the cave for a full year. The resulting product possesses the texture of cream cheese and a slightly sweet, powerfully rich cake that can be used like truffles to transform a mundane bowl of vegetables into a flavor symphony.

In Naha, we met Yukie Miyaguni, a *sensei,* or honored expert in Yakuzen, the practice of using food as medicine. She made us a killer miso vegetable soup and an astounding sweet bread, created by steaming instead of baking. We also met a mother-and-daughter team—owners of the Daiichi Hotel—who, each morning for breakfast, produce a 50-dish fantasia of traditional Okinawan foods. The combined calories of the entire meal: 560.

Realizing that some of our recipes may be a touch exotic for the American palate (though not mine!), we persuaded chef Toyokawa to take traditional Okinawan ingredients and create modern, easy-to-make recipes. So, if you want to ease into the world of Asian blue zones cooking, you might start with miso soup (page 106), tofu stir-fry (page 97), or my favorite, simple purple sweet potatoes mashed with coconut milk (page 119). You'll be a fast convert. *

FLAVOR PROFILE

These flavor pairings help form the framework for Okinawa's most popular dishes. You can use these compatible flavors to help enhance a variety of different meals.

* * *

dashi + soy sauce + scallions

miso + dashi + tofu

miso + dashi + scallions

garlic + soy sauce + sesame oil

ginger + soy sauce

ginger + scallions

turmeric + soy milk

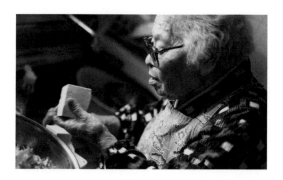

Yukiko Nakaima, 89 YEARS OLD

Eighty-nine-year-old Yukiko Nakaima invited us into her kitchen to show us how to simmer Okinawan squash and make a plant-based version of the otherwise porky national dish, *goya champuru* (page 94). She stood about four feet eight inches tall but commanded the kitchen like a drill sergeant, banging out five dishes in a half hour. Then she insisted we eat them all, refusing any excuse to decline, despite the fact she'd made enough food to serve 10 people.

Okinawa is the tropical southern-
most group of islands in Japan.

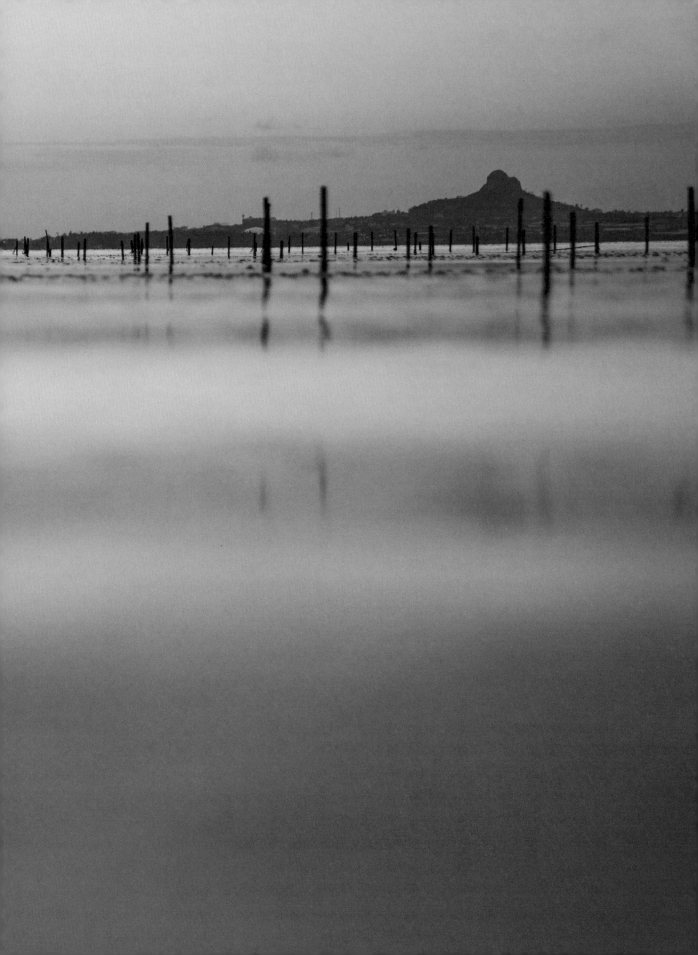

Okinawan Champuru Four Ways

Champuru means "something mixed" in the Okinawan language, and it can refer to this dish or sometimes to Okinawan culture: a blend of Ryuku, Japanese, Chinese, and Southeast Asian cultures and cuisines. The stir-fried dishes usually consist of tofu with vegetables, meat, or fish; the most recognizable version on the island today includes tofu, bitter melon, and egg.

GOYA CHAMPURU

TOTAL COOK TIME: 25 MINUTES | **MAKES 3 SERVINGS**

1 bitter melon, cut in half lengthwise, seeded, and thinly sliced

2 teaspoons salt

2 tablespoons vegetable or soybean oil

2 teaspoons minced garlic

1 teaspoon chili flakes

2 tablespoons soy sauce

1 tablespoon rice wine vinegar

1 teaspoon sugar

Place sliced bitter melon in a colander over the sink or a bowl. Sprinkle salt over slices and drain for 10 minutes.

Rinse bitter melon and squeeze to remove bitter liquid. Pat dry with paper towels.

In a sauté pan, heat oil over medium-high heat.

When oil is hot, add garlic and chili flakes. Stir-fry for about a minute, making sure not to burn.

Add bitter melon and stir-fry for 2-3 minutes.

Turn off heat and toss with soy sauce, vinegar, and sugar until well coated.

10-MINUTE VEGGIE CHAMPURU (right)

TOTAL COOK TIME: 10 MINUTES | **MAKES 3 SERVINGS**

1 tablespoon sesame oil

1 pound tofu, drained and cut into 1-inch cubes

1 clove garlic, minced

1 carrot, julienned

1 bunch greens, chopped stems and leaves divided (spinach, kale, or broccoli are all good options)

1 cup bean sprouts

1 tablespoon soy sauce

Heat oil in a sauté pan over medium heat and stir-fry tofu for about 2 minutes until lightly browned. Remove tofu from pan.

Add garlic, carrots, stems of greens, and stir-fry for 2 minutes.

Add green leaves and sprouts and browned tofu to pan. Stir-fry to combine for 2 more minutes.

Add soy sauce and stir to coat.

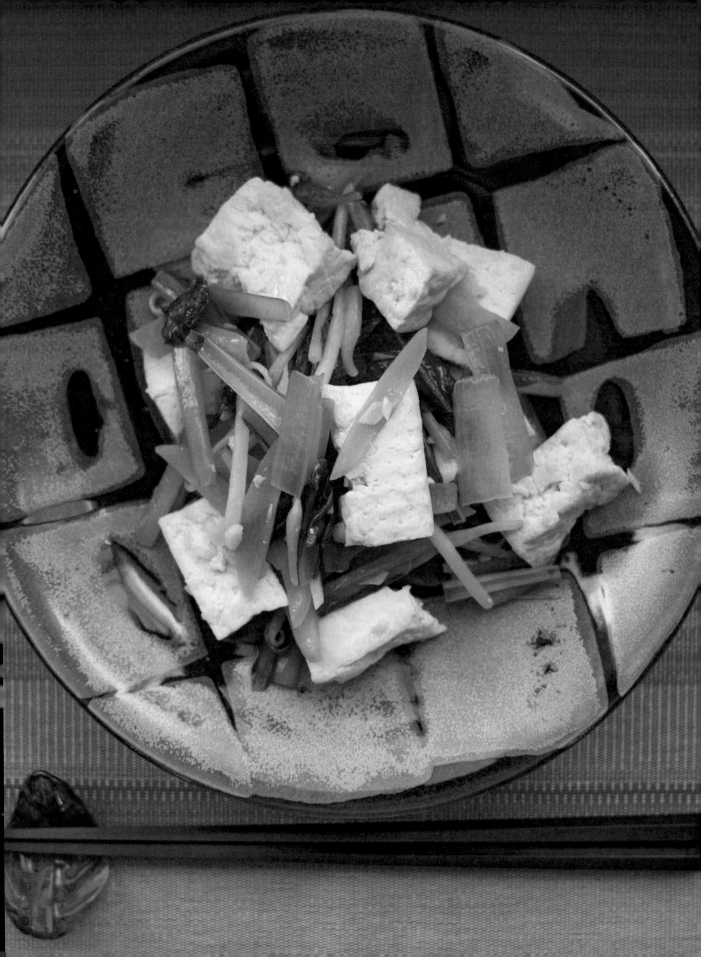

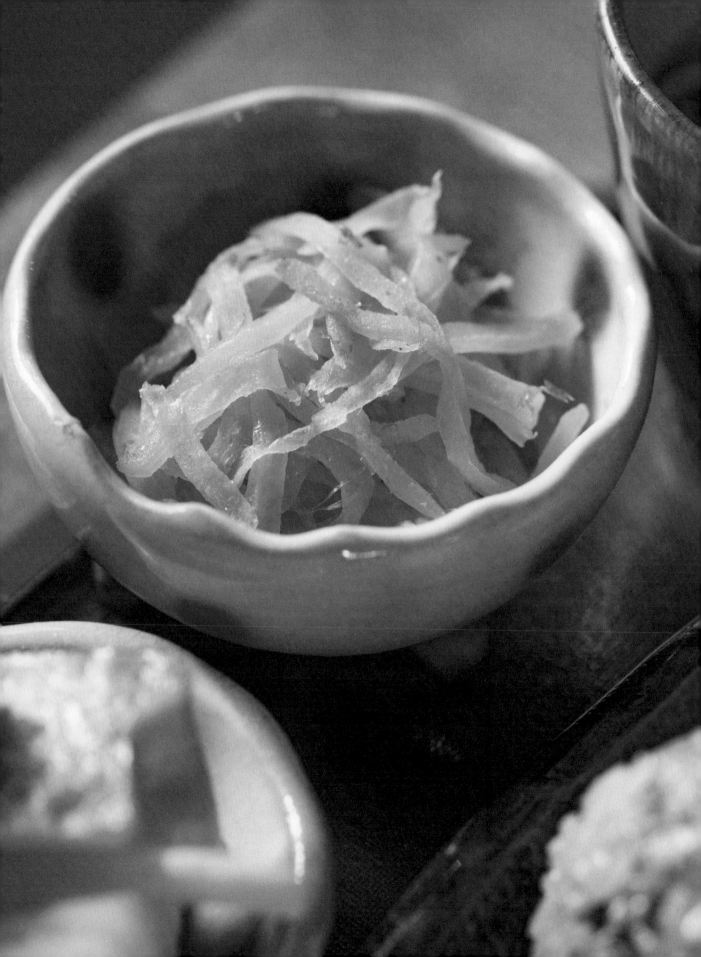

(Okinawan Champuru Four Ways continued)

TOFU AND VEGGIE CHAMPURU

TOTAL COOK TIME: 15 MINUTES | MAKES 3 SERVINGS

4 cups mustard greens or Swiss chard

1 teaspoon salt

7 ounces extra-firm tofu (half a block) cut into 1-inch cubes

2 tablespoons vegetable or soybean oil, divided

Soy sauce

In a large bowl, lightly salt greens and knead with hands.

Chop greens into 1-inch pieces. Wring out pieces over the sink to remove excess water.

In a sauté pan, sauté tofu over medium heat in 1 tablespoon oil for 2-3 minutes per side, or until it's lightly browned. Set aside.

In same pan, sauté greens over medium heat in remaining oil, stirring constantly until soft.

Add tofu back into the pan and toss gently to combine. Season to taste with soy sauce.

GREEN PAPAYA CHAMPURU (left)

TOTAL COOK TIME: 15 MINUTES | MAKES 2 SERVINGS

1 large young (green) papaya, pitted and peeled

1 tablespoon water

1½ cups dashi broth (page 105)

1 tablespoon vegetable oil

1 tablespoon soy sauce

Grate papaya into strips.

In a large sauté pan, sauté papaya in 1 tablespoon of water over high heat for 1 minute, stirring constantly.

Add dashi and oil, continuing to stir to combine.

Bring to simmer and continue to cook until most of the liquid is gone but papaya is not dried out.

Immediately remove from heat and season with soy sauce.

Sweet and Spicy Carrot Medley

TOTAL COOK TIME: 15 MINUTES | MAKES 2 SERVINGS

Carrots, though nutritionally dense, can often be a bore when served on their own. This Okinawan preparation, featuring seasonings and influences from Japanese, Chinese, and Southeast Asian cuisine, is simple but transformative (though you can easily Americanize it by using vegetable broth for the dashi). Filled with subtle, delicious flavors, it's well worth adding to your repertoire!

It should be noted that Okinawan carrots, long and light yellow in color, are a staple of the island (carrot soup is another popular delicacy). Residents have even devised a special carrot mandoline to help create delicious variations with this multi-faceted vegetable!

2 carrots, peeled and grated into long strips

1 small sweet onion, julienned

1 tablespoon sesame oil

3 tablespoons dashi (page 105) or vegetable broth

1 teaspoon mirin

1 teaspoon cooking sake (optional)

1 to 2 teaspoons chili paste (or red pepper flakes)

In a sauté pan over medium heat, lightly sauté the carrots and onion in oil.

Add dashi or broth and cook until absorbed, tossing gently to combine, about 2 minutes.

Add the mirin, sake (if using), and chili paste or red pepper flakes to taste and mix to combine, cooking for another minute.

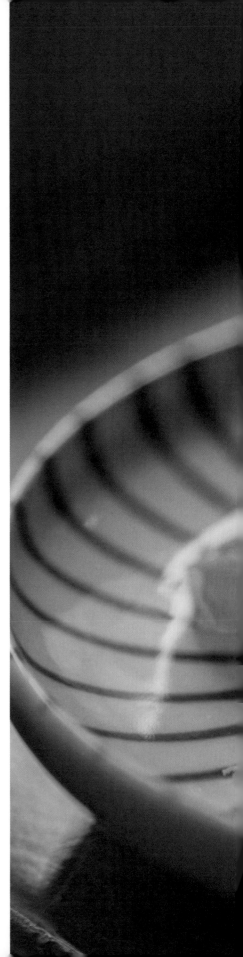

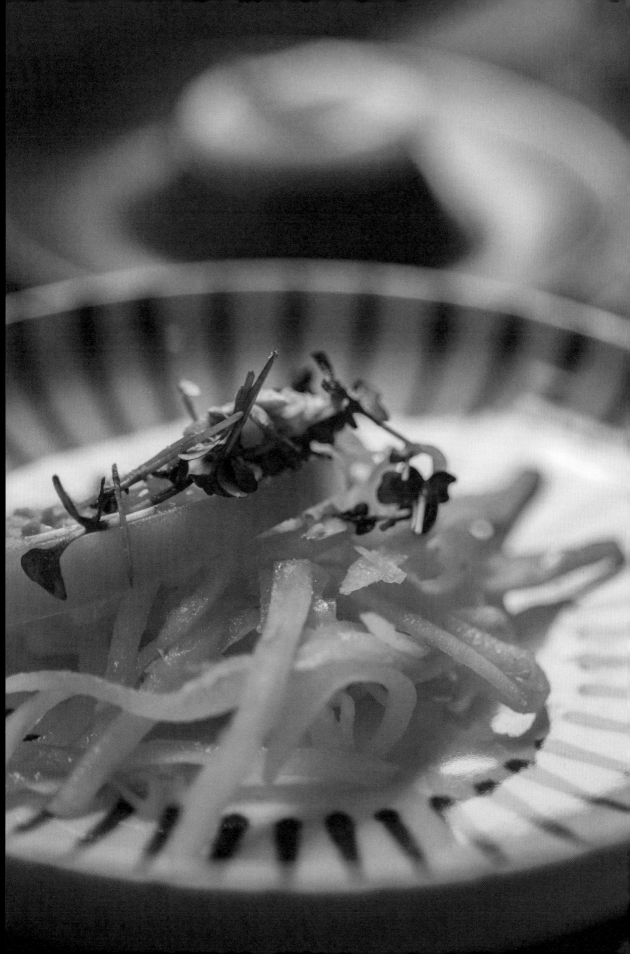

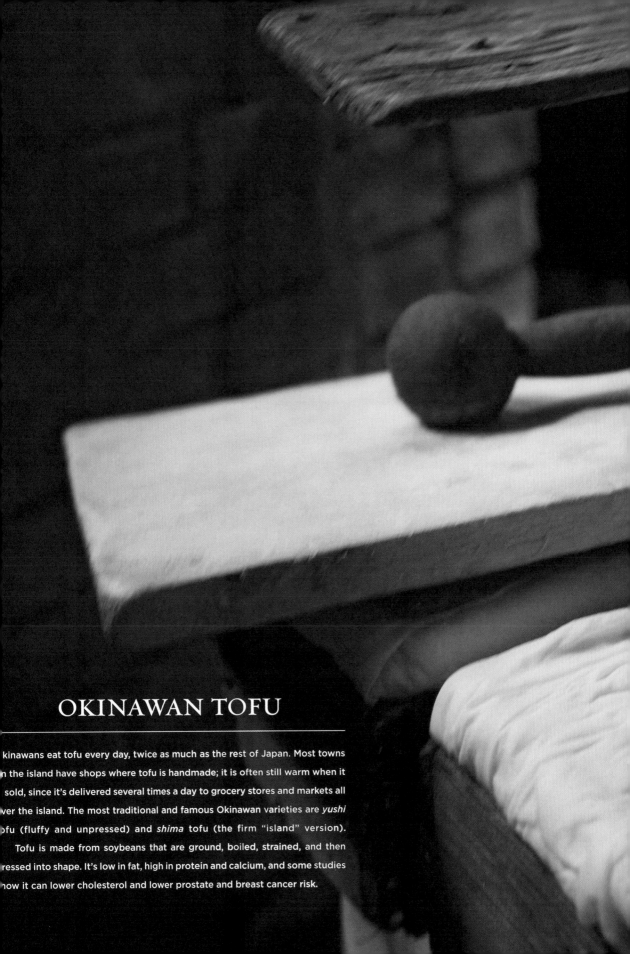

OKINAWAN TOFU

kinawans eat tofu every day, twice as much as the rest of Japan. Most towns
n the island have shops where tofu is handmade; it is often still warm when it
 sold, since it's delivered several times a day to grocery stores and markets all
ver the island. The most traditional and famous Okinawan varieties are *yushi*
ofu (fluffy and unpressed) and *shima* tofu (the firm "island" version).

   Tofu is made from soybeans that are ground, boiled, strained, and then
ressed into shape. It's low in fat, high in protein and calcium, and some studies
how it can lower cholesterol and lower prostate and breast cancer risk.

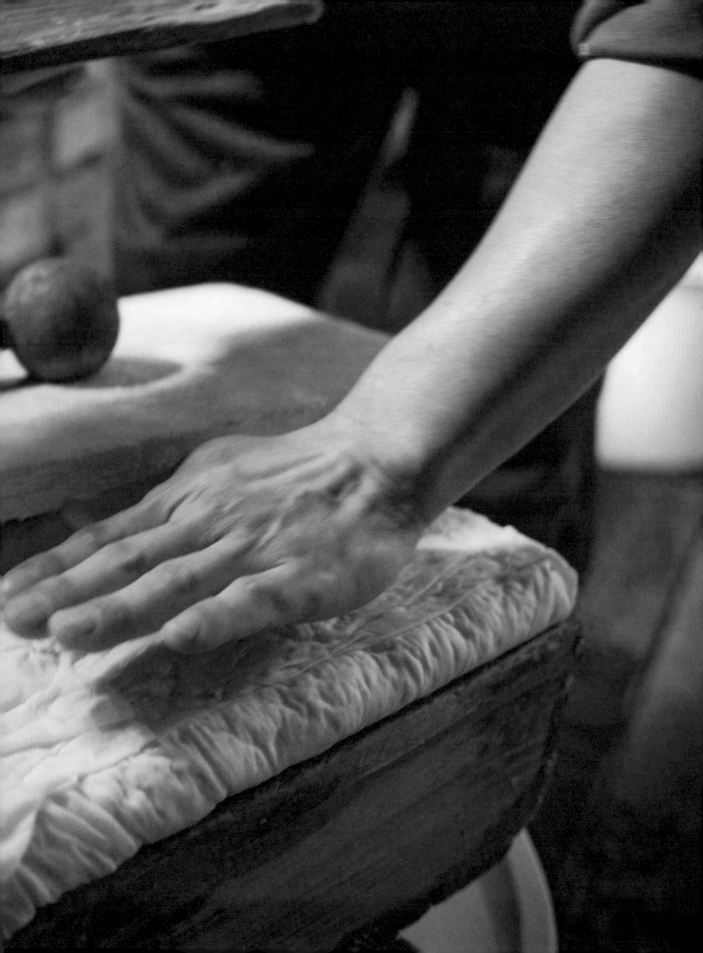

Sweet Potato and Onion Hash

TOTAL COOK TIME: 25 MINUTES | MAKES 2 SERVINGS

In this sweet-savory potato dish, try to use white sweet potatoes, which are less sugary than the orange version. The onions add a lot of flavor with a dash of their own sweetness. This is another simple recipe that we found to be shockingly good. You can serve it as a side to a meal with soup and rice, as they do in Okinawa, or even enjoy it as a snack or a light meal. A staple of the traditional Okinawan diet, sweet potatoes are rich in fiber and essential minerals and vitamins.

2 cups white sweet potatoes, peeled and cut into medium dice

1 cup thinly sliced onion (about half an onion)

½ cup julienned carrots (about 1½ carrots)

1 teaspoon salt

1 tablespoon vegetable oil

1 cup dashi broth (page 105)

1 cup chopped scallions, both white and green parts

2 tablespoons soy sauce, plus more if needed

In a large sauté pan, stir-fry sweet potatoes, onion, and carrots over medium-high heat with salt in oil for 2-3 minutes.

Add dashi broth, cover, and lower heat to simmer until potatoes are tender, about 10 minutes.

Turn off heat; add scallions and soy sauce to taste.

Note: For a simpler version of this dish, steam purple, white, or orange sweet potatoes until soft. Toss with 1 tablespoon of vegetable oil, chopped scallions, and a dash of salt.

Okinawan Glazed Greens

TOTAL COOK TIME: 10 MINUTES | MAKES 4 SERVINGS

Okinawan centenarians generally eat greens, often grown in the nutrient-rich soil of their year-round gardens, every day for most of their lives. The greens are used for cooking, and the herbs for both medicinal and culinary purposes. Besides being a continuous source of fresh vegetables, gardening is also a source of daily physical activity and exercise with a wide range of motion. The outdoor exposure provides a regular dose of vitamin D from the sun and gardening has been shown in studies to reduce stress and improve overall mood.

Use this quick and easy recipe to whip up any type of green vegetable with the probiotic power of miso. You can create variations with green beans, sautéed kale, or bok choy for a delicious side dish.

8 cups chopped greens like spinach, mizuna, or mustard greens

⅓ cup citrus juice (orange or lime)

2 tablespoons white miso

2 tablespoons mirin (sweet rice wine), plus more if needed

Parboil the greens by heating water to a boil, adding the greens, and removing after 1 to 2 minutes, once the greens have turned a bright color.

Drain greens. Over the sink, lightly squeeze greens between your hands to remove excess water.

In a mixing bowl, whisk together citrus juice, white miso, and mirin.

Add greens to the bowl and mix with hands. Season to taste with more mirin.

Sweet and Savory Taro

TOTAL COOK TIME: 15 MINUTES | MAKES 2 SERVINGS

Before eating this, I never imagined this hairy-looking tuber could taste so good. With a flavor similar to kettle cooked popcorn (but less sweet), it's a tasty side dish.

1 medium taro, peeled and cut into small 2-inch wedges

2 tablespoons vegetable oil

1 tablespoon sugar

1 tablespoon cooking sake

2 tablespoons mirin

Preheat oven to 400 degrees.

Toss taro wedges with vegetable oil and place on a baking sheet in a single layer. Bake for 20 minutes.

Meanwhile, mix sugar, sake, and mirin in a small sauce pot and heat until sugar is dissolved.

While taro is still hot, toss with sweet sauce in a large mixing bowl until coated.

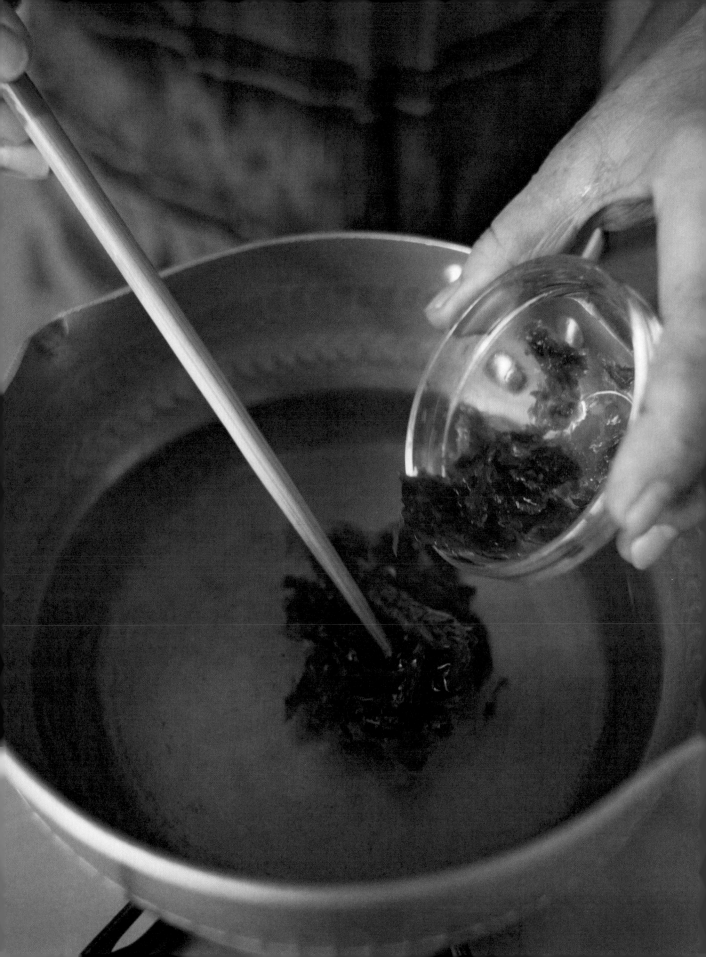

Dashi Broth

TOTAL COOK TIME: 20 MINUTES | MAKES 4 SERVINGS

This seaweed broth is the base of almost every Okinawan dish; it's used in soup, stews, steamed vegetables, and even to enrich the flavors of stir-fries. Okinawan dashi uses either bonito flakes, kelp, or both as its base. I recommend making a big batch and freezing it so you can use it for anything or everything.

For thousands of years, Okinawans have taken in their essential minerals (sodium, calcium, potassium, iodine) by using seaweed in their cooking. Kelp, one of the cornerstones of Okinawan (and Japanese) cooking, gives many dishes a rich umami flavor.

KELP (KOMBU) DASHI (left)

1 ounce *kombu* (a 4-inch x 6-inch piece of kelp)

5 cups water

¾ cup dried bonito flakes

Wipe off white layer on kelp with dry cloth. Soak *kombu* overnight in water.

Drain *kombu* and combine with 5 fresh cups of water in a soup pot.

Heat until just before boiling. As soon as the liquid boils, strain *kombu* out.

Add bonito flakes and bring dashi broth to a boil, skimming top if necessary.

When dashi boils, reduce heat to simmer immediately; let simmer for 30 seconds.

Remove from heat and let bonito flakes sink to the bottom, about 10 minutes.

Strain dashi into a bowl.

Use dashi immediately or store in the refrigerator for up to one week.

MUSHROOM DASHI

4 cups water

1 ounce *kombu* (4-inch x 6-inch piece of kelp)

5 dried porcini mushrooms, soaked in water for 1 hour

Rinse off the *kombu* with water.

Boil water and reduce to simmer.

Add *kombu* and mushrooms to pot and let simmer on low for 15-20 minutes.

Strain and reserve broth.

Miso Soup Two Ways

MISO SOUP WITH VEGGIES (right)

TOTAL COOK TIME: 25 MINUTES | MAKES 6 SERVINGS

This rich broth is a heartier, less salty version of the miso soup you get in sushi restaurants around the world, with the addition of an alluring variety of textures. The daikon gives it a satisfying crunch; the oyster mushrooms add a meaty element. Miso soup is central to Okinawan cuisine and is usually enjoyed as part of every meal, including breakfast. As in the rest of Japan, an everyday meal in Okinawa consists of miso soup and rice with seasonal side dishes.

⅛ small daikon radish (both roots and leaves), peeled, quartered, and thinly sliced

1 small carrot, peeled and sliced to same size as the radish

½ cup chopped Chinese cabbage (like Napa or bok choy)

½ cup sliced oyster mushrooms

6 cups dashi broth (page 105)

3 tablespoons red miso

1 tablespoon vegetable oil

⅓ cup cubed tofu

½ cup chopped sweet potato leaves (or other greens)

In a soup pot, combine all ingredients except tofu and greens and bring to a boil.

Immediately turn down heat and simmer for about 15 minutes, or until daikon is soft.

Add tofu and greens at the very end and immediately turn off heat.

RED MISO SOUP WITH SPINACH AND TOFU

TOTAL COOK TIME: 15 MINUTES | MAKES 2 SERVINGS

This staple soup for centenarians is often cooked for breakfast and then reheated for lunch and dinner. It's made distinctive with a base of richly fermented red miso and only takes about five minutes to make. Red miso is aged for a year or more—and as a fermented food, it provides the gut with beneficial bacteria.

2 cups dashi broth (page 105)

2 tablespoons red miso

3 tablespoons drained and crumbled firm tofu

1 cup Okinawan spinach (edible *Gynura,* can substitute with other spinach)

½ cup chopped green onion

Heat dashi broth to a low simmer.

Add all other ingredients, whisk until miso is dissolved, then simmer for 3 minutes.

Serve with rice.

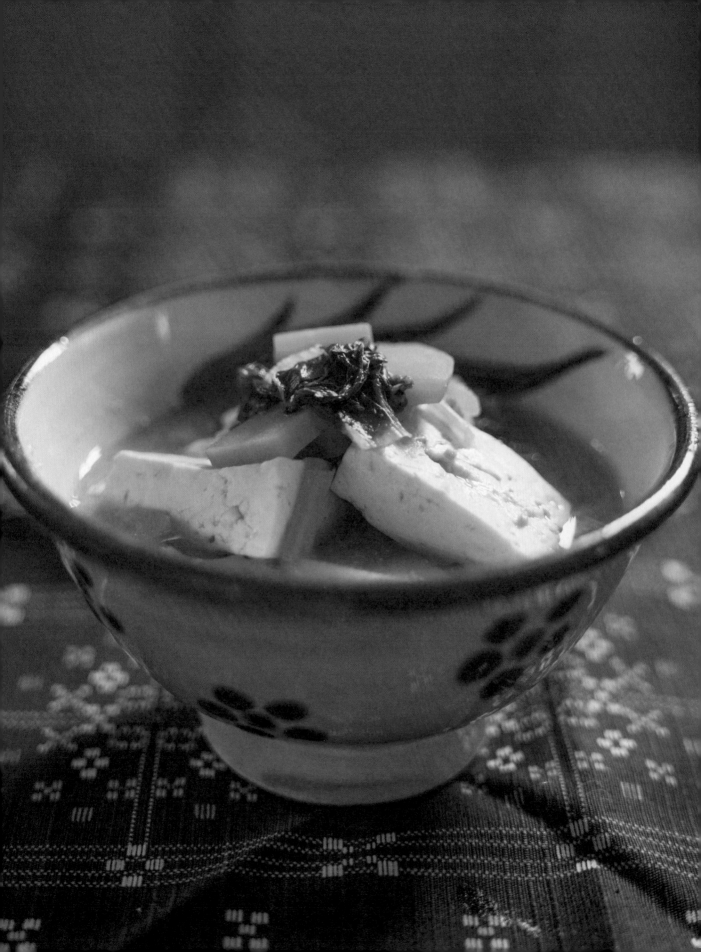

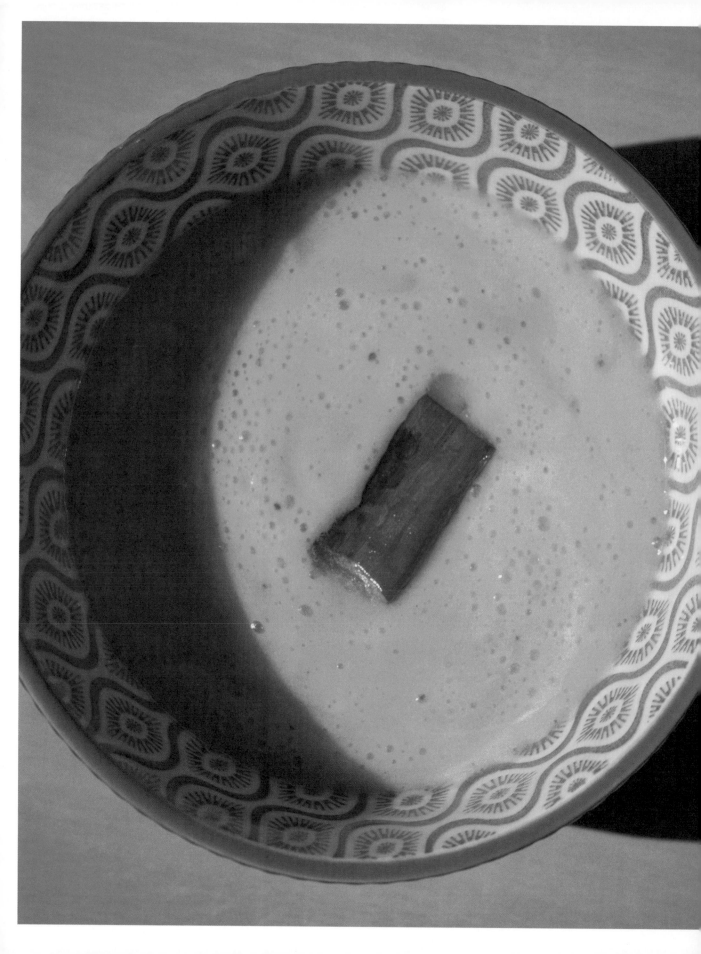

Cream of Pumpkin Soup (left)

TOTAL COOK TIME: 30 MINUTES | MAKES 2 SERVINGS

Okinawans make this soup from kabocha, or Japanese pumpkin—a good substitute is acorn or butternut squash. The result is a silky, slightly sweet soup that takes about 20 minutes to whip up if you have an immersion blender or food processor. You can also make this in a flash with canned pumpkin puree, which is usually a blend of pumpkin and orange squash.

½ pound acorn or butternut squash, peeled, seeded, and cut into large chunks

¼ cup chopped leeks (or onion)

1 tablespoon vegetable oil

1¾ cups unsweetened soy milk

1 teaspoon cumin seed

1 teaspoon dried turmeric

1 teaspoon salt, plus more if needed

Place a steamer tray into a pot with about 2 inches of water. Bring water to a boil and steam squash until soft, about 15 minutes.

In a soup pot, stir-fry leeks in vegetable oil until soft but not browned, about 3-4 minutes.

Add soy milk, steamed squash, and spices and simmer for 15 minutes.

Blend all together with an immersion blender or in a food processor (in batches, if necessary) until smooth. Add salt to taste.

Simmered Okinawan Pumpkin

TOTAL COOK TIME: 35 MINUTES | MAKES 2 SERVINGS

We traveled to Ogimi, ground zero of world longevity, for this recipe. We got this recipe from 89-year-old Yukiko Nakaima, who spent the afternoon cooking the most amazing Okinawan longevity foods for us. When I asked the secret to her vitality, I expected she'd talk about her purple potatoes or miso-braised squash. "Optimism," she said wagging a finger at me, "I say yes to everything."

½ *shima* pumpkin (or kabocha or other squash), cut into 1-inch chunks

2 cups dashi broth (page 105)

1 teaspoon soy sauce

Put all ingredients in a medium soup pot. Bring to a boil and immediately reduce heat to simmer.

Simmer all ingredients together for about 20-30 minutes until tender.

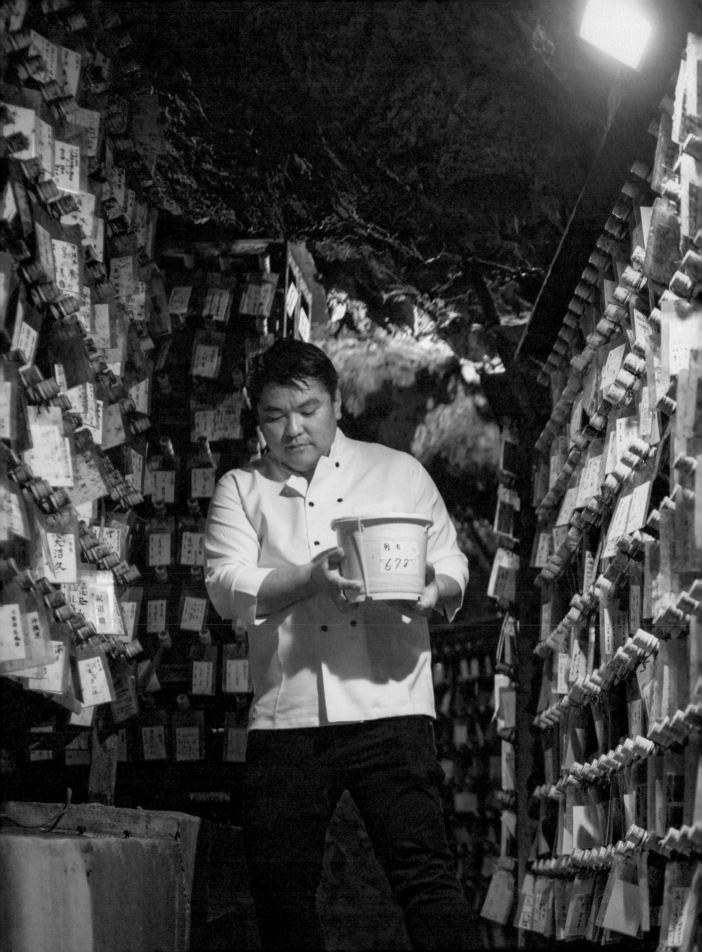

UNDERGROUND STORAGE

This limestone cave in Okinawa stores aging sake, *awamori,* and tofu. Awamori is an alcoholic drink unique to Okinawa and is made by distilling long grain (Thai) rice. Bottles are placed here by customers for a fee to age for periods of 5, 12, and 20 years. Okinawan tofu is also aged here, for periods from three months to one year. A combination of the two—*tofuyo,* made of tofu soaked in awamori—also resides here; people describe its taste and texture as similar to cream cheese or sea urchin. Fermented foods, now known to be rich in probiotic bacteria good for our intestinal health and immune system, feature in Okinawan cuisine in the forms of miso, fermented tofu, soy sauce, sake, and awamori.

Tofu Steak With Miso Mushrooms

TOTAL COOK TIME: 20 MINUTES | MAKES 2 SERVINGS

This recipe is adapted from *The Okinawa Program* (a plan authored by the scientists of the Okinawan Centenarian Study), but we asked Sensei Yukie Miyaguni, head of a cooking school in Okinawa, to spice it up. This is a perfect main dish that will delight vegetarian friends and even satisfy meat eaters. Soybean-based foods, including miso and tofu, are key staples in the traditional Okinawan diet, which is high in nutrients and antioxidants but low in calories and fat.

½ pound firm tofu, sliced into four square pieces

1 tablespoon all-purpose flour

1 tablespoon vegetable or soybean oil

1½ cups shiitake mushrooms

1 tablespoon mirin

1 teaspoon grated ginger

1 tablespoon red miso paste

¼ teaspoon red pepper flakes

1 tablespoon sesame oil

½ cup chopped leeks or green onion

Cherry tomato halves, for garnish

Coat the wet tofu with flour.

In a sauté pan over medium-high heat, brown tofu in vegetable or soybean oil for 3-4 minutes per side.

In separate pan, sauté mushrooms, mirin, ginger, miso, and pepper flakes in sesame oil over medium heat for 3-4 minutes or until the mushrooms are cooked.

When done, turn off heat and add leeks or green onion to the pan, mixing to combine.

Place two pieces of tofu per plate and cover with seasoned mushrooms.

Garnish with cherry tomato halves.

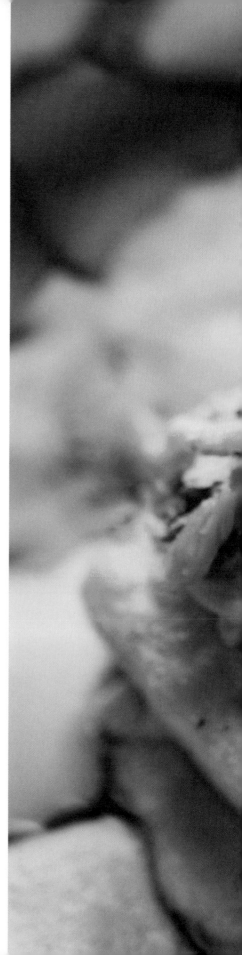

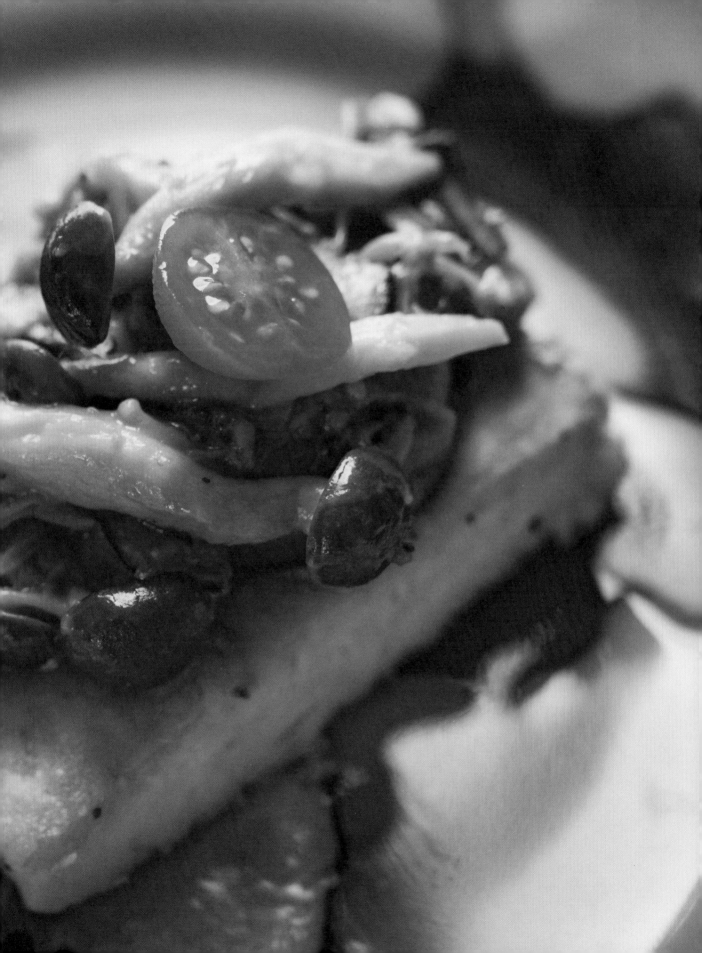

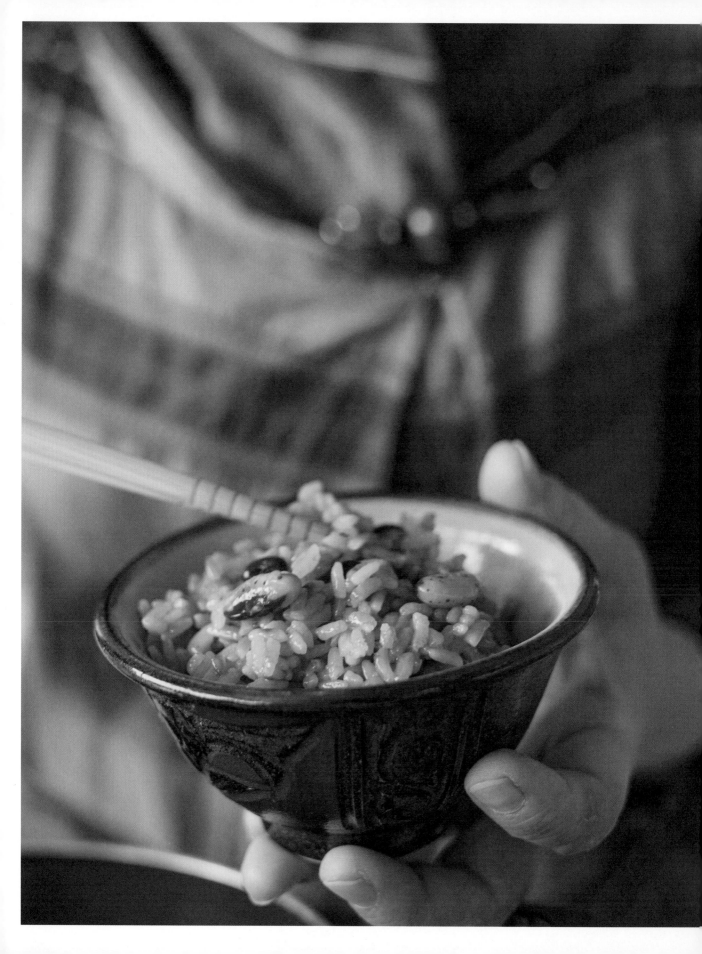

Okinawan Beans and Rice (left)

TOTAL COOK TIME: 70 MINUTES | MAKES 2 SERVINGS

The Okinawan version of beans and rice is called *aka kashichi*. This nutty, subtle dish—deceptively simple and surprisingly good—is a common ancestor offering at Okinawans' twice-monthly visits to the cemetery. Glutinous rice, which is used to make mochi, was traditionally used only for special occasions. Even though this has been historically a celebratory dish, it is today also commonly eaten during lunch or dinner.

1 cup sweet rice (glutinous rice)	Soak rice in cold water for 30 minutes.
1½ cups water, plus more for soaking rice and beans	Boil soaked beans for 1 hour until tender, drain and rinse. If using canned, skip this step but drain and rinse beans.
1 tablespoon dried kidney beans, soaked for 4 hours	If cooking with a rice cooker, add sweet rice and beans to rice cooker with water and salt. Cook according to manufacturer's instructions.
1 tablespoon dried black beans, soaked for 4 hours	If cooking on the stovetop, add rice and beans to a medium pot. Bring to a boil uncovered and then immediately reduce to a low simmer. Cover with a lid and cook for about 30 minutes.
Pinch of salt	
1 teaspoon black sesame seeds	Fluff rice with a fork before serving to separate grains.
	Add sesame seeds and salt. Serve hot.

Savory Rice Porridge

TOTAL COOK TIME: 25 MINUTES | MAKES 2 SERVINGS

This warm, soothing, and savory rice porridge (called *kandaba jushi*) restores energy; Okinawans often cook it for children, the elderly, and people recovering from illness. But it's not just medicinal—it often replaces rice in the traditional Okinawan meal of rice, miso soup, and vegetables.

½ cup medium-grain white rice	Add rice, miso, greens, and dashi to a soup pot and bring to a boil.
2½ tablespoons miso	Reduce to simmer immediately and cook for about 15 minutes or until rice is soft.
3 cups dark greens like sweet potato leaves (*kandaba*), spinach, beet tops, or rainbow collard greens	Add salt to taste before serving.
2 cups dashi broth (page 105)	
Salt (optional)	

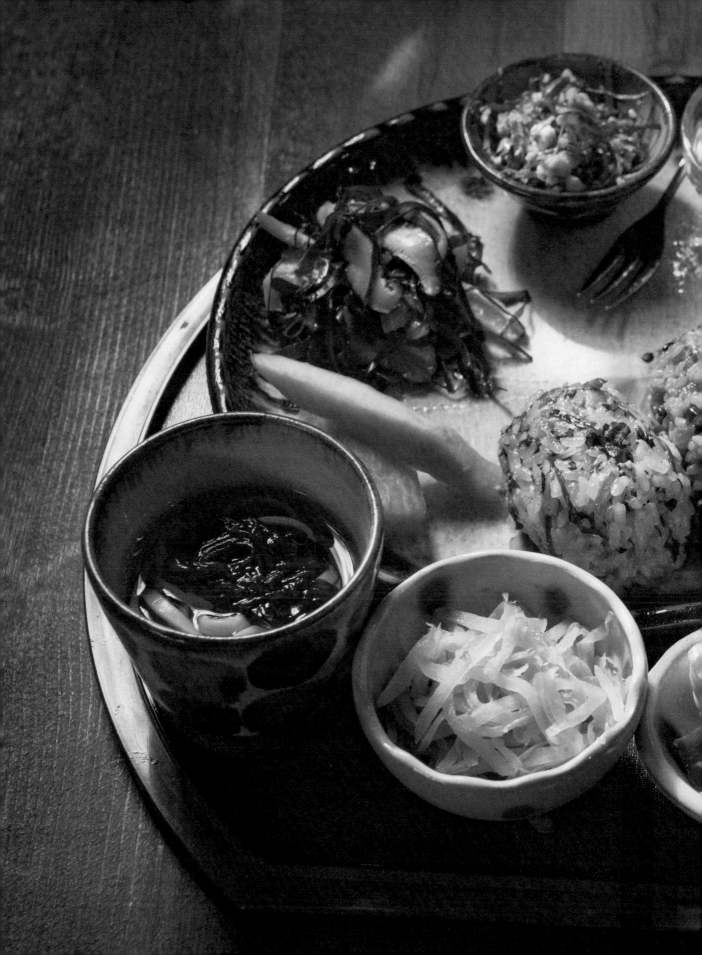

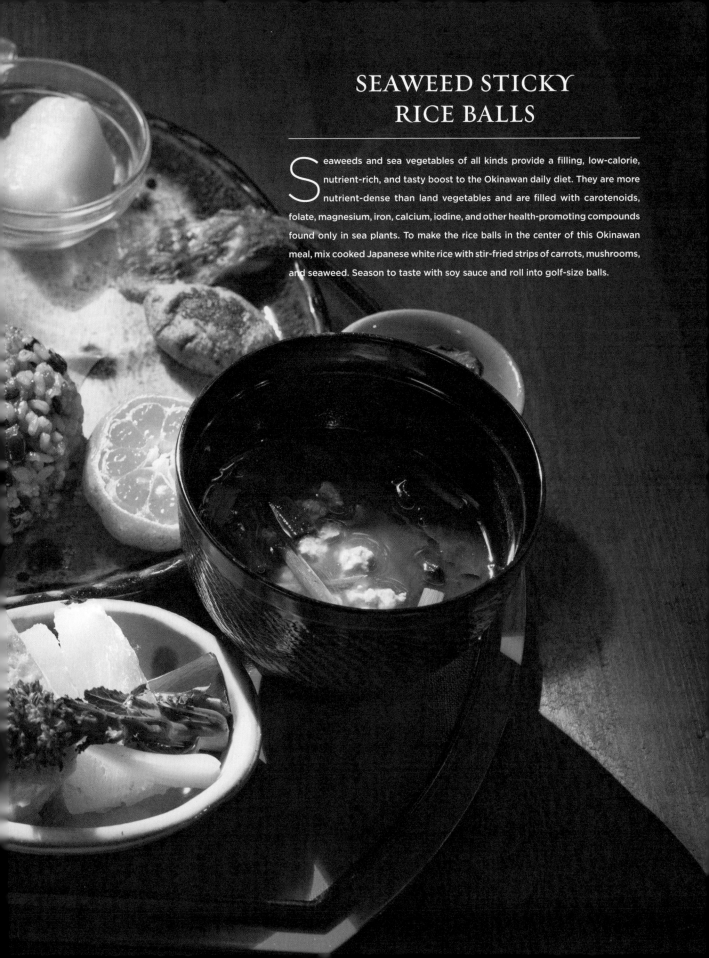

SEAWEED STICKY RICE BALLS

Seaweeds and sea vegetables of all kinds provide a filling, low-calorie, nutrient-rich, and tasty boost to the Okinawan daily diet. They are more nutrient-dense than land vegetables and are filled with carotenoids, folate, magnesium, iron, calcium, iodine, and other health-promoting compounds found only in sea plants. To make the rice balls in the center of this Okinawan meal, mix cooked Japanese white rice with stir-fried strips of carrots, mushrooms, and seaweed. Season to taste with soy sauce and roll into golf-size balls.

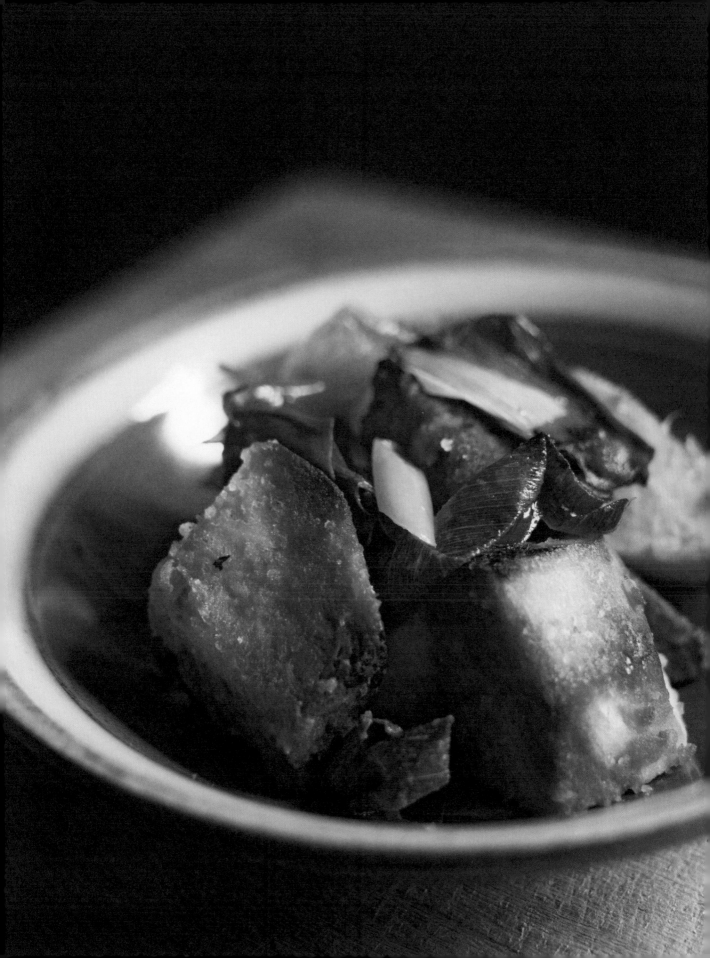

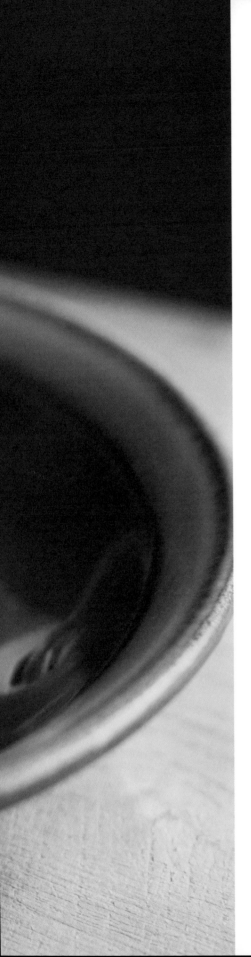

Steamed Purple Sweet Potatoes

TOTAL COOK TIME: 25 MINUTES | MAKES 3 SERVINGS

One of the pillars of the Okinawan diet, Okinawan *imo* is a supercharged purple sweet potato, a cousin of the common yellow-orange varieties that has been an island staple since the 17th century. Despite its saccharine flavor, it does not spike blood sugar as much as a regular white potato. Like other sweet potatoes, it contains an antioxidant called sporamin, which possesses a variety of potent antiaging properties. The purple version contains higher levels than its orange and yellow cousins.

This superfood is high in complex carbs, has a surprisingly low glycemic load, and packs an antioxidant punch with anthocyanin (the compound that makes blueberries blue). Okinawans typically serve sweet potatoes steamed, which perfectly renders their creamy texture and sweet flavor.

The best places to find purple sweet potatoes are Asian markets, but they are also sold through online grocers. If this proves difficult, you can swap in any other type of sweet potatoes. Here's a coconut version of my own invention, which I served—to rave reviews—to a *New York Times* food critic.

1 pound purple sweet potatoes, peeled and cut into 2-inch cubes

One 13.5-ounce can or carton of organic coconut milk

Steam potatoes for 10-15 minutes until tender. Remove from heat and let rest with lid on for 3-4 minutes.

In a large bowl, mash sweet potatoes lightly with coconut milk.

Note: The potatoes can be boiled rather than steamed, but they will lose some of their essential nutrients in this process.

Three-Minute Okinawan Rice Noodle Bowl

TOTAL COOK TIME: 15 MINUTES │ MAKES 4 SERVINGS

Somen are thin, white wheat noodles that people eat with a dipping sauce in other parts of Japan. In Okinawa, it's more common to stir-fry them or add them to soup. Since they require only 2-3 minutes of boiling time, they make for quick, satisfying appetizer or entrée dishes. You can combine this with seasoned bitter melon or veggie *champuru* (both on page 94) to make a heartier *somen champuru* recipe.

1 pound *somen* noodles

2 tablespoons sesame oil, divided

1 cup firm tofu, drained and cut into 1-inch chunks

¼ cup chopped garlic chives (or scallions)

Soy sauce

Cook noodles for 2-3 minutes, according to package directions.

Drain and mix noodles with sesame oil so they don't stick together.

In a large sauté pan, heat ½ tablespoon of sesame oil over medium-high heat and brown tofu.

When tofu is browned, add chives and *somen* noodles to the pan and mix well.

Season to taste with a splash or two of soy sauce.

Iced Banapple Turmeric Smoothie

TOTAL COOK TIME: 5 MINUTES | MAKES 1 SERVING

Turmeric, which has recently been celebrated for its immune-boosting properties, has figured prominently in the Okinawan diet for hundreds of years. Okinawans use it as both a cooking spice and a tea, and scientists have started to study it for its anticancer, anti-inflammatory, and antiaging properties. Its main compound, curcumin, has shown in both clinical and population studies to slow the progression of dementia—a reason why Okinawans may suffer much lower rates of Alzheimer's disease than Americans.

Turmeric regulates FOXO3 (a gene associated with longevity that reduces inflammation in the body), making our cells more efficient. Traditionally, Okinawans sliced and dried turmeric and then steeped it to make tea. But today most people rely on powdered turmeric for their daily cooking and drinking. You can enjoy this smoothie as a snack, a light meal, or even a dessert.

1 ripe banana

1 apple, cored and cut into a few pieces

1 teaspoon turmeric powder

1 cup vanilla soy milk

5 cups of ice

Blend all ingredients in a high-speed blender. Serve immediately.

Foamy Golden Milk

TOTAL COOK TIME: 5 MINUTES | MAKES 2 SERVINGS

The best way to enjoy turmeric is with black pepper, since it increases the spice's anti-inflammatory compound curcumin. Fat is necessary for better absorption, but you don't have to go crazy: A cup of coconut, cashew, or almond milk for this latte has more than enough to do the trick.

2 cups coconut, cashew, or almond milk (unsweetened and unflavored)

1 teaspoon turmeric powder

1 teaspoon vanilla extract

¼ teaspoon ground cinnamon

Pinch ground black pepper

Honey or agave (optional)

In a small soup pot, heat all ingredients except for sweetener over low-medium heat. Stir as needed.

Use an electric frother or whisk to create a foamy consistency.

Remove from heat and divide into two mugs. Sweeten with honey or agave, if using.

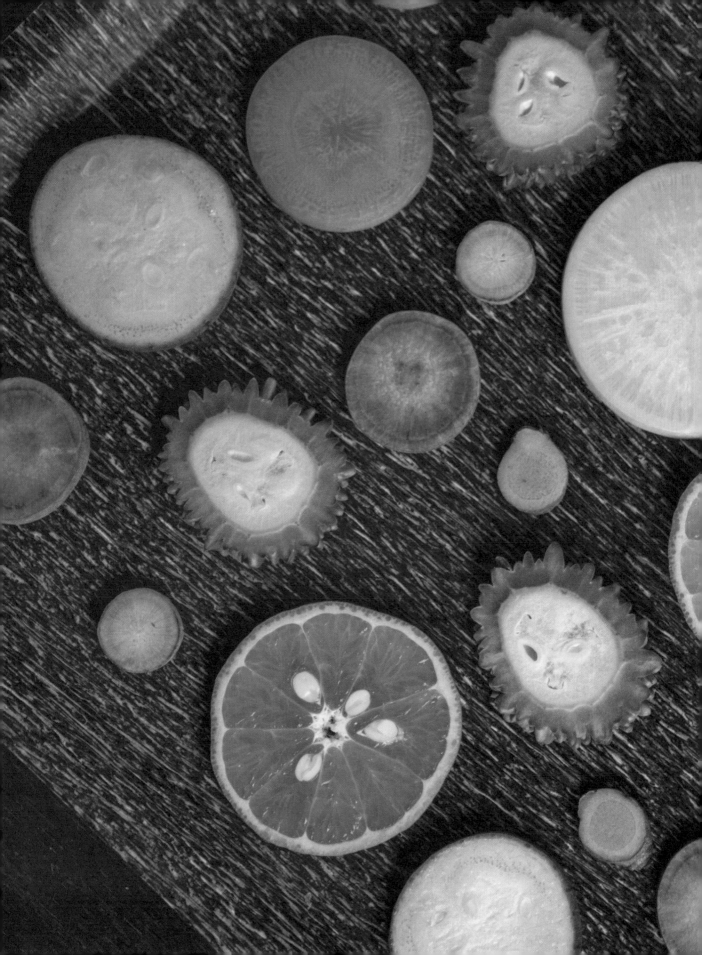

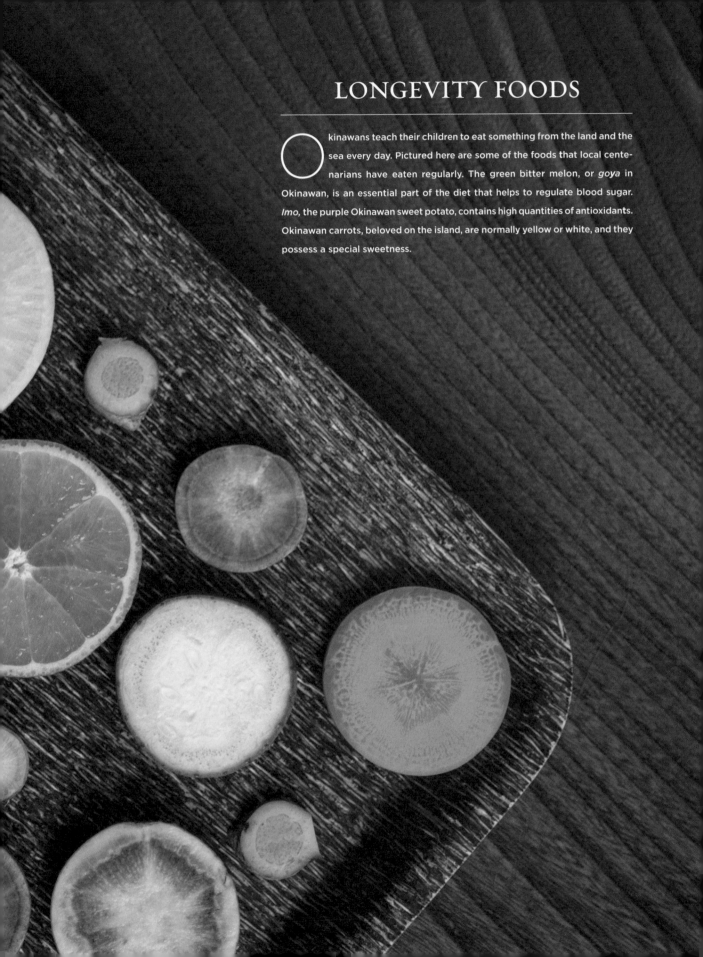

LONGEVITY FOODS

O kinawans teach their children to eat something from the land and the sea every day. Pictured here are some of the foods that local centenarians have eaten regularly. The green bitter melon, or *goya* in Okinawan, is an essential part of the diet that helps to regulate blood sugar. *Imo*, the purple Okinawan sweet potato, contains high quantities of antioxidants. Okinawan carrots, beloved on the island, are normally yellow or white, and they possess a special sweetness.

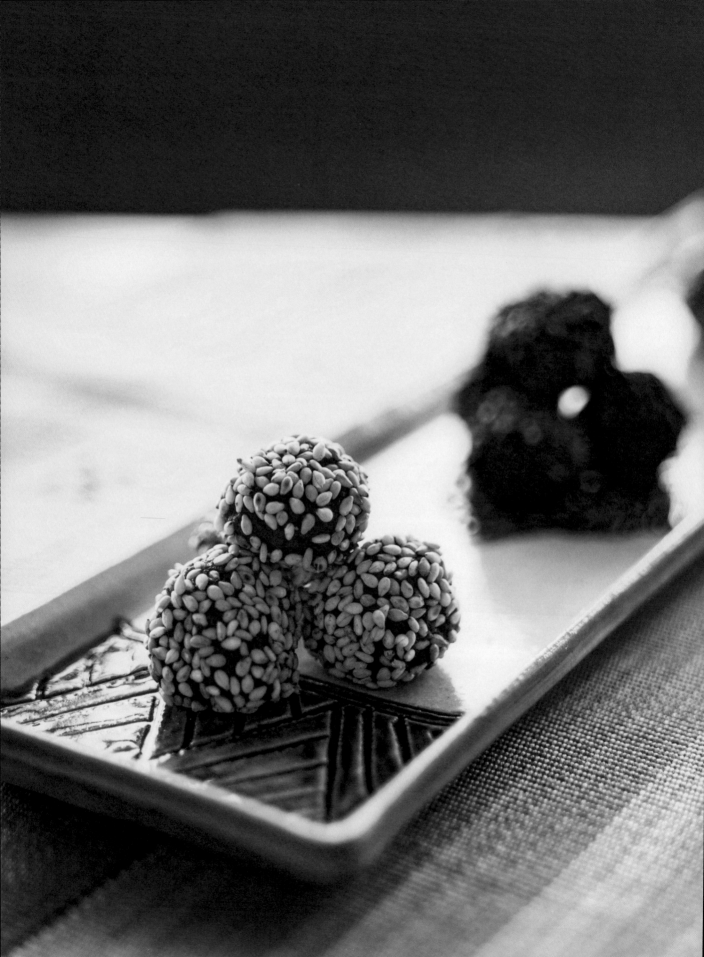

Sweet Potato Bites (left)

TOTAL COOK TIME: 10 MINUTES | MAKES 3 SERVINGS

Sweet potatoes accounted for 60 percent of the Okinawan diet until about 1950. This slightly sweetened preparation is delicious and can serve as a dessert or a snack. On our last visit to Okinawa, we watched the potatoes cooking and were uninspired until Jordan, a Hawaiian who lives on the island, produced two packages of macadamia nuts from his backpack. We ground them up, rolled the sweet potatoes into balls, and rolled the balls into the nuts. Voilà!

1 pound (about 3) white, orange, or purple sweet potatoes, peeled and cut into cubes

1 tablespoon brown sugar

⅓ cup ground peanuts, macadamia nuts, or sesame seeds

Dash of cinnamon

Boil or steam the potatoes until tender, then mash potatoes with sugar.

Once cool enough to handle, roll potatoes into walnut-size balls.

On a clean surface, spread a layer of ground nuts of your choice or sesame seeds. Gently roll the potato balls in the nuts to coat.

Powder with cinnamon to serve.

Okinawan Sweet Bread (next page)

TOTAL COOK TIME: 25 MINUTES | MAKES 5 SERVINGS

Since most Okinawan kitchens lacked ovens until very recently (and many still do), residents tend to steam, rather than bake, traditional desserts. Steaming bread produces a spongy, angel food cake–like texture, which is at once sweet and pleasing. This Okinawan sugar cake, called *agarasa,* is a famous local specialty that can be enjoyed as a dessert, as a snack, or with morning coffee or tea. It's traditionally made with Okinawan black sugar, which has a caramel flavor that is unmistakable.

1 cup brown sugar

¾ cup hot water

2 cups all-purpose flour

2 teaspoons baking powder

⅔ cup soy milk

In a large bowl, mix brown sugar and hot water until sugar dissolves.

Add flour, baking powder, and soy milk to the dissolved brown sugar. Mix until you get a crumbly texture.

Spoon the dough into a loaf pan, cupcake tin, or ramekins.

Steam for about 15 minutes in a steamer basket, or until a toothpick comes out clean.

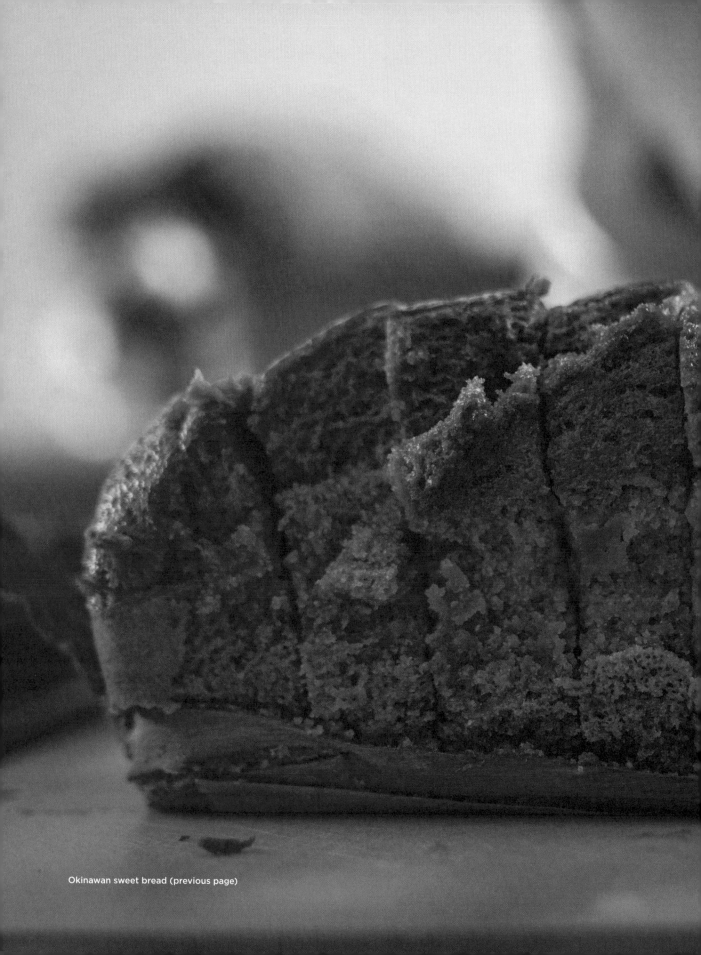

Okinawan sweet bread (previous page)

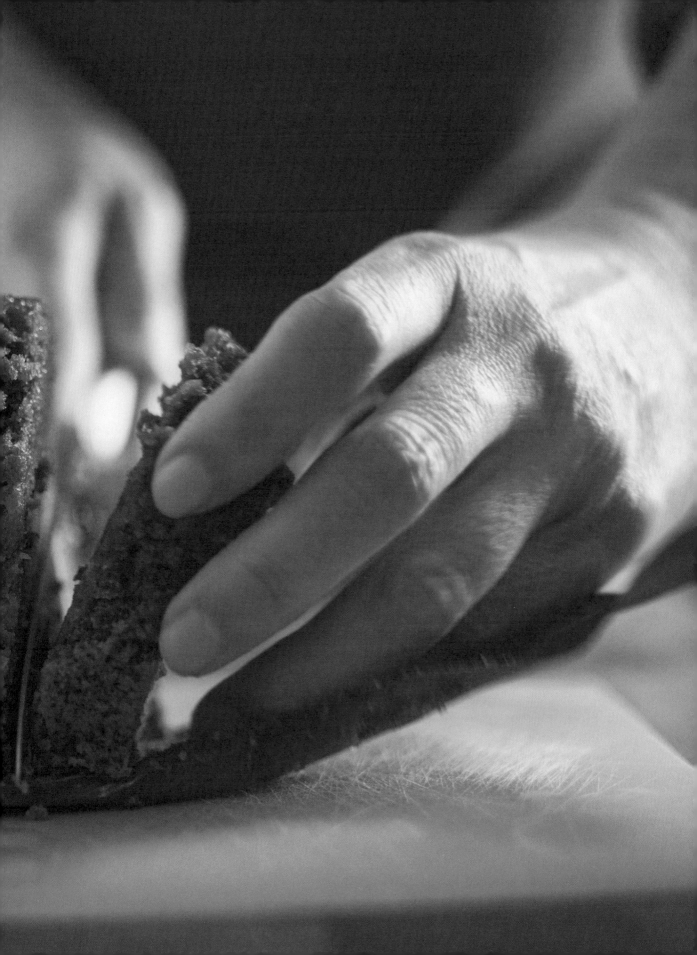

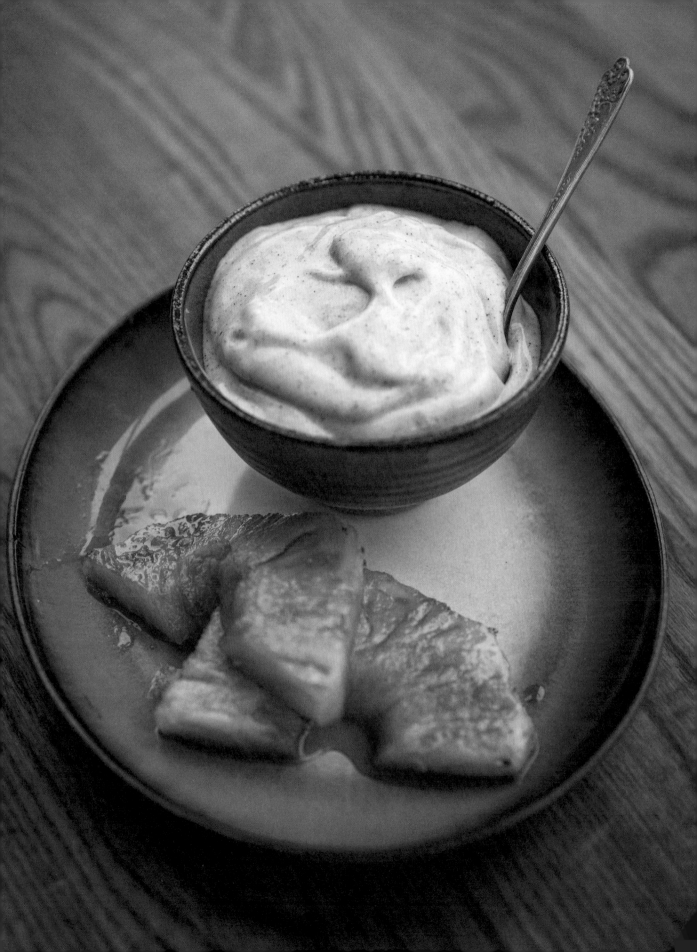

Chinese Five-Spice Banana Ice Cream With Roasted Pineapple

TOTAL COOK TIME: 15 MINUTES | MAKES 4 SERVINGS

This incredibly easy and dairy-free ice cream is refreshing at any time of year. (And if you don't have time to roast the pineapple, the ice cream is also delicious on its own.)

In 2014, NCH Healthcare System, a world-class operation in Naples, Florida, brought in the Blue Zones Project to fulfill its 10-year vision to make the region a healthier and happier place to live. NCH became the first hospital system in the United States to become Blue Zones certified, and now more than 250 other businesses, restaurants, schools, faith-based communities, and country clubs in the region have also been Blue Zones certified.

Three towns in this region are named among the top 10 healthiest in the country, and Naples is the first community in the country to ever take the top spot in the Gallup-Sharecare Well-Being Index three years in a row. Well-being has also improved across the counties, with remarkable improvements in the amount of fruits and vegetables residents are eating and how much they exercise, as well as marked reductions in daily stress.

CHINESE FIVE-SPICE BANANA ICE CREAM

4 ripe frozen bananas, sliced

4 to 5 teaspoons Chinese five-spice powder*

Coconut or nut milk, as needed

Roasted pineapple (see below)

Combine bananas and spice in a food processor and blend. Occasionally scrape down the sides and continue to blend until smooth, approximately 3-5 minutes. If you need to thin it a little, add a couple teaspoons of coconut or nut milk at a time, making sure not to add too much.

Scoop into a bowl and enjoy immediately as soft-serve ice cream.

For firmer ice cream, place in an airtight freezer-safe container and freeze for at least 1 hour.

Top with roasted pineapple, if using.

*Chinese five-spice powder is usually a blend of cinnamon, cloves, fennel, star anise, and Szechuan peppercorns.

OVEN-ROASTED PINEAPPLE

8 pineapple rings, sliced about ½-inch thick

¼ cup brown sugar

Preheat oven to 350 degrees.

Taste the pineapple first to decide how much sugar you need. You can use much less if it's very ripe and sweet.

Place the slices of pineapple on a foil-lined cookie sheet and top with brown sugar. Roast for 20 minutes or until golden.

Serve over banana ice cream or eat on its own.

✳ By Chef Lisa Fidler, FineMark National Bank & Trust, Blue Zones Project Southwest Florida

Sweet red peppers grow in
the backyards of Nicoyans.

CHAPTER THREE

Nicoya

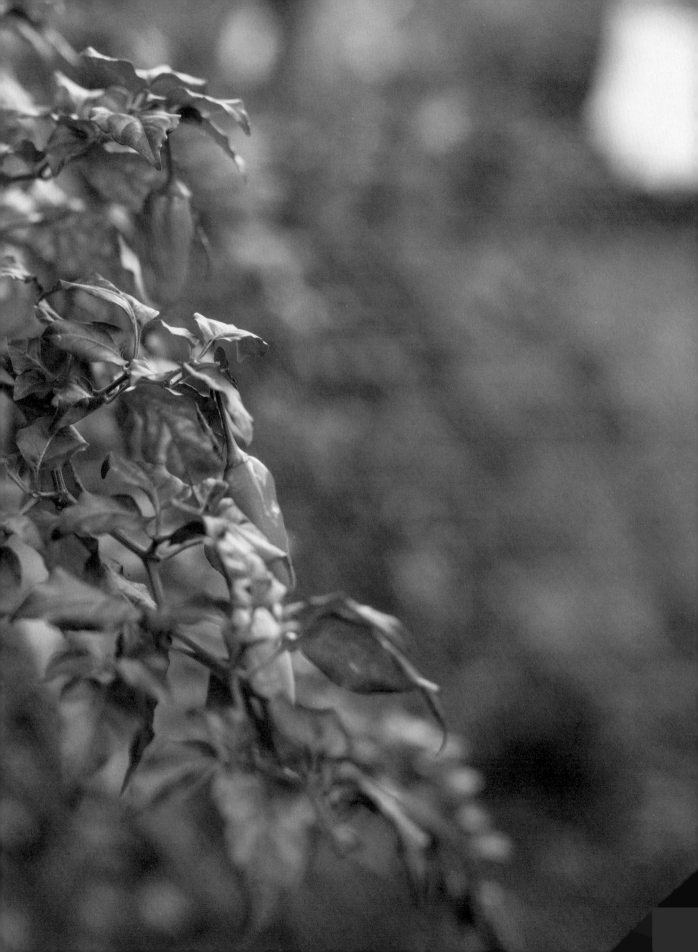

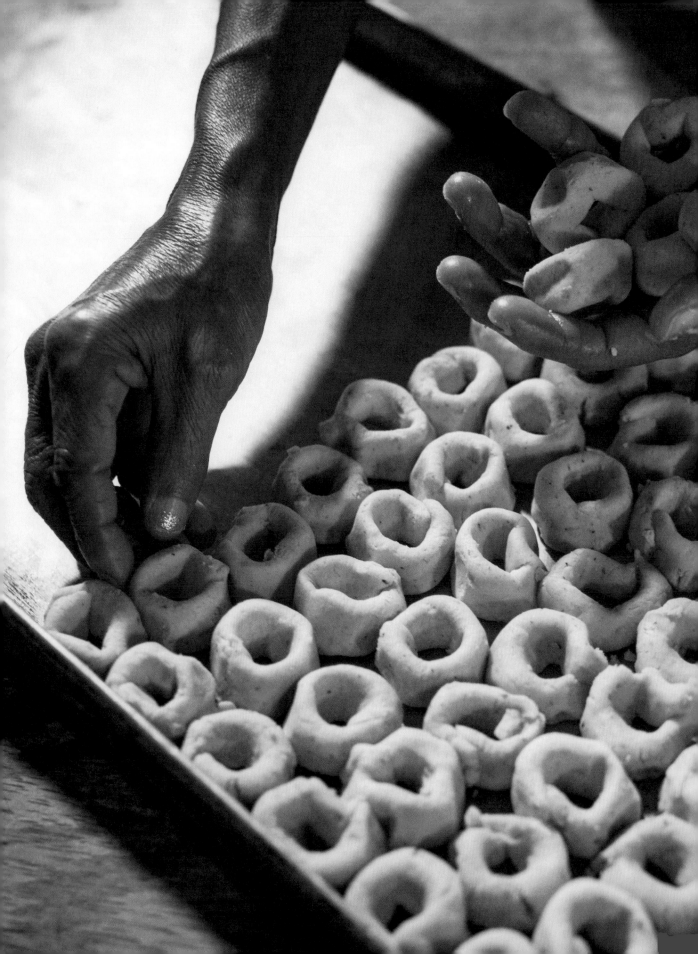

Nicoya, Costa Rica

may have found the world's healthiest breakfast. • In a tucked-away corner of Nicoya, Costa Rica, under a vaulted red-tiled roof blackened with smoke, a dozen or so women of the Cooperativa Nicoya wake each morning at 4:00 a.m. They stoke wood fires in long clay ovens, put cauldrons of spicy beans to boil, and mix corn dough (*nixtamal*) with wood ash, according to an ancient technique dating back at least 8,000 years. One of the women, Maria Elena Jimenez Rojas, pinches off a

golf ball–size piece of dough on a piece of waxed paper and rotates it with mechanical precision into a perfectly round patty. She slaps it onto a hot clay plate, or *comol*. It roasts briefly as it expands to a puffy disc before collapsing into a perfect tortilla.

At the other end of the wood stove, three other women mix beans with onions, red peppers, and local herbs. The beans cook slowly for about an hour to tender perfection and are then mixed with rice to produce the uniquely Costa Rican *gallo pinto*—rice and beans (page 151).

At 6 a.m., the first customers file in, most of them market vendors or laborers. They take seats on benches at long green tables. Cooperativa waitresses, wearing simple dresses and flip-flops, serve giant cups of weak local coffee, steaming plates of the *gallo pinto,* and baskets of warm tortillas. As muddy ranchero music plays from a distant radio, customers fill their tortillas with beans topped with chilero hot sauce (page 160). This is arguably the most perfect food combination ever, and for some it brings forth tears of joy.

The corn tortillas, chewy with a nutty flavor, are an excellent source of

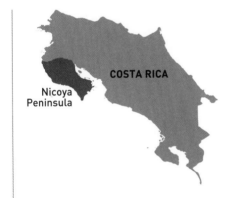

COSTA RICA

Nicoya
Peninsula

A woman lays Costa Rican doughnuts (page 166) on a baking sheet, preparing them for the oven.

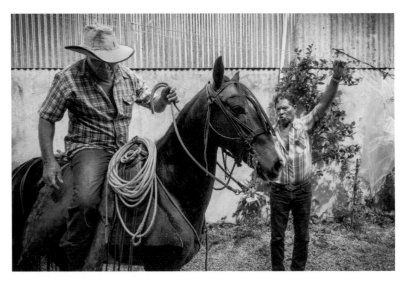

A neighbor lifts a clothesline so his friend, on horseback, can get into his backyard.

whole-grain, low-glycemic complex carbohydrates. The wood ash breaks down the corn's cell walls, making niacin bioavailable and freeing amino acids so the body can absorb them.

The black beans contain the same pigment-based anthocyanins (antioxidants) found in blueberries. They're rich, colon cleansing, blood pressure lowering, and insulin regulating, and they are filled with folates like potassium and B vitamins to boot. The bean-and-rice combination creates a whole protein, which is to say all the amino acids necessary for human sustenance.

The coffee here, made from a local strain of "pea berry" beans, provides a boost of antioxidants plus metabolism-boosting caffeine. The chilero, made with vinegar, carrots, and searingly hot peppers, offers a probiotic boost to the breakfast along with curcumin, a compound shown to possess anti-oxidant, anti-inflammatory, and anticancer properties.

Total cost of the breakfast: $4.23. A very fair price to discover Nicoya's secrets to longevity.

THE TRADITIONAL Chorotega people of Nicoya, Costa Rica, have been eating essentially this same breakfast for millennia. Not coincidentally, they're living longer than anyone else in the Americas (and by some measurements, the world). Men here have about a three-fold better chance of reaching a healthy age 90 than North Americans do. Even more interesting, Stanford geneticist David Rehkopf and Costa Rican demographer Luis

Rosero-Bixby have examined the telomeres (the DNA tips that are a rough marker of biological age) of Nicoyans and found that they are the longest of all people in Costa Rica. Indeed, their bodies may be a decade younger than their chronological age would suggest. And the people with the longest telomeres of all? The poorest in the community: those most likely to subsist on beans, tortillas, chilero, and black coffee.

That's not to say these are the only regional dishes that explain Nicoya's exceptional longevity. This blue zones community is a 100-mile-long strip that runs along the spine of the Nicoya Peninsula and does not include the tourist beach developments typical of Costa Rica's coasts. It is mostly dry pastureland, interspersed with ever diminishing forests. Until about 50 years ago, people here were mostly subsistence farmers or ranch hands, supplementing their corn and bean diet with tropical fruits, garden vegetables, and occasionally wild game and fish.

The most essential longevity ingredient here, as in all blue zones areas, is good taste. A uniquely Latin American flavor palette emerged with less of the spicy heat of Mexico but more character than the rest of Latin America. Hearty soups and stews made with local produce (yuca, *ayote,* peppers, cilantro) marry with Old World standards (onion, garlic, carrots) to create a

Ginger, yuca, tomatoes, peppers, and plantains are just some of the rich and healthful ingredients available in Nicoyan markets.

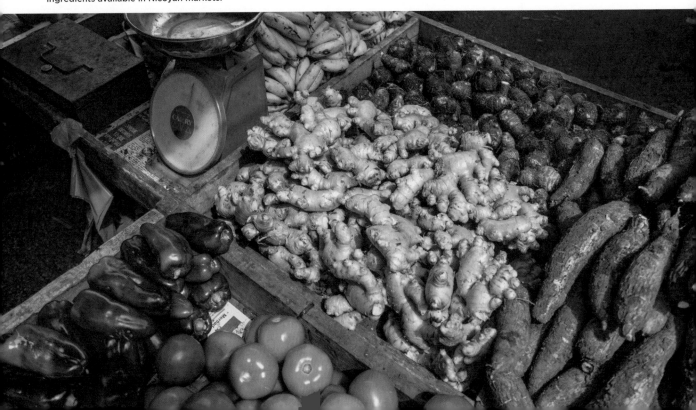

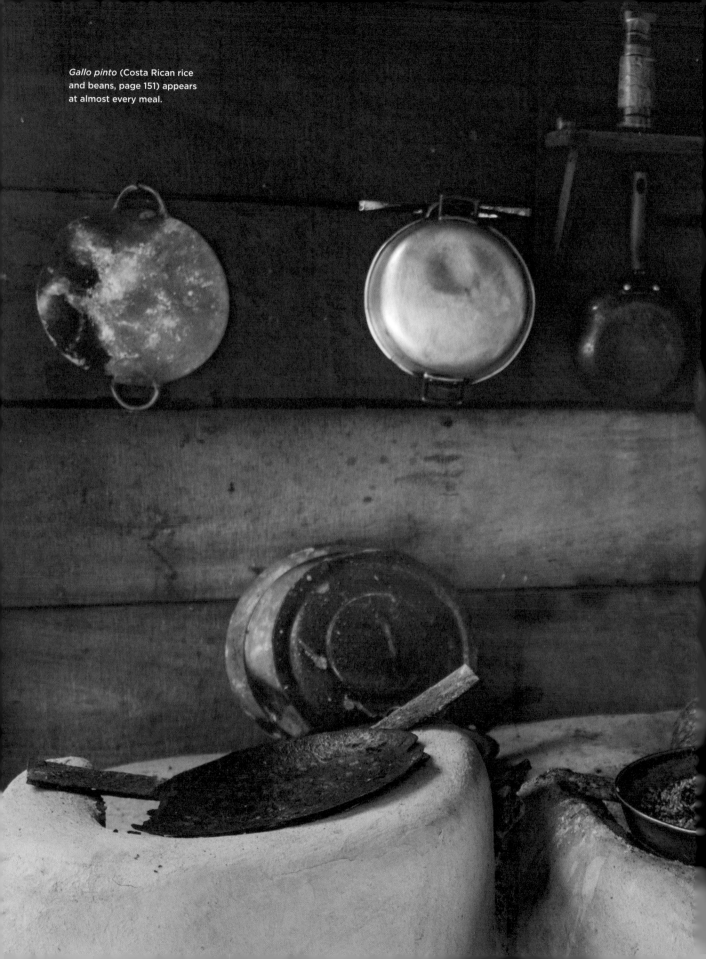

Gallo pinto (Costa Rican rice and beans, page 151) appears at almost every meal.

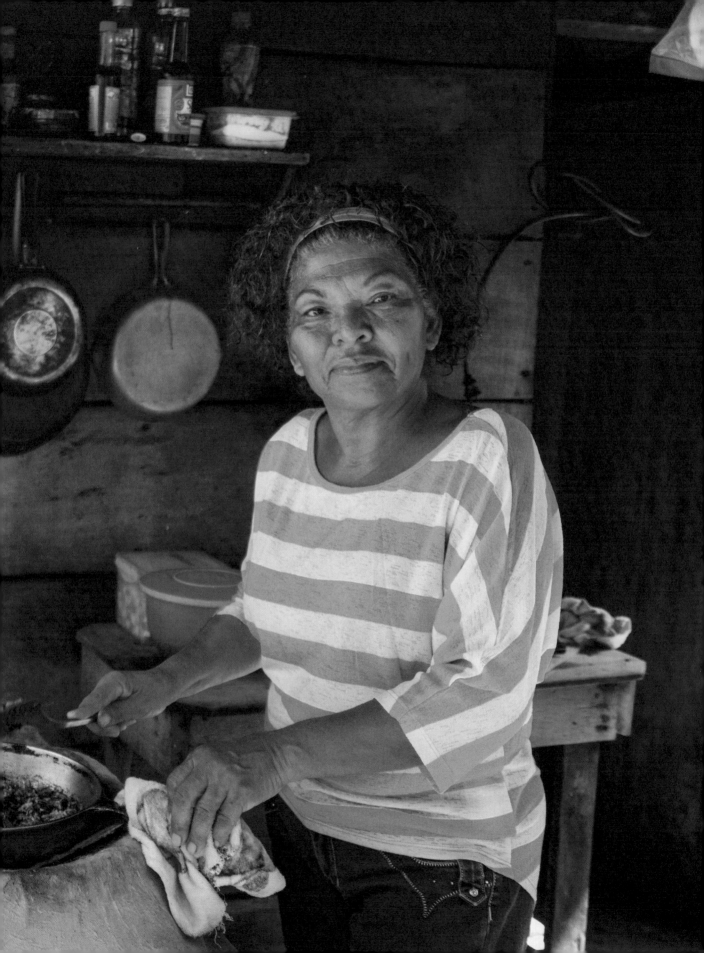

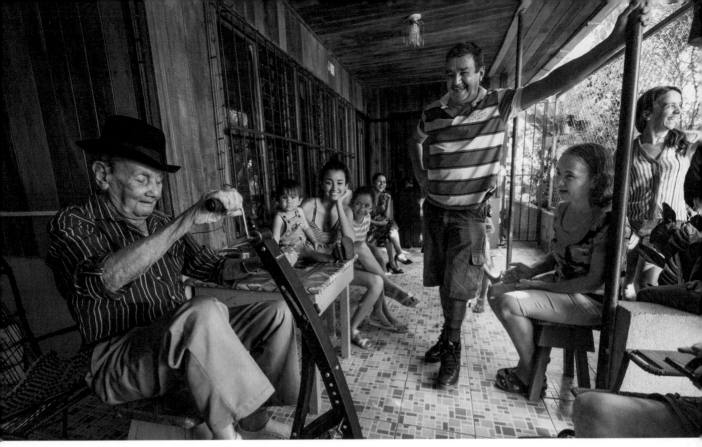
A centenarian rides his exercise machine surrounded by his extended family.

uniquely Tico (as Costa Ricans refer to themselves) flavor. Easy access to abundant fruit from home gardens (papaya, coconut, avocado, pineapple) is a year-round enhancement to the longevity diet.

As in other blue zones areas, a web of mutually supporting factors also helps contribute to Nicoyans' overall longevity. When I led a National Geographic Expedition here in 2008, we found that the water that leaches through Nicoya's mineral-rich subsoil is abundant with magnesium and calcium, perhaps explaining stronger bones and healthier hearts. We also noted people's strong connection to family, reliance on their God to get them through the tough times, and daily low-intensity physical activity (like walking and gardening) come into play.

NO ONE REPRESENTS the Nicoyan ideal better than Jose Bonifacio, a 100-year-old cowboy who stills ride his horse every morning. For our visit, his daughter and granddaughter have prepared lunch for us. In an outdoor kitchen, over a wood-fired *fogón* oven, they prepare chunky vegetable soup (page 148), a veggie hash with corn and onions (page 144), hearts of palm with herbs and garlic (page 161), creamy lima beans and herbs, and fried green plantains (page 155). They serve it all with plastic mugs of shockingly refreshing *horchata* (page 173) and citrus fresco.

Next, we travel to the heart of the Nicoya blue zone area: Santa Cruz. There we spend an afternoon with Doña María Rangel, her daughter Gioconda y Anabelle Rangel, and her son-in-law Carlos.

In their sprawling, cacophonous backyard kitchen of open-flame stoves, pots, and corn grinders, the multigenerational family cooks eight dishes for us. At our feet are two toddlers, the family dog, and a platoon of pecking chickens. In the mornings, the family runs a commercial handmade tortilla business. But for us, they spread their wings and whipped up a butternut squash soup (page 149), lima beans and herbs, and an amazing hearts of palm ceviche (page 156), which was a dead ringer for its fishy cousin.

Finally, we pay a visit to our old pal Jose Guevara, whom I first met when I took Dr. Mehmet Oz to Nicoya in 2011. He was 100 then. Now at 106, he was still wielding a machete and singing songs. He lives in a compound of sorts with his daughters Susana (74) and Leonor (70), who care for him—not out of obligation, but out of joy. They've nicknamed their father "cutie."

On a steamy afternoon, we watched the sisters prepare their father's favorite dishes (besides rice and beans). Over an open flame they made their version of *gallo pinto,* a brilliant zucchini stew with cornmeal, and a bean, potato, and onion stew (page 163). Before Jose and I dug in, he clasped his hands and gave thanks to the Lord. I did too—not just for the food, but for inspiration like him. Jose had worked as a lumberjack for much of his life, waking at four o'clock each morning and knocking off at 3 p.m. He'd actually done a good bit of thinking about his longevity and boiled it down to three secrets: Start your day with fruit, eat beans at every meal, and practice absolute honesty.

Words to live by, methinks. *

FLAVOR PROFILE

The flavor pairings below are the foundation of the most popular Nicoyan dishes. You can use these arresting combinations to enhance a variety of different meals.

* * *

beans + corn + squash

garlic + cilantro + *culantro coyote*

garlic + onions + mini sweet peppers

lime + cilantro + onion

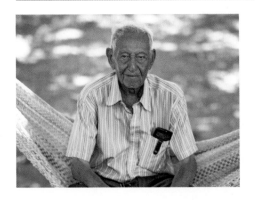

Jose Bonifacio, 100 YEARS OLD

Cowboy Jose Bonifacio is probably the coolest of the 300 or so centenarians I've interviewed. We arrive early, waiting for him in the cool shade under the 100-year-old mango trees in his courtyard. He trots up on a horse wearing blue jeans, a checkered shirt, and a jaunty-angled cowboy hat. He dismounts with a bounce and welcomes us warmly with a handshake and a half-toothed smile. He's lived in the same house his whole life, now with four generations of descendants. At 100, he still recites romantic poems and professes his love of women.

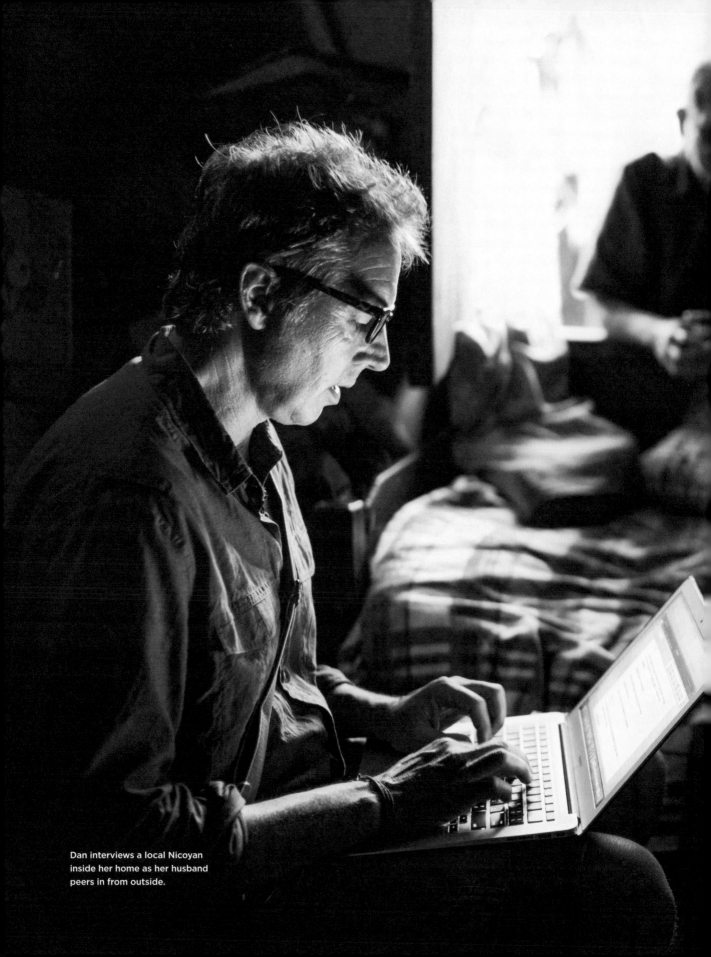
Dan interviews a local Nicoyan inside her home as her husband peers in from outside.

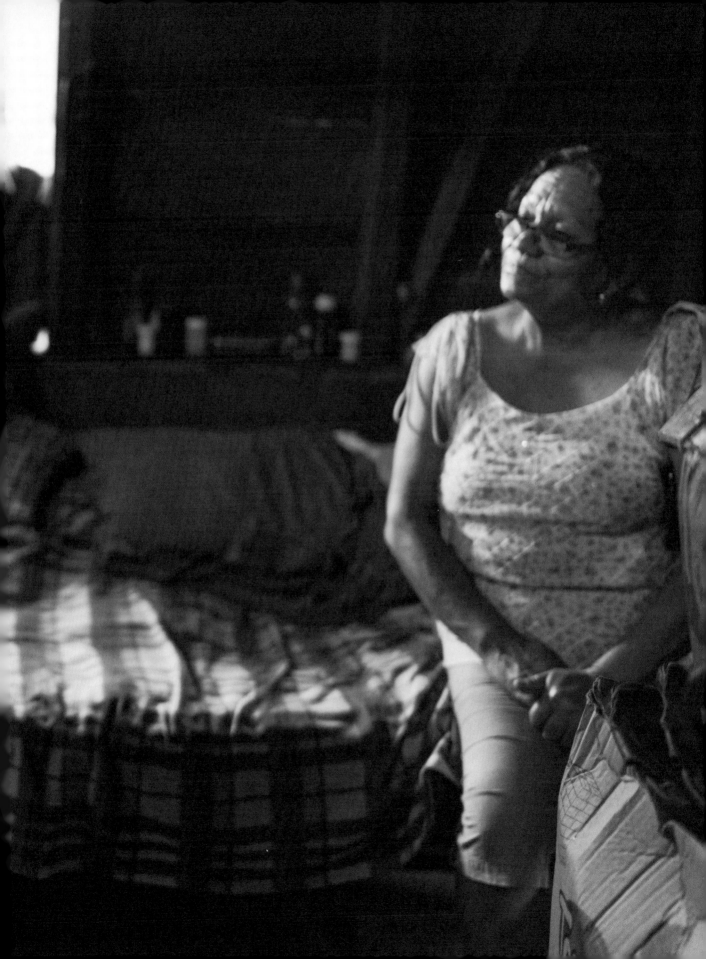

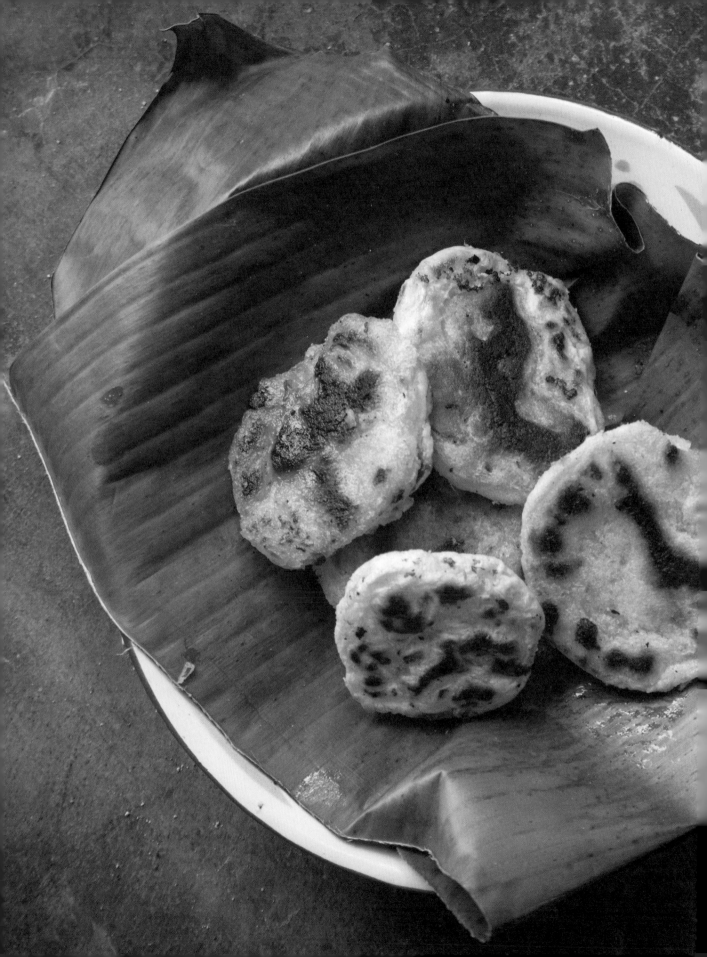

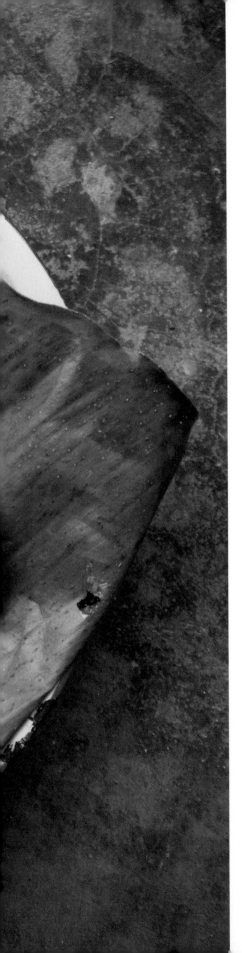

Yuca Cakes

TOTAL COOK TIME: 50 MINUTES | MAKES 4 SERVINGS

Yuca, or *cassava,* is like the potato of Costa Rica—it can be mashed, fried, boiled, or baked. This root vegetable is traditionally a staple food for families, since it's delicious, versatile, and inexpensive. These savory yuca cakes are slightly nutty in flavor: a tasty, traditional dish enjoyed throughout the Nicoya Peninsula. A good source of fiber, vitamin C, folate, B vitamins, and potassium, yuca also has a low glycemic index.

This delightful *enyucado* recipe can be enjoyed as a snack or dressed up into a full meal. You can enjoy the simple preparation as is or customize it if you prefer. Herbs and spices like garlic and chili pepper, as well as other vegetables such as onion, scallions, or celery, can be used in these savory patties. You can also garnish with toppings like avocado, cashew cream, hot sauce, or sweeten them with jam or honey.

1½ pounds yuca (can substitute with sweet potato), peeled

2 mini sweet red peppers,* seeded and finely chopped

1 *culantro coyote* leaf (page 147), finely chopped

½ teaspoon salt

1 tablespoon extra-virgin olive oil

Boil the yuca about 30 minutes, until soft. Drain the yuca and mash in a medium bowl.

Add peppers, culantro, and salt and mix to combine.

When cool enough to handle, roll mixture into plum-size balls, then flatten with your palm or the back of a spoon.

In a frying pan, heat 1 tablespoon of olive oil over medium-high heat.

Add yuca patties to oil. Do not crowd them in the pan; work in batches if necessary. Fry 3-4 minutes on each side, until browned and crispy. Remove to a paper towel–lined plate and serve hot or warm. (Alternatively, you can bake the patties on a baking sheet at 350 degrees for 15 minutes.)

*You can find the sweet red peppers (see photo pages 130–131) used in the Nicoya region of Costa Rica in American grocery stores in packs labeled "mini sweet peppers" or at Latin markets. But if you can't track them down, you can swap in one red or yellow bell pepper instead.

Veggie Hash With Corn and Onions

TOTAL COOK TIME: 25 MINUTES | MAKES 4 SERVINGS

Picadillo is the consummate Costa Rican comfort food and is popular throughout all of Latin America. It's similar to a potato hash, as all the ingredients are chopped into small pieces. The name comes from the Spanish word *picar*, which means "to chop." Costa Rican versions also include the names of the main vegetables involved such as *picadillo de ayote* (squash), and *picadillo de palmito* (hearts of palm).

    Picadillo de chayote is an authentic and easy Costa Rican family dish, whether you enjoy it as a filling for tortillas or pair it with soup and rice to make a hearty meal.

1 large chayote squash, peeled, pitted, and diced

3 ears corn, kernels removed, or ½ pound frozen sweet corn kernels

3 sweet red or yellow peppers, seeded and diced

½ sweet onion (like Vidalia), minced

4 teaspoons cilantro

4 teaspoons chopped *culantro coyote* (page 147)

1 celery stalk, diced

2 cloves garlic, minced

1 cup water

1 teaspoon achiote paste*

Salt and pepper (optional)

In a large sauté pan or pot, combine all ingredients together, including salt and pepper to taste, if using; cook over medium heat until there is about a ¼ cup of "gravy" at the bottom of the pan, about 15-20 minutes.

*Achiote paste is a cooking condiment used to add red color and a mild chili flavor to dishes. You can find it in a Mexican or Latin market or at an online retailer. It is often sold as a spice cake and is a mix of achiote and several other spices. If you can't find it, use mild chili powder with a squeeze of lime instead, or paprika for color.

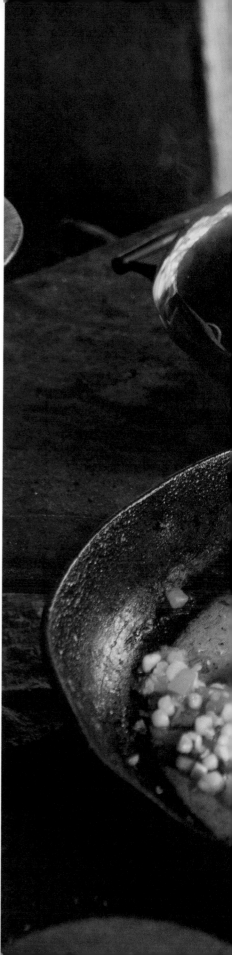

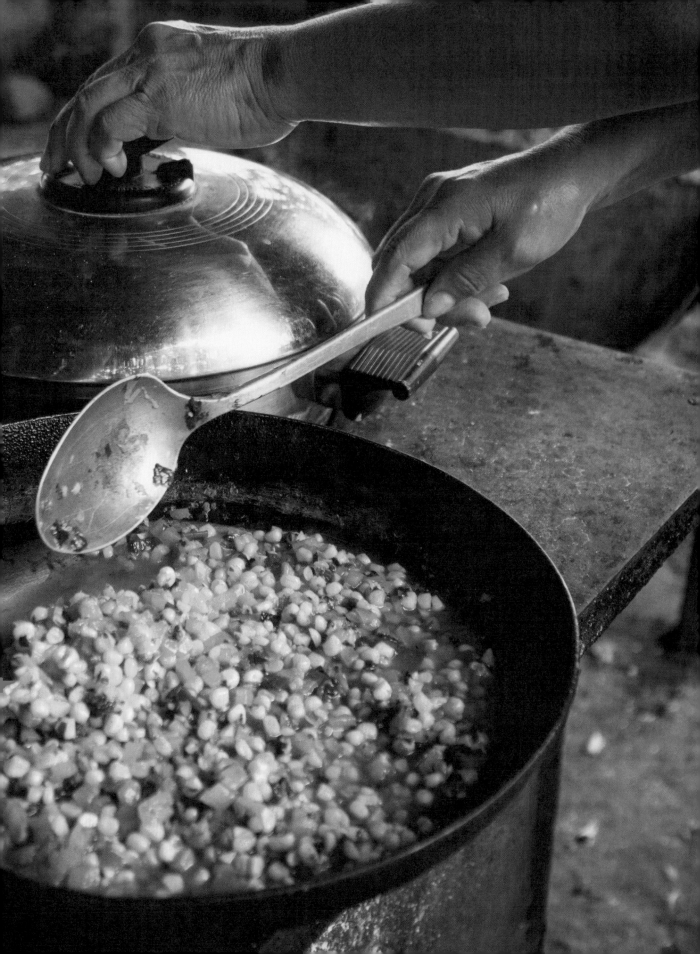

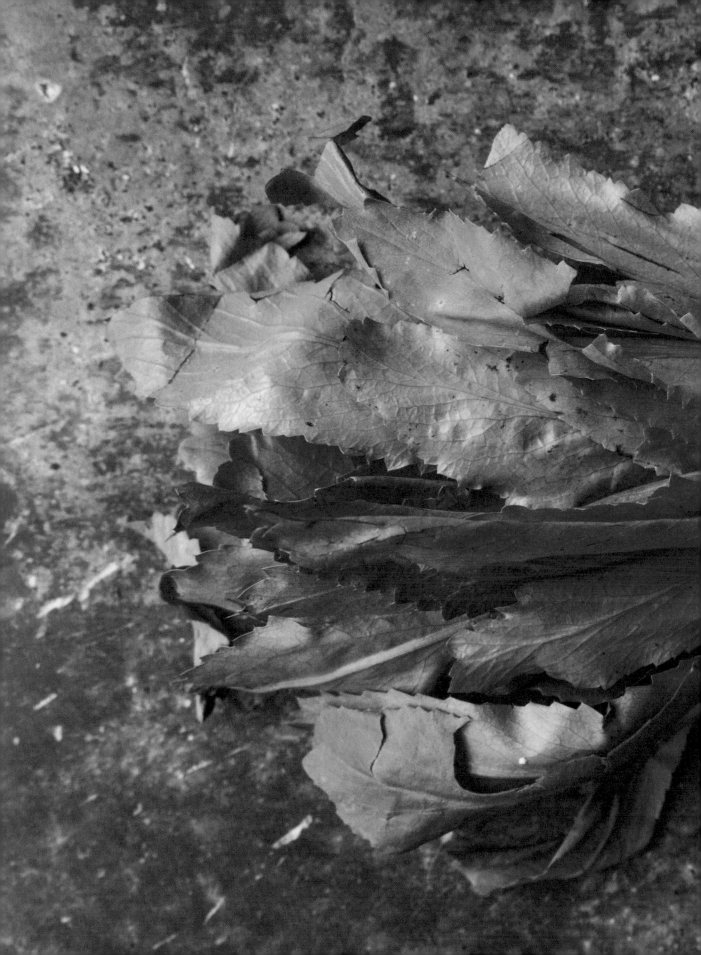

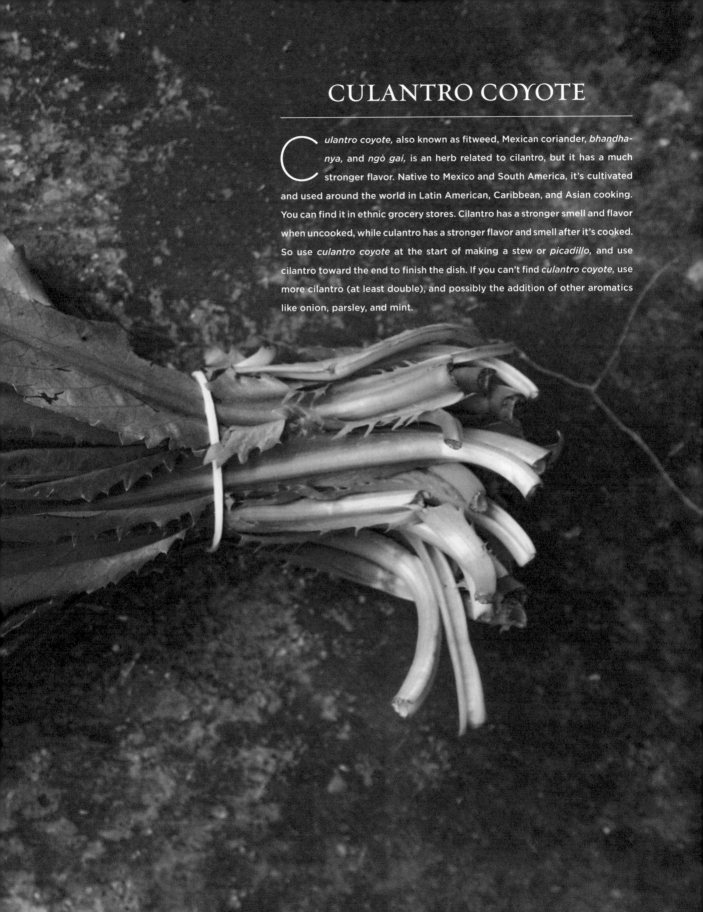

CULANTRO COYOTE

Culantro coyote, also known as fitweed, Mexican coriander, *bhandha-nya*, and *ngò gai*, is an herb related to cilantro, but it has a much stronger flavor. Native to Mexico and South America, it's cultivated and used around the world in Latin American, Caribbean, and Asian cooking. You can find it in ethnic grocery stores. Cilantro has a stronger smell and flavor when uncooked, while culantro has a stronger flavor and smell after it's cooked. So use *culantro coyote* at the start of making a stew or *picadillo,* and use cilantro toward the end to finish the dish. If you can't find *culantro coyote,* use more cilantro (at least double), and possibly the addition of other aromatics like onion, parsley, and mint.

Nicoya Chunky Tropical Vegetable Soup

TOTAL COOK TIME: 45 MINUTES | MAKES 8 SERVINGS

This tasty soup—almost a stew—called *sopa de yuca* is a savory mix of both familiar and exotic tropical vegetables. Hearty and satisfying, it's a particularly welcome treat during cold days; it will warm you through and through. Since this recipe contains so many different types of vegetables, feel free to swap in what you have on hand.

Ayote is a hard, black squash that becomes deeply sweet and flavorful when cooked, but you can easily use butternut squash. Feel free to omit the yuca if you can't find it easily, or substitute with sweet potato or white potato. Serve with brown rice or some crusty bread.

The biggest secret of the Nicoyan diet is the "three sisters": beans, corn, and squash. Since at least 5000 B.C., Mesoamericans have cultivated these staples in *milpas* fields. This almost perfect agricultural system also amounts to an almost perfect food combo: rich in complex carbohydrates, protein, essential fatty acids, calcium, and niacin.

1 tablespoon extra-virgin olive oil

2 cloves garlic, minced

1 small onion, diced

2 chayote squash, peeled and cut into ½-inch dice

2 pounds yuca, peeled and cut into ½-inch dice

3 small yellow squash or zucchini, peeled and cut into ½-inch dice

3 potatoes, peeled and cut into ½-inch dice

3 carrots, peeled and cut into ½-inch dice

1 *ayote* squash, peeled, seeded, and cut into ½-inch dice

4 sweet peppers, seeded and diced

1 celery stalk, chopped

3 to 4 quarts vegetable broth

Salt (optional)

Heat the oil in a soup pot; add garlic and onion and stir-fry for 3-4 minutes.

Add the rest of the ingredients through the broth to the pot; cover and cook on low heat until the vegetables are soft, about 30-40 minutes.

Season with salt to taste before serving. Serve with *gallo pinto* (page 151) and corn tortillas (page 152) for a full meal.

Creamy Butternut Squash Soup

TOTAL COOK TIME: 40 MINUTES | MAKES 4 SERVINGS

Squash, one of the oldest crops in Costa Rica, grows everywhere in the country. The pre-Columbian people used it as an essential ingredient but also as a way to thicken their soups (along with grains, corn, and potatoes). The soups were mostly meatless until the Spaniards arrived in the 16th century.

This creamy but creamless soup, *crema de ayote,* is a versatile dish with just a few ingredients, perfect for making as a hearty meal to enjoy all week. It brings out the core Costa Rican flavors of cilantro and sweet pepper for a zesty variation on our more mild and creamy vegetable soups in the United States.

1 pound butternut squash, peeled, seeded, and coarsely chopped

4 sweet red peppers, seeded and coarsely chopped

1 teaspoon chopped cilantro

1 teaspoon chopped *culantro coyote**

½ onion, minced

1 cup vegetable broth

Salt and pepper (optional)

In a soup pot, combine all ingredients through the broth and bring to a boil; then reduce heat immediately to a low simmer. Cook until the squash can be easily mashed with a spoon or fork, about 30 minutes.

Use a wooden spoon or potato masher to mash squash until soup is creamy and smooth. Add salt and pepper to taste.

Serve with a dollop of cashew cream (page 277), if desired.

*See a description of *culantro coyote* on page 147. If you don't have it, add 2 teaspoons chopped fresh cilantro and 2 more tablespoons minced onion.

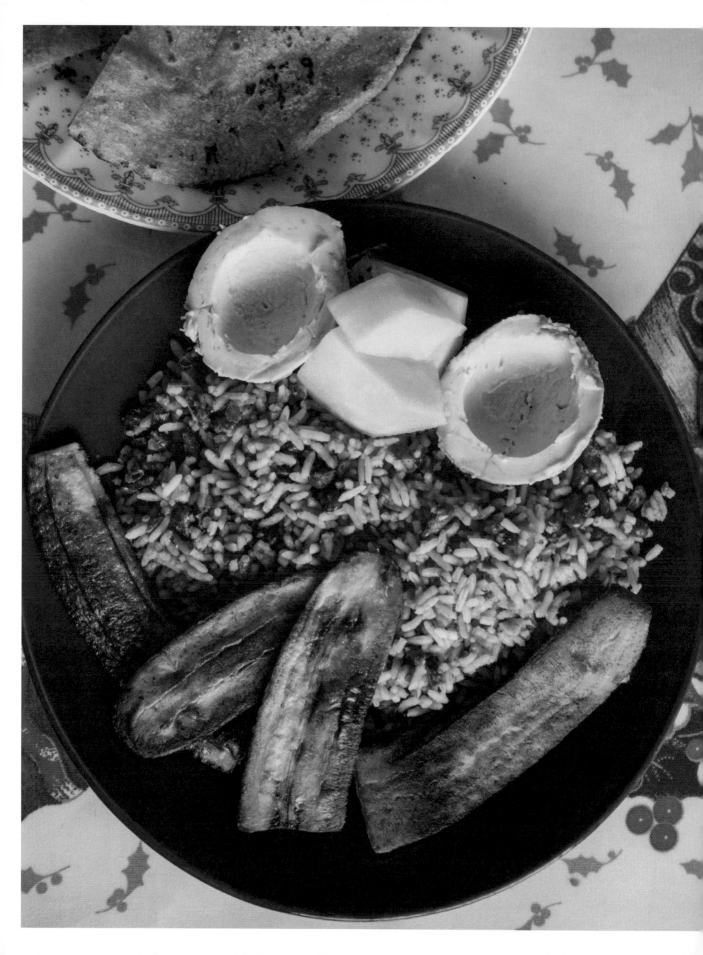

The Casado Plate (left)

The traditional lunch of all Ticos is called a casado. It comes in countless variations depending on the day, the kitchen, or the *soda* (local restaurant), but it's always built around rice and beans. *Casado* means "married," and the dish is a marriage of bright flavors and colors. Common casado plate additions are fried plantains, sliced avocados, a fried egg, corn, *picadíllos,* and sliced vegetables.

COMPONENTS OF A TYPICAL CASADO PLATE:

Gallo Pinto (below)

Hearts of Palm Ceviche (page 156)

Fried Green Plantains (page 155)

Chilero Hot Sauce (page 160)

Nixtamal Tortillas, for serving (page 152)

Optional toppings: corn, sliced avocado, chopped cilantro, lettuce, tomatoes

Jose Guevara's Gallo Pinto

TOTAL COOK TIME: 20 MINUTES | MAKES 3 SERVINGS

I last visted Jose Guevara in Costa Rica in 2015 when he was he was 105 years old and gave me this recipe, his version of Costa Rican rice and beans, or *gallo pinto.* The genius of the Costa Rican kitchen is its ability to make a humble bean dish so delicious that you could eat it every day (in fact, many Ticos, as Costa Ricans refer to themselves, eat it for breakfast, lunch, and dinner). It's often topped with eggs and Salsa Lizano (a bottled condiment, slightly sweet and acidic, that you can find on every restaurant table).

1½ tablespoons vegetable oil

1 onion, chopped

1 clove garlic, minced

2 tablespoons Worcestershire sauce

1½ cups cooked black beans (or one 8-ounce can black beans, drained)

3 cups cooked long-grain white rice

Salt and pepper (optional)

½ avocado, sliced, for topping (optional)

Chilero hot sauce (optional garnish) (see page 160)

Chopped cilantro (optional garnish)

In a large skillet, heat oil over medium heat. Add onion and sauté until it starts to soften, about 4 minutes.

Add garlic and cook for another 5-7 minutes, or until vegetables are browned.

Add Worcestershire sauce and beans; turn heat to low and stir. Cook for 2-3 minutes more.

Add rice and stir to combine. Cook and stir until rice and beans are evenly distributed and are heated through. Season with salt and pepper to taste.

Top with sliced avocado, hot sauce, and chopped cilantro, if desired.

Nixtamal Tortillas

TOTAL COOK TIME: 15 MINUTES | **MAKES 5 SERVINGS**

Nixtamal refers to corn that has been soaked and partially cooked with wood ash or lime (calcium hydroxide). This ancient Mesoamerican process increases the nutritional value of corn; the ancient Aztec discovered the positive effects of calcium hydroxide on this grain when they ground their corn against riverbed limestone thousands of years ago.

Lime or ash releases the amino acid niacin in corn, which helps to reduce bad cholesterol and increase good cholesterol and also aids in digestion. Corn itself is high in fiber, folate, and vitamins B and C.

You can buy your *nixtamal* corn flour (called masa harina) from the ethnic food aisle, from Mexican or Latin groceries, or online.

2 cups masa harina

¼ teaspoon baking soda

1½ cups warm tap water,
  plus more as needed

Plastic wrap

Waxed paper, as needed

In a large bowl, whisk the masa harina and baking soda together. Add water and stir until a soft dough forms (if the mixture won't form a soft ball of dough, add warm water in 1 tablespoon increments until it will). Cover with plastic wrap and set aside for 5 minutes.

On a clean, dry work surface, knead dough gently for 1 minute. Divide it into 16 equal balls, each about the size of a small plum.

Roll out dough between pieces of waxed paper into 6-inch rounds.

Set a griddle or cast iron skillet over high heat until smoking.

Set dough on the griddle and cook for 30 seconds. Flip with kitchen tongs and cook until lightly toasted, with tiny bubbles in the tortilla, about 30 more seconds. Work in batches.

Transfer to a clean kitchen towel and wrap gently. Serve warm.

Technique tip: Cool any unused tortillas to room temperature and store in the refrigerator, tightly wrapped in a kitchen towel, for up to 1 day. Reheat on a baking sheet 4 to 6 inches from a heated broiler for 10 seconds.

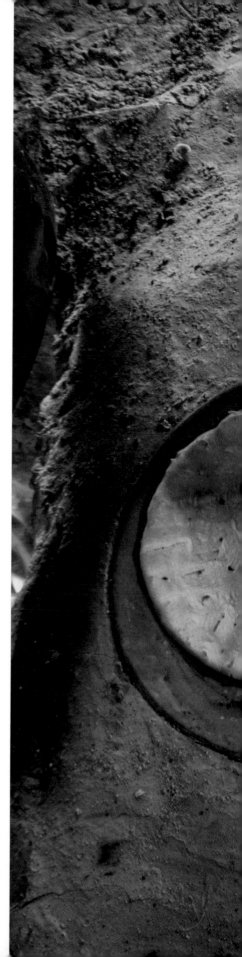

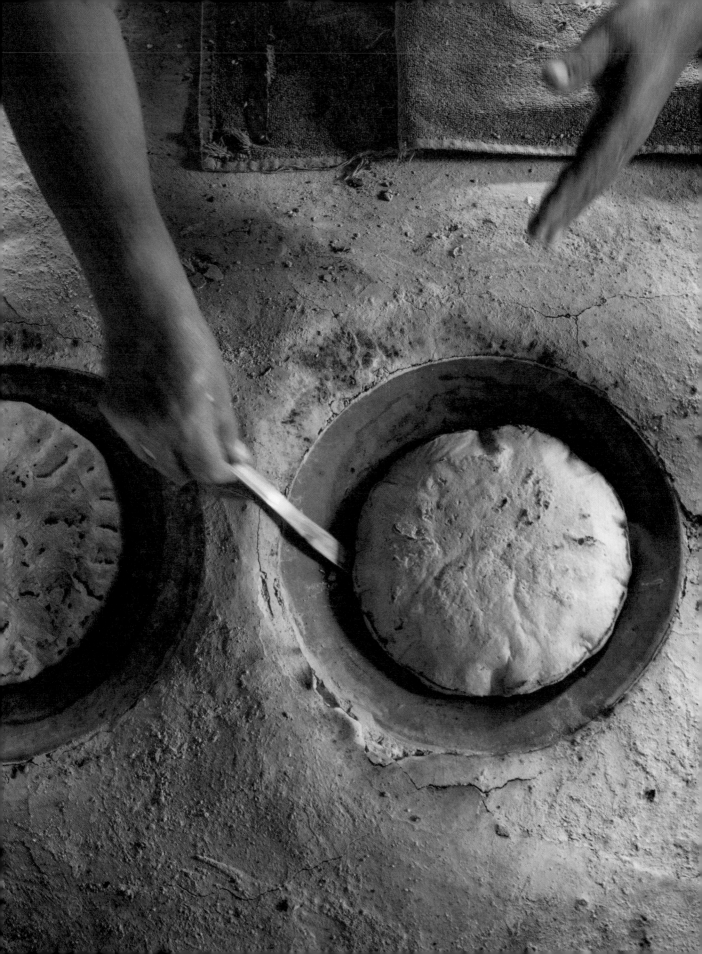

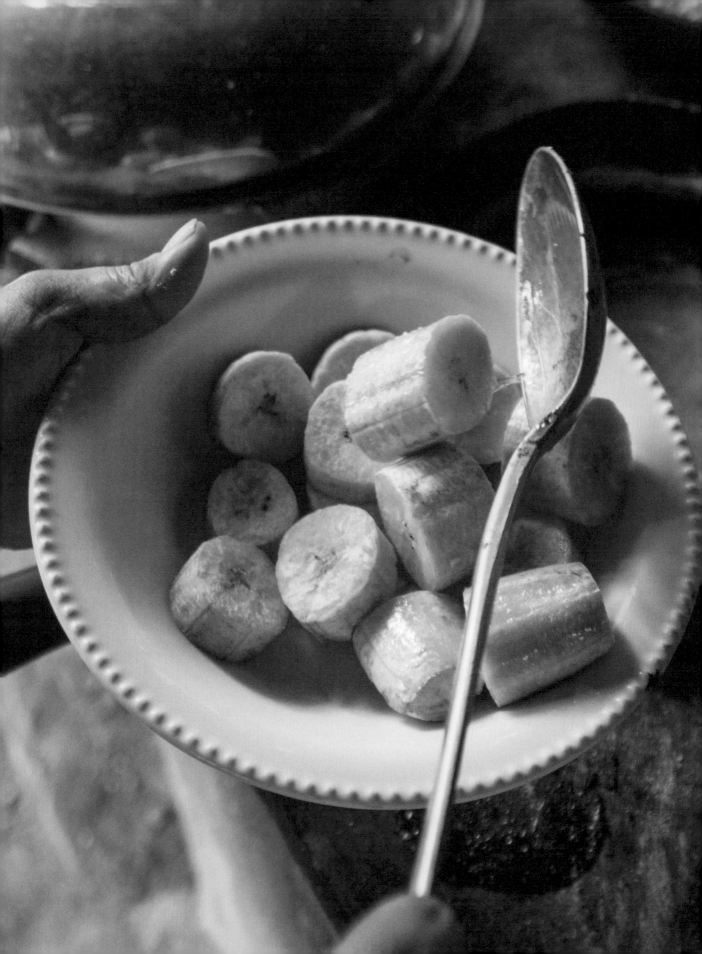

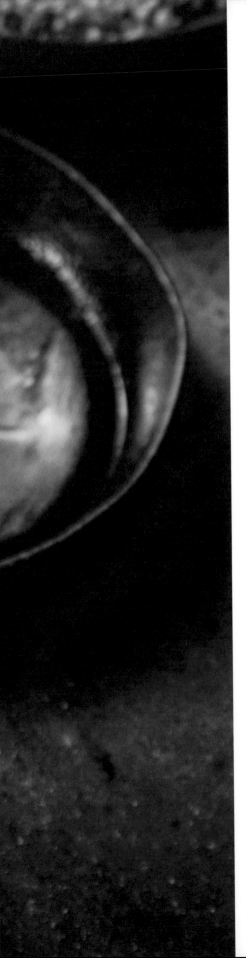

Fried Green Plantains

TOTAL COOK TIME: 30 MINUTES | MAKES 4 SERVINGS

A traditional Costa Rican comfort food, these twice-fried *patacones* are the perfect versatile snack or side, which you can enjoy alone, with toppings, or with dipping sauces. Plantains look like oversize bananas and are typically cooked before they are eaten. Green plantains are unripe, and potatolike in texture; they taste like a bitter potato when eaten raw. Rich in vitamins A and C, potassium, and fiber, they are a versatile ingredient; Costa Ricans fry, boil, bake, and grill them. They are often fried into *patacones* or chopped into *picadillos* (similar to a hash).

Vegetable oil

4 green plantains, each cut on an angle into 4 to 5 pieces

Salt (optional)

In a deep fry pan, heat about 1 inch of vegetable oil on medium-high heat until it's hot. (To test oil temp, dip the handle of a wooden spoon into the oil. When the oil bubbles around the stick, it's ready for frying.)

In batches, fry plantain pieces about 2-3 minutes on both sides, until lightly golden. Remove plantains from pan and drain on a plate covered with 2 or 3 paper towels.

While still warm, use the bottom of a glass to flatten the fried plantain pieces until they are about ¼-inch thick.

Heat oil again and return flattened plantain rounds into the oil. Fry until both sides are golden brown, about 2-3 minutes per side. Drain on a paper towel–lined plate.

Season with salt to taste and serve with refried beans, cashew cream (page 277), or chilero hot sauce (page 160) for dipping.

Hearts of Palm Ceviche

TOTAL COOK TIME: 10 MINUTES | **MAKES 3 SERVINGS**

Of all recipes I tasted in Costa Rica, this one delighted me the most. I used to love fresh fish ceviche but have stopped eating it because of sustainability and health concerns about eating fish. But this recipe brings all the cool citrus flavor and texture of the traditional ceviche I used to eat, with none of the health or environmental risks.

Hearts of palm are harvested from the inner core of certain palm trees, and Costa Ricans eat them cooked or in salads. Easy to enjoy and prepare, they are rich in immune boosters vitamin C and zinc. This ceviche is traditionally made with searingly hot habanero peppers, but you can substitute with sweet or mild peppers if you're spice averse.

1 cup hearts of palm, sliced into small rounds (use fresh, canned, or jarred)

1 small sweet onion (like Vidalia), quartered and sliced

2 small sweet red peppers, cut into ¼-inch dice

¼ small habanero pepper, seeded and minced

1 tablespoon chopped fresh cilantro

Juice of 1 to 2 limes

1 teaspoon salt

Pepper (optional)

Combine ingredients through cilantro in a bowl, drizzle with lime juice, and add salt; toss to combine.

Season with pepper, if desired, and serve immediately. Enjoy alone or served with popcorn, plantain chips, or tortilla chips.

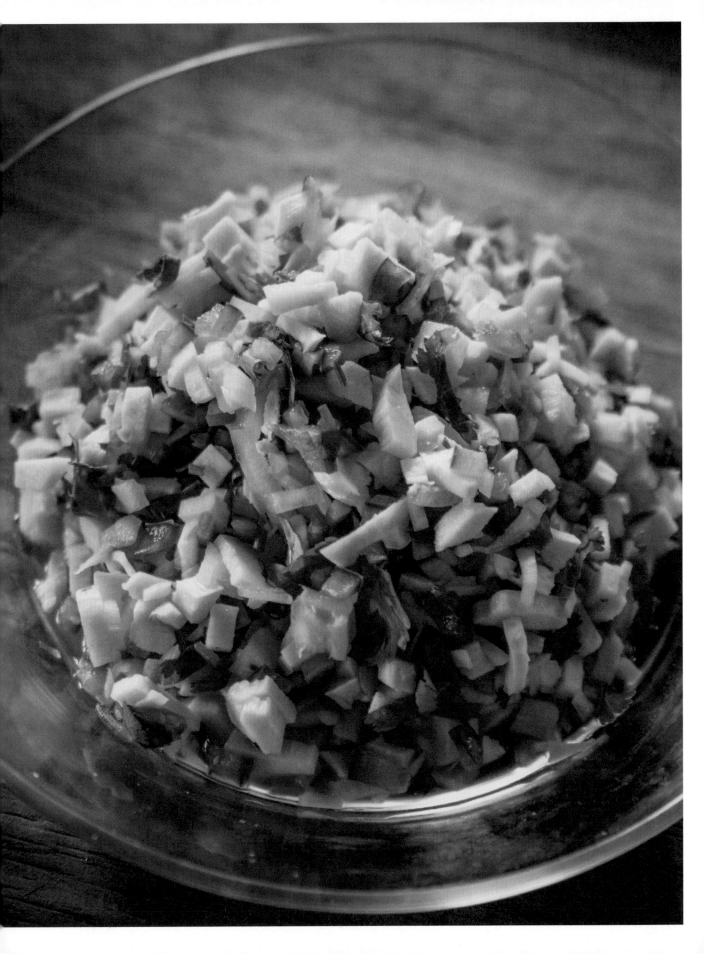

NICOYAN DIET STAPLES

Nicoyans enjoy beans, rice, and corn at almost every meal; squash, peppers, and different tubers like potatoes and yuca also make daily appearances in all types of dishes. Papaya trees grow like weeds on the peninsula, so locals enjoy them year-round, along with a bounty of other colorful fruits including plantains, mangoes, guava, zapote, pineapple, peach palms, and lemons and limes. They also choose to enhance the flavor and nutrient density of their meals with anti-inflammatory herbs and spices like ginger, cilantro, *culantro coyote,* and garlic.

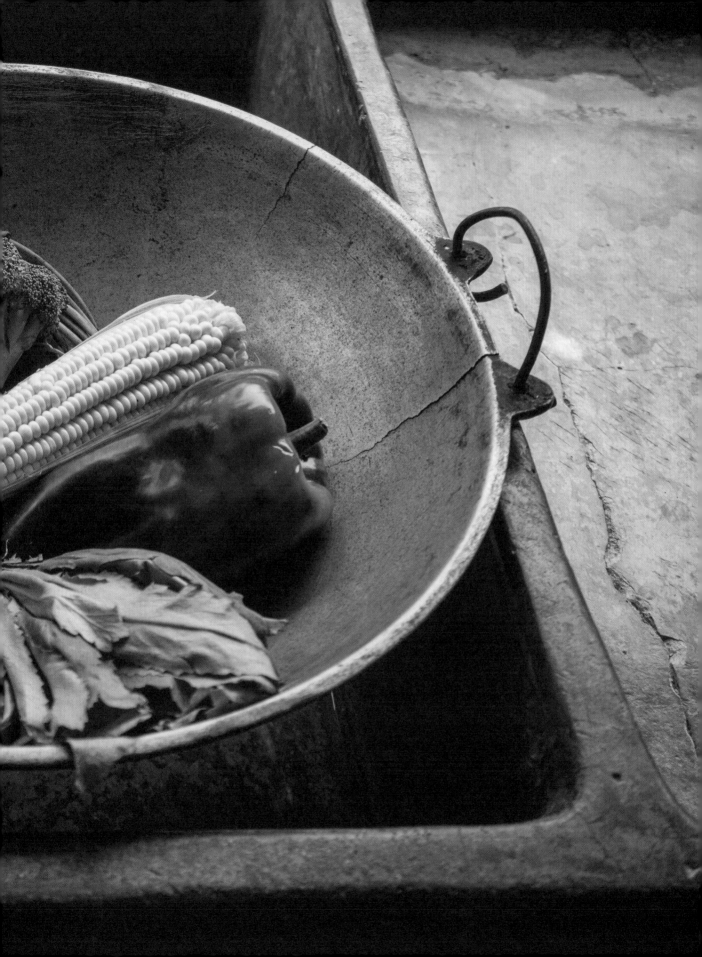

Chilero Hot Sauce

TOTAL COOK TIME: 20 MINUTES, PLUS PICKLING TIME | MAKES 24 SERVINGS

Probably the most popular Costa Rican condiment, chilero's tangy-spicy flavor is addicting, spicy, and slightly sweet. The veggie-packed, peppery sauce enlivens almost every type of food here, including rice, beans, and stews, and it gives dishes a kicking finishing touch. The best part? It's surprisingly easy to make and is an excellent substitute for Tabasco and other bottled hot sauces. The vinegar gives it a probiotic boost, and the vegetables and chili peppers add to its antioxidant and antibacterial properties.

Costa Ricans often refer to themselves as Ticos—individual males are Ticos and females are Ticas, but the general population is Tico. Each has his or her own chilero recipe, so it can sometimes be searingly hot. But every version centers around chili peppers, vinegar, and sugar. You can experiment with different vegetables, including onions, cauliflower, broccoli, and green beans, as well as your own comfort level of spiciness.

2 carrots, peeled and sliced into ¼-inch rounds

4 small sweet onions (like Vidalia), halved and sliced

2 cucumbers, sliced into ¼-inch rounds

1 head cauliflower, stem removed and florets cut into bite-size pieces

4 red or green (or combination) bell peppers, seeded and sliced into strips

6 jalapeño peppers, finely chopped (remove most of the seeds if you prefer a milder sauce)

8 spicy chili peppers (like habanero), finely chopped (remove most of the seeds if you prefer a milder sauce)

1 tablespoon salt

24 ounces white vinegar

Quickly parboil carrots and onions by boiling water and dropping them in for 1 to 2 minutes, until their color turns bright. Drain and pat dry.

Sprinkle all vegetables with salt.

Fill clean wide-mouth glass pickling bottle(s) or jar(s) with vegetables; then pour vinegar into bottles, pushing down vegetables until vinegar covers them entirely.

Allow the chilero to sit at room temperature (not in the sun) for at least a day before using. Two or three days is better.

Store for 2 to 3 months in the refrigerator.

Hearts of Palm Picadillo

TOTAL COOK TIME: 35 MINUTES | MAKES 4 SERVINGS

This much-overlooked vegetable adds a surprisingly meaty texture to both hot and cold dishes. Its mild taste makes it a blank canvas for all types of flavors, making it easy to transform into sweet, spicy, or tangy dishes. You can find hearts of palm raw in some markets, but they are also available canned or jarred. They look like very plump white artichoke stalks (without the tips).

2 pounds hearts of palm
  (can use canned or jarred)

3 red or yellow mini sweet
  peppers, seeded and diced

4 teaspoons chopped cilantro

4 teaspoons *culantro coyote*

1 stalk celery, diced

2 cloves garlic, minced

½ sweet onion (like Vidalia),
  minced

1½ cups of water, divided

Salt and pepper (optional)

In a large sauté pan over medium heat, combine first seven ingredients (through onion) with ½ cup water.

Stir once in a while, if needed, and add ½ cup water at a time until all water has evaporated, about 25 minutes. Turn down heat to medium-low, if needed, to avoid burning.

Season with salt and pepper to taste. Serve warm alone, or as a component of a casado plate.

Blue Zones Green Papaya

TOTAL COOK TIME: 15 MINUTES | MAKES 4 SERVINGS

Costa Rica is rich in fruits and vegetables, and papaya trees grow everywhere in Nicoya. Both green and ripe papaya are staples in the local cuisine in both sweet and savory dishes. This refreshing salad makes the perfect side to a stew or beans and rice dish.

1 tablespoon extra-virgin olive oil
  or vegetable oil

3 red, orange, or yellow sweet
  peppers, seeded and sliced into
  strips

1 small sweet onion (like Vidalia),
  halved and thinly sliced

1 clove garlic, minced

2 pounds green papaya, peeled
  and julienned

3 large *culantro coyote* leaves
  (page 147), coarsely chopped

Corn tortillas

1 tablespoon coarsely chopped
  fresh cilantro, for topping

Chilero hot sauce (opposite)

In a medium pan, sauté peppers, onion, and garlic in oil over medium-high heat for 4-5 minutes, until onion is translucent.

Reduce heat to medium-low, add papaya and *culantro coyote* and cook 4-6 more minutes or until veggies are well combined and cooked through, stirring frequently to make sure the mixture doesn't burn.

Serve in corn tortillas with cilantro and chilero hot sauce.

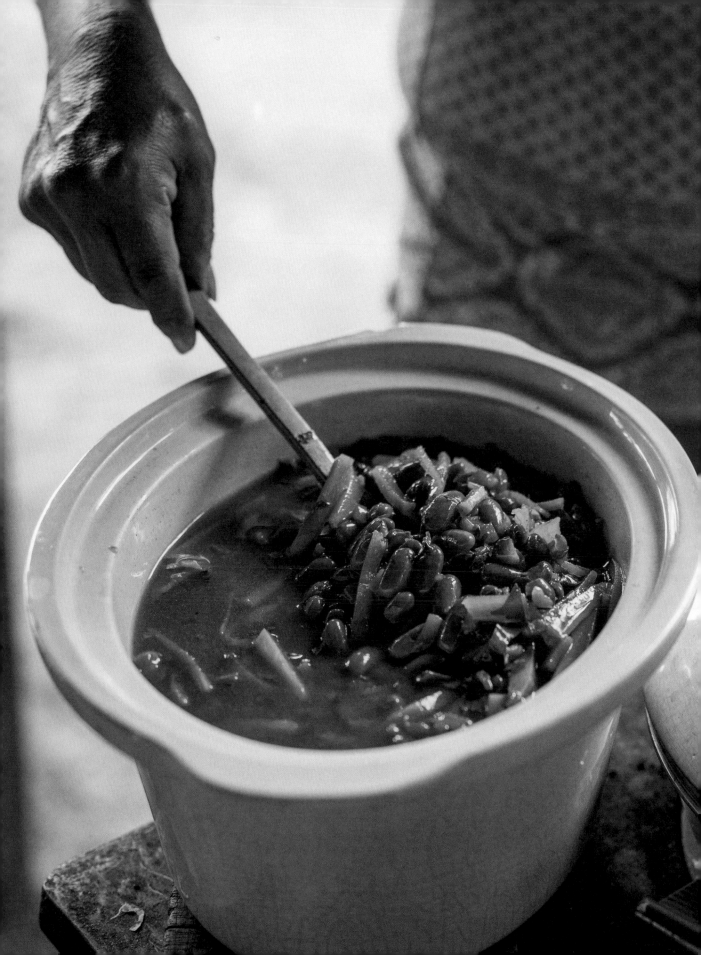

Bean Soup Three Ways

Featured in almost every Nicoyan meal, black beans contain high levels of anthocyanins, the important flavonoids in red onions and blueberries, and have 10 times the antioxidants of an equivalent serving of oranges. These hearty, one-pot meals are staples in Costa Rican kitchens, but should also find their place on the American dinner table. They are easy to make, high in nutritious vegetables and spices, and cost less than $1 a serving. Rich and hearty, they will serve as a main meal paired with corn tortillas or rice. You can do as the Nicoyans do—make a large batch of bean soup and then enjoy it all week.

TENDER BEAN, POTATO, AND ONION STEW (left)

TOTAL COOK TIME: 1 HOUR | MAKES 6 SERVINGS

1 pound dried kidney beans, soaked overnight (or three 15-ounce cans, drained)

1 cup low-sodium vegetable broth

1 chayote squash, diced

½ carrot, peeled and diced

3 red, orange, or yellow sweet peppers, seeded and diced

2 large potatoes, peeled and diced

2 teaspoons chopped *culantro coyote* (page 147)

1 small onion, diced

2 cloves garlic, minced

Salt and pepper (optional)

If using dried beans, drain and rinse the beans; discard the soaking water.

Place beans in a large pot and add vegetable broth. Add water, as necessary, to cover beans. Bring broth to a boil; then immediately turn down to simmer. Cook for 25 minutes.

Stir in the rest of ingredients; cook for about 25 more minutes, or until beans are tender, stirring occasionally to keep from burning.

Add salt and pepper to taste before serving. Enjoy alone or with tortillas or rice.

BLACK BEAN AND POTATO SOUP

TOTAL COOK TIME: 35 MINUTES | MAKES 10 SERVINGS

½ chayote squash (about 1 cup), diced

½ large carrot, peeled and minced

2 large potatoes, peeled and diced

2 teaspoons chopped *culantro coyote* (page 147)

1 small sweet onion (like Vidalia), diced

2 cloves garlic, minced

4 cups low-sodium vegetable stock

2 pounds black beans, cooked (or six 15-ounce cans, drained)

Salt and pepper (optional)

In a large stock pot, combine all ingredients. Bring stock to a boil; then lower heat and simmer for 25 minutes.

Take 2 cups of soup and blend in a blender or with immersion blender, until combined but still chunky. Add back into soup pot and stir to combine. Add salt and pepper to taste.

Serve hot with rice, corn tortillas, or crusty bread; or top with a dollop of cashew cream (page 277).

(Bean Soup Three Ways continued)

VEGETABLE SOUP WITH RICE

TOTAL COOK TIME: 40 MINUTES | MAKES 3 SERVINGS

8 cups water

4 cups low-sodium vegetable broth

1 cup rice

1 sweet onion (like Vidalia), minced

3 cloves garlic, minced

1 chayote squash, cubed

1 carrot, peeled and cut into ¼-inch rounds

1 white sweet potato, peeled and cubed

1 *tiquisque,** peeled and cubed

Salt and pepper (optional)

In a soup pot, combine all ingredients and bring to a boil.

Reduce heat to a low simmer and cook for 30 minutes, or until rice is cooked through.

Add salt and pepper to taste before serving.

*Tiquisque is a variety of taro common in Costa Rica. It looks like a hairy, ugly potato and is often sold in Latin or other ethnic markets. If you can't find it at nearby stores, feel free to substitute with potatoes.

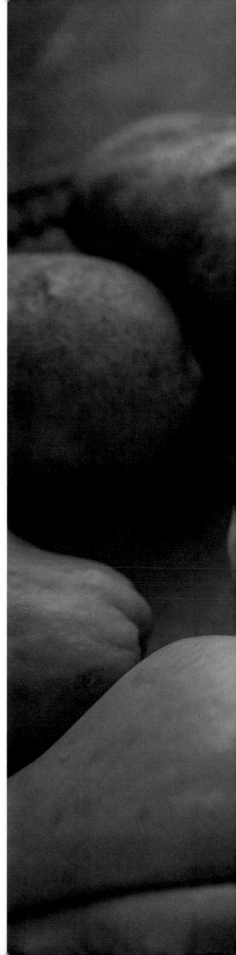

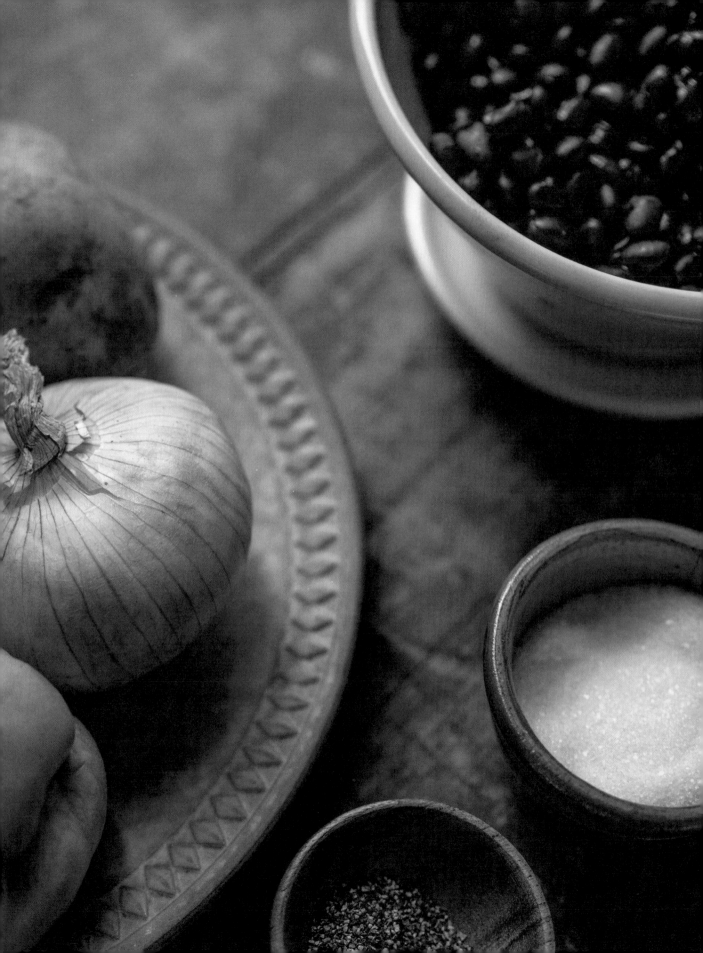

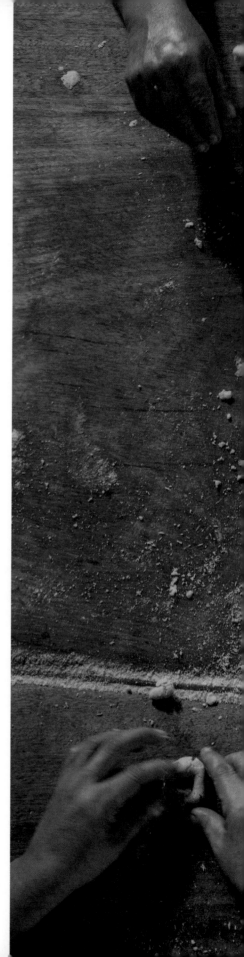

Costa Rican Baked Doughnuts

TOTAL COOK TIME: 1 HOUR | MAKES 10 SERVINGS

These cornmeal doughnuts (*bizcochos*) are usually deep fried with cheese, but this lighter version is baked and made sweeter with creamed corn. Enjoy these traditional treats for snacks, breakfast, or dessert, and you can even adjust the toppings to make it a sweet or savory dish. These are a combination of corncake, muffin, and doughnut, so you can make them into a savory meal with salsa, avocados, jalapeños, and hot sauce, or bring out their sweetness with a dollop of syrup and fresh fruit.

2 cups masa harina

1½ teaspoons salt

3 tablespoons brown sugar

1 cup warm water

⅓ cup creamed corn

1 teaspoon vanilla

Preheat oven to 350 degrees.

In a large bowl, mix masa harina, salt, and sugar together. Add the warm water in small batches, mixing with your hands.

After water is combined, add rest of ingredients, mixing with your hands to combine.

When dough forms, pinch off thumb-size pieces and roll between your hands.

Form small palm-size tubes and close them to form rings.

Place rings on greased baking tray and bake for about 35 minutes, or until golden brown.

Allow to cool before enjoying.

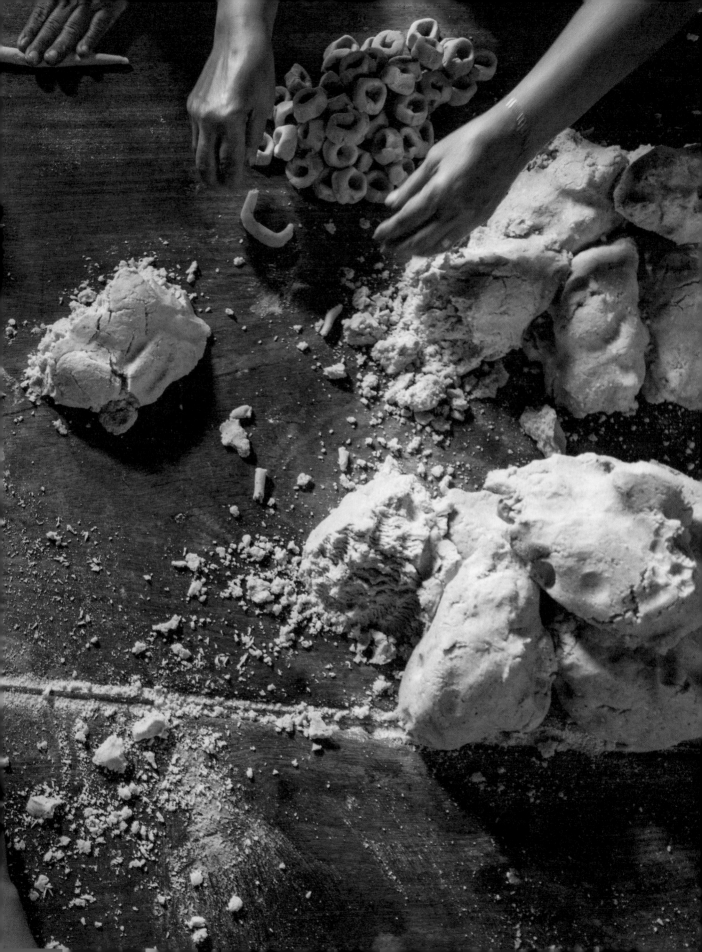

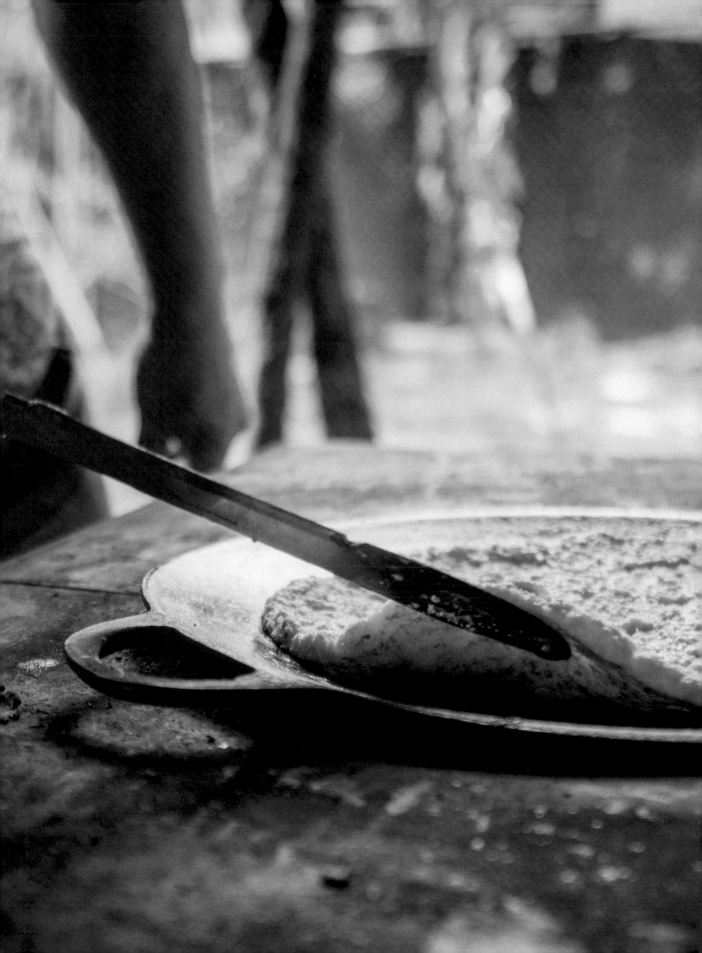

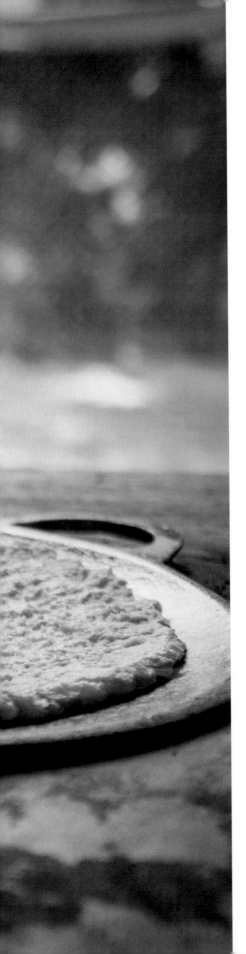

Sweet Corncakes

TOTAL COOK TIME: 20 MINUTES | MAKES 3 SERVINGS

These simple, traditional corn pancakes are a healthy substitute for the flour-and-egg pancakes commonly served in the United States. The sweet, toasty cakes don't require a slathering of syrup, and they have more fiber, fewer calories, and less fat than their American counterparts. As in all the other blue zones regions outside the United States, Costa Rican breakfasts are very similar to lunches and dinners.

4 cups fresh sweet corn kernels (or two 16-ounce cans, drained)

3 tablespoons water

1 teaspoon salt

2 tablespoons granulated sugar

Vegetable oil for frying

Honey, fruit, cinnamon, or cashew cream (page 277) for optional topping

Blend corn, water, salt, and sugar in a blender until mostly smooth.

Heat a pan over medium-high heat and coat with a thin layer of oil.

Cook the batter like pancakes, spooning approximately ¼ cup onto the pan and spreading into circles.

Reduce heat to low, let the corncakes brown, and then flip over and cook until golden and browned.

Continue cooking in batches, covering the finished corncakes on a plate to keep them warm.

Serve with honey and fruit. These are also delicious topped with cinnamon or cashew cream.

Tico Tropical Salad

TOTAL PREP TIME: 15 MINUTES | MAKES 4 SERVINGS

In the tropical Nicoya Peninsula, locals have year-round access to fresh fruits and vegetables, which might explain some of their extraordinary longevity. Indeed, tropical fruits offer more heart-healthy potassium and folate than the more common citrus fruits do. This sweet and exotic mix will provide you with a daily dose of phytonutrients and fiber.

1 cup papaya, peeled, seeded, and cut into ½-inch dice

2 bananas, cut into ½-inch dice

2 cups melon (any variety, like honeydew or watermelon), cut into ½-inch dice

1 cup pineapple, peeled, cored, and cut into ½-inch dice

1 tablespoon honey

Juice of ½ lime

Chopped nuts or shredded coconut (optional)

In a large bowl, mix fruit together.

In a separate small bowl, whisk together honey and lime juice until combined. Then pour over fruit and gently mix to distribute dressing.

Top with chopped nuts or shredded coconut, if desired, and serve cold.

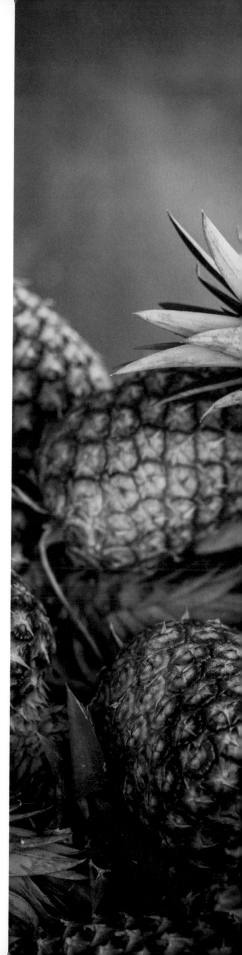

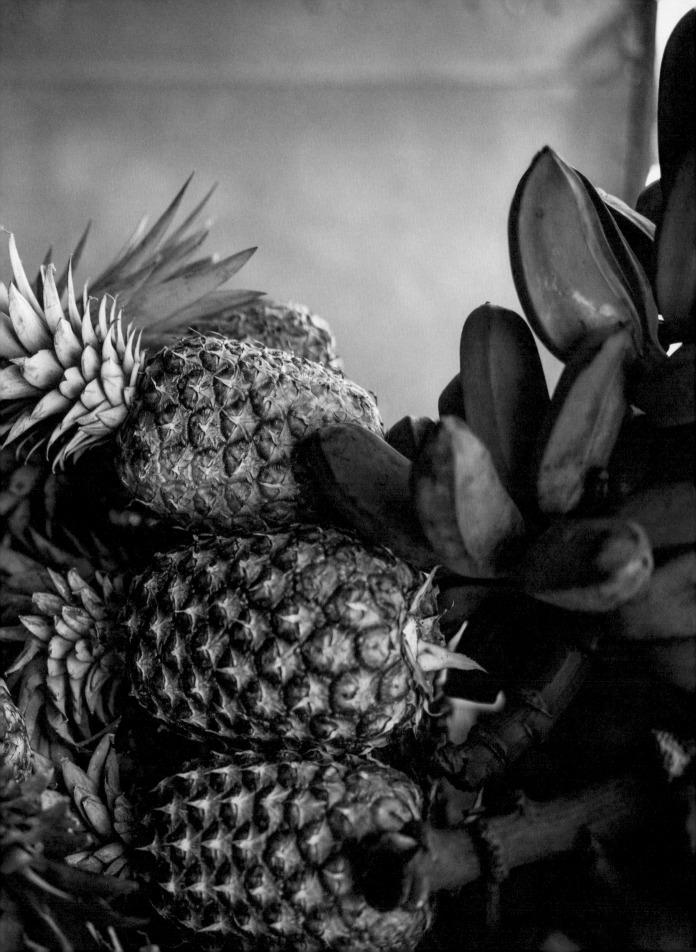

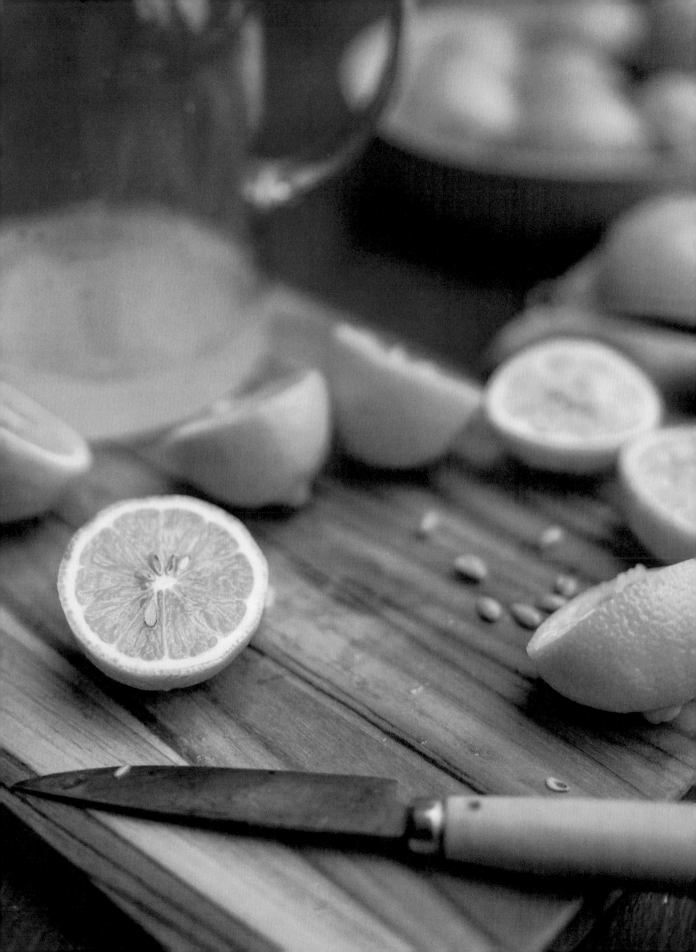

Lemonade With Chan Seeds

TOTAL PREP TIME: 30 MINUTES | MAKES 3 SERVINGS

Nicoya has the hottest climate of all of the blue zones, so hydration is important. This drink, *chan con limon,* was one of my favorite ways to quench my thirst with delicious flavors. Chan seeds look and act like chia seeds but come from a different plant. They are enjoyed throughout Costa Rica and other parts of Central and South America for their taste and texture (and are known digestive aids, due to their fiber and antioxidant content). You can find chan seeds in Latin American grocery stores and at online retailers, and you can also substitute chia seeds if you wish.

Juice from 6 lemons

1 cup granulated sugar

1 quart plus 1 cup water

3 tablespoons chan seeds (or chia seeds)

Squeeze lemon juice into a large container or pitcher with 1 quart of water.

Add seeds to pitcher and let soak for 20 minutes or more, until they've expanded.

In a separate bowl, stir sugar with 1 cup of warm water until dissolved. Add to lemon juice mixture; stir well to combine.

Serve over ice, if desired.

Horchata

TOTAL PREP TIME: 12 HOURS | MAKES 10 SERVINGS

The Costa Rican version of *horchata* is creamy, cinnamon-infused, simple, and refreshing. Serve over ice on a hot day or just enjoy as a complement to spicy dishes.

4 cups long-grain rice

10 cups water, divided

2 teaspoons ground cinnamon or 4 sticks cinnamon

1 teaspoon ground nutmeg

About 1 cup granulated sugar

Soak rice overnight in 4 cups of water with cinnamon sticks (if using).

In the morning, remove cinnamon sticks and blend the rice with soaking water in a blender or with an immersion blender, about 1 to 2 minutes, or until the mixture is blended but not smooth.

Strain mixture into a large pitcher, pressing with a spoon to extract as much liquid as possible. Discard the rice pulp.

Stir in the remaining 6 cups of water, nutmeg, ground cinnamon (if using), and sugar to taste.

Chill before serving or serve over ice.

Cinnamon, Rice, and Vanilla Shake (right)

TOTAL COOK TIME: 35 MINUTES | MAKES 10 SERVINGS

Chilled grain drinks like this shake, or *resbaladera,* are popular throughout Central and South America. Enjoy this over ice on a hot day or as a dessert or snack similar to a milkshake or smoothie.

1 cup long-grain white rice

3 cups water

1 cinnamon stick

2 cups vanilla-flavored rice or soy milk

3 teaspoons vanilla extract

½ cup granulated sugar

Place rice, water, and cinnamon stick in a saucepan and bring to a simmer over medium to medium-high heat. Cook for about 20 minutes or until rice is tender. Remove from heat and let cool.

Remove cinnamon stick and pour mixture into blender; blend on low, gradually adding in milk until just combined.

Strain the thick, blended liquid into a pitcher or large container, using a spoon to press down solids and squeeze out as much liquid as possible.

Add vanilla extract and sugar, stirring to combine. Add water or more milk to create the consistency you like.

Refrigerate until well chilled, then serve.

Sipping Sweet Corn Custard

TOTAL COOK TIME: 30 MINUTES | MAKES 12 SERVINGS

This traditionally hot corn drink, called *chicheme* and typical of the Guanacaste region of Costa Rica, can be made with white or the more traditional purple corn flour or cornmeal. It's custardy, creamy, and smooth with a hint of spice from the ginger. Even though Nicoyans enjoy this as a hot beverage on cold days and a refreshing iced drink on hot days, you can also make and eat this as a soup. Its taste and consistency are very similar to sweet corn chowder.

1 pound cornmeal

3 one-inch pieces of ginger, peeled and sliced

4 cups water

4 cups vanilla soy, rice, almond, or coconut milk

¼ cup granulated sugar

Ground cinnamon or nutmeg (optional)

In a saucepan, bring all ingredients to a boil, then reduce heat immediately to low.

Simmer for 20 minutes, stirring occasionally as the liquid thickens. Add more milk if you prefer a thinner drink.

Remove ginger pieces before serving.

Serve hot, or wait for it to cool and enjoy over ice.

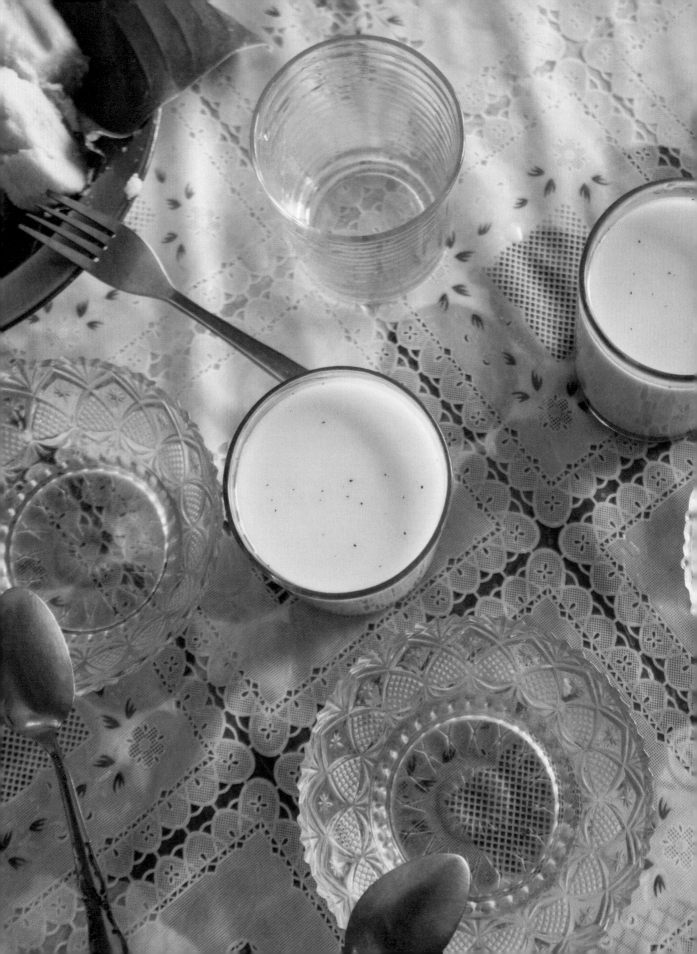

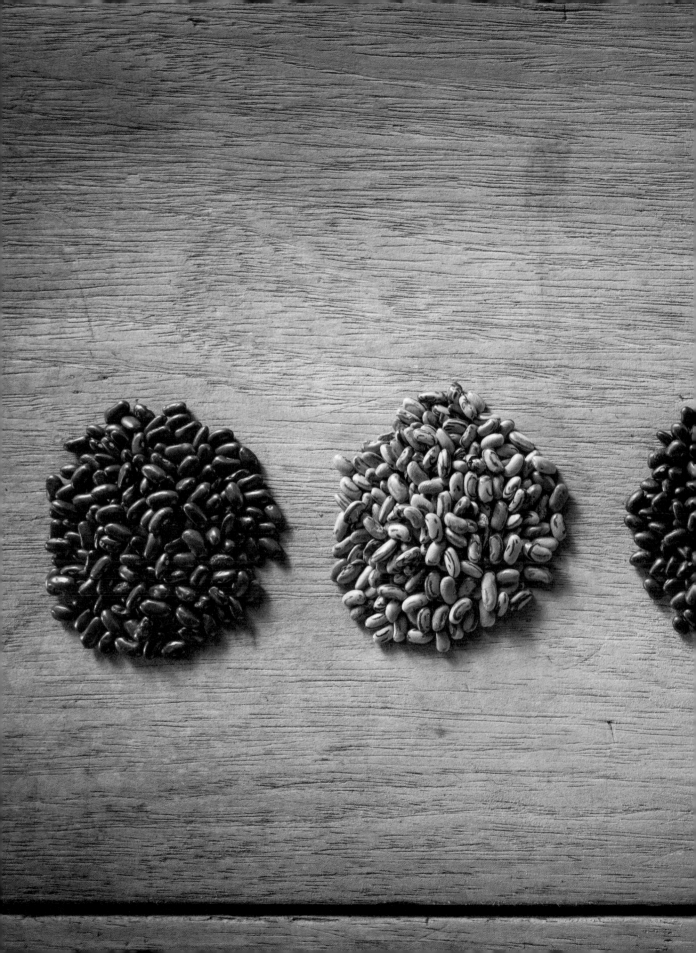

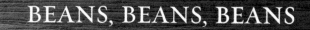

BEANS, BEANS, BEANS

Nicoyans eat beans every day, and often at every meal including breakfast. Paired with corn tortillas and squash, they make the perfect meal, rich in fiber, complex carbohydrates, protein, calcium, and niacin. Just as in all other blue zones regions, Nicoyans benefit from the healthful properties of beans, including their properties that help reduce cholesterol, decrease blood sugar levels, and increase healthy gut bacteria.

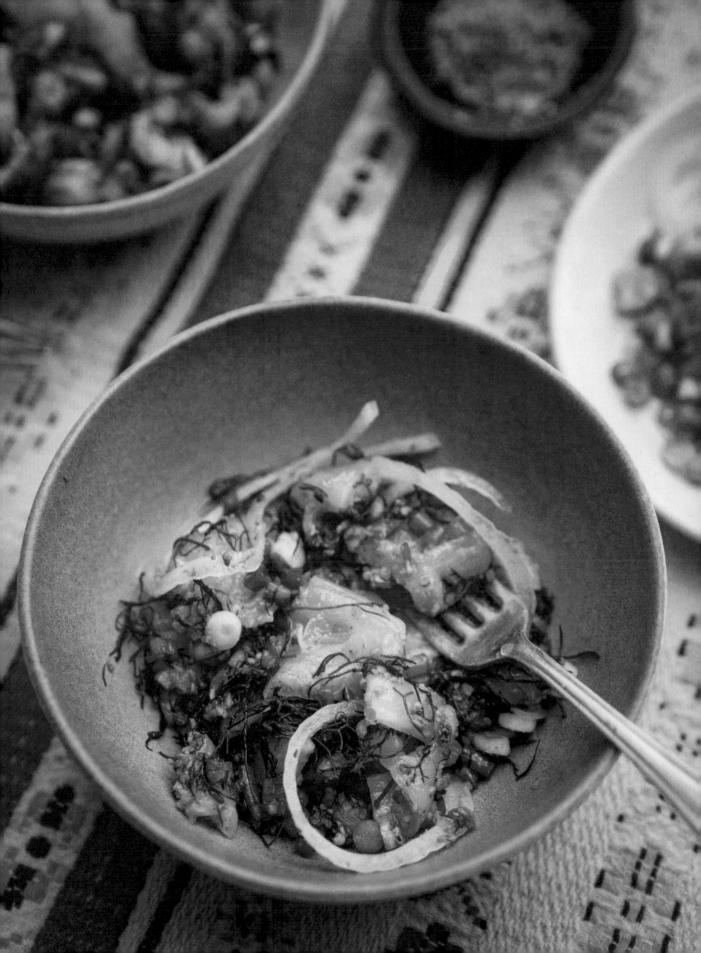

Breadfruit (Ulu) Poke

TOTAL PREP TIME: 20 MINUTES | MAKES 8 SERVINGS

Breadfruit (*ulu*) is a staple food in Hawaii, the Caribbean, South Asia, and Polynesia. It's similar to jackfruit and has a mild flavor and consistency similar to potatoes and taro, which means it's also versatile and easy to use in many different dishes. You can find it in Caribbean, Hawaiian, and some Asian grocery stores, or canned at online grocers.

The Blue Zones Project launched in Hawaii in 2014, brought to the state by HMSA (Hawaii Medical Service Association), the state's largest health plan, which covers more than half of Hawaii's population. In Hawaii, Blue Zones Project works in eight communities across three islands—Hawaii Island, Maui, and Oahu. Hawaii Island is the first county in the country to receive a Blue Zones designation.

Thousands of volunteers and dozens of schools, grocery stores, restaurants, employers, and faith-based organizations are taking part in Blue Zones Project to make the healthy choice the easy choice in their community.

Hawaii is currently ranked first in well-being and happiness compared with other states in the nation.

1 whole steamed *ulu* (breadfruit),* skinned, cored, and cubed (about 8 cups), or two 16-ounce cans breadfruit, drained

½ cup sweet onion, finely sliced into rounds

2 cups *ogo* (Hawaiian seaweed) or other seaweed, chopped

1½ cups scallions, finely sliced

¾ cup sesame seed oil

3 tablespoons *inamona***

Salt (optional)

In a large mixing bowl, combine cubed *ulu,* most of the onion (reserving some for garnish), 1½ cups *ogo* (reserving ½ cup for garnish), and 1 cup scallions (reserving ½ cup for garnish).

Add sesame seed oil and toss to coat evenly.

Add *inamona* and salt to taste.

Garnish with reserved onion, *ogo,* and scallions. Serve immediately.

*You can substitute with jackfruit.
**Inamona* is a Hawaiian condiment made from roasted candlenuts and salt. If you can't find it, substitute with sea salt to taste and toasted sesame seeds and chopped macadamia nuts or pine nuts.

✳ By Chef Kealoha Domingo, Nui Kealoha, Blue Zones Project Hawaii

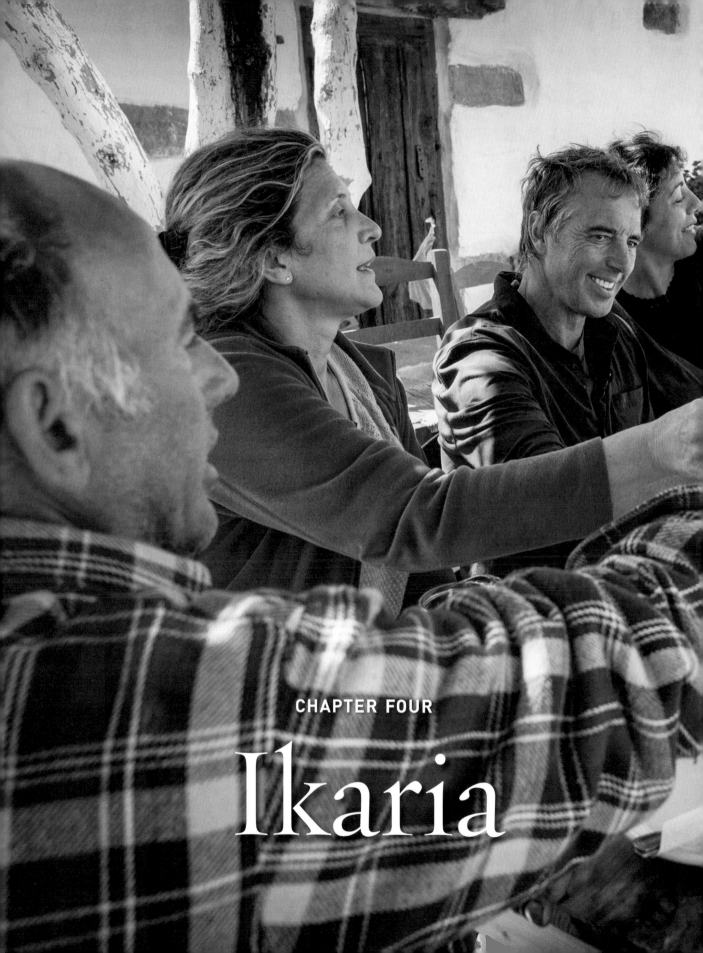

CHAPTER FOUR

Ikaria

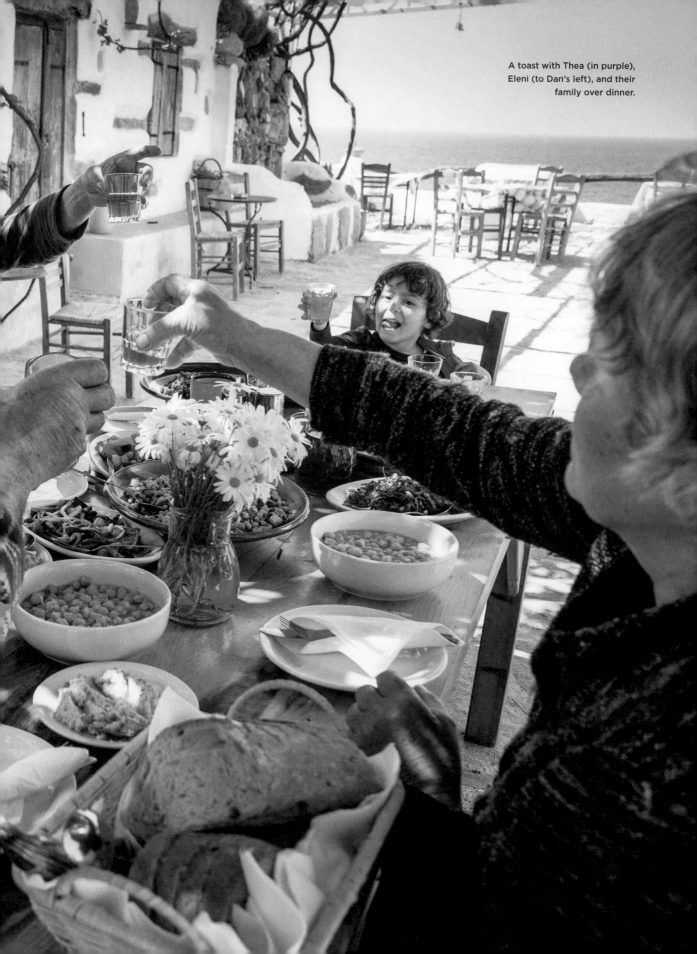

A toast with Thea (in purple), Eleni (to Dan's left), and their family over dinner.

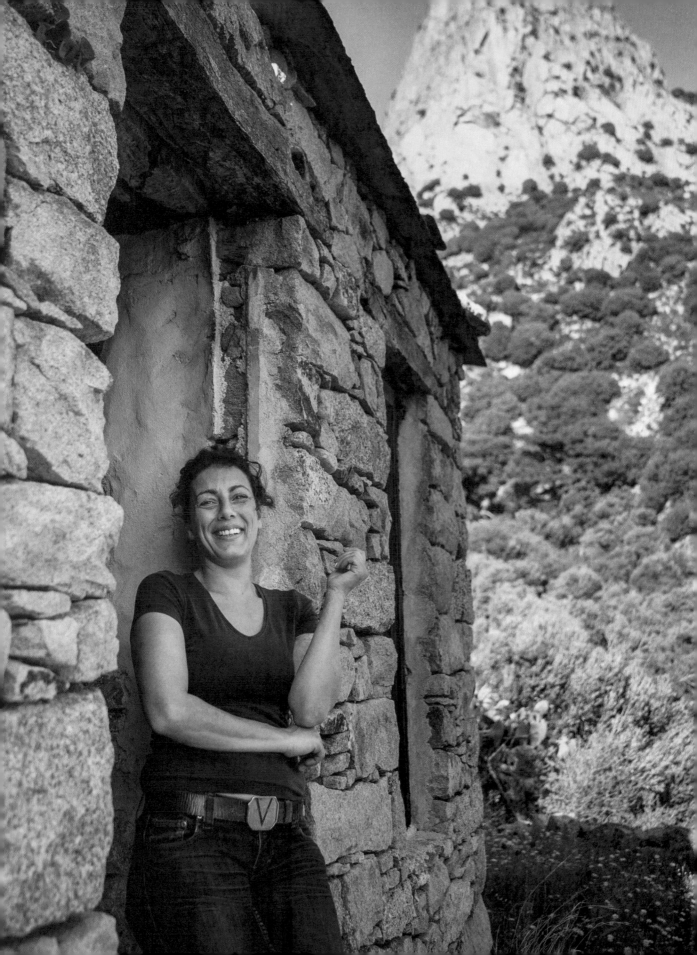

Ikaria, Greece

I t's late afternoon at Thea's Guesthouse in the vortex of Greece's blue zones region. Two windows look out over an herb-and-conifer-covered slope and a turquoise sea beyond. Inside, over the murmur of gossip, clamoring pans and laughter ring out from the kitchen. Athina Mazari, a husky, handsome woman of 60, shuttles between 10 or so dishes in various stages of preparation: She stirs a fennel-and-bean stew, spreads chickpeas on a baking pan, slices a bunch of arugula into a

potato salad, and stuffs eggplants with savory veggies and herbs. Her daughter, Eleni Karimalis, a bronzed Phoenician beauty with knee-high boots, low-rise jeans, and raven hair skewered into a bun, chops zucchini with a severe staccato pluck. Athina's three-year-old granddaughter, Anthiopi, stands on a stool with a celery baton and issues singsong commands to her mother and grandmother.

Thea Parikos, looking like a robust version of Botticelli's Venus in a pink cardigan, rolls out phyllo dough for a savory *horta* pie of fragrant greens. The air is thick with herby aromas, simmering olive oil, and the aura of strong women who possess a legendary command of not only their men but also centuries-old culinary tradition.

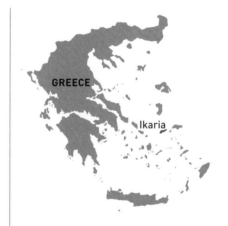

WE'RE ON IKARIA in far eastern Greece, a 99-square-mile island that rises steeply out of the sea like an emerging brontosaurus. Lashing winds and the island's rocky, wave-beaten coasts have repelled visitors since the time of Christ, leaving Ikarians alone to incubate their own unique culture and cuisine. The result is a population that lives about eight years longer than

Eleni Karimalis, our host in Ikaria, stands in front of an abandoned home while taking us on a hike.

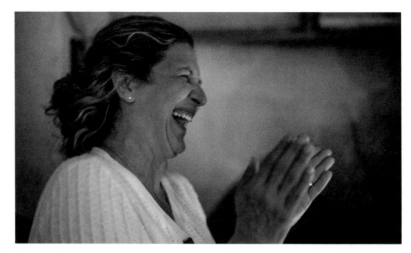

Thea, a welcoming host, laughs over dinner, proof that meals should always be shared.

the average American, with half the rate of heart disease and nearly a fifth the rate of dementia.

Much can be attributed to the Ikarians' strong, stress-shedding sense of identity. People here identify as Ikarians first and then, reluctantly, as Greeks. This outsize camaraderie engenders an environment of mutual care that has gotten Ikaria through the famines and economic hardships of the past centuries. Loneliness, an affliction that studies show can shave up to eight years off life expectancy, is rare in Ikaria: If you don't show up for church or the village festival, neighbors will be pounding on your door. Narrow village streets are always nudging Ikarians into social interaction.

As in Sardinia, Italy, women here bear much of the stress of daily life, allowing their men to spend more time playing dominoes and futilely discussing politics. This stress disparity probably explains why on both islands, men and women live uncharacteristically and equally long lives. (Women outlive men in almost every society in the world.) In the United States, for every one male centenarian there are five female centenarians. On both blue zones islands, the ratio is closer to 1:1. Also as in Sardinia, Ikarians traditionally live in mountain villages, where every trip to the store or to a friend's house occasions an uphill walk. This routine exercise—as opposed to, say, scheduling biweekly visits to the gym—goes a long way in extending life expectancy.

Most Ikarians belong to the Greek Orthodox church, a religion that calls for more than 200 days of fasting a year. This habit may bring some of the benefits of caloric restriction and lower oxidative stress on the body. Fringier pundits point to the high concentration of mildly radioactive radon in parts of the island, which may impart some homeopathic longevity benefits.

For my money, traditional herbs and the island's unique variant of the Mediterranean diet explain most of the Ikarian longevity advantage.

THE IKARIAN DIET, like that found on many other Mediterranean islands, includes a generous dose of vegetables and olive oil as well as lower amounts of dairy and meat products. It is a remote place, however, and the local diet is unique from other Greek and nearby islands because of its focus on beans and legumes (especially chickpeas and lentils), wild greens, goat's milk, and smaller amounts of fish.

Most of the food eaten in Ikaria is harvested from seasonal gardens, which provide the purest form of the Mediterranean diet in the world. Winter beds are robust with lettuce, cabbage, broccoli, green onions, cauliflower, leeks, green peas; summer plots feature arugula, tomatoes, peppers, green beans, eggplant, cucumbers, zucchini, and varieties of citrus fruits. Olives and dried beans, mostly chickpeas, black-eyed peas, and lentils—along with foraged asparagus, wild onions, cockles, and occasionally fish and meat (mostly goat and pork during festivals)—feed people between growing seasons.

Ikarians love to gather and eat the 100 or so varieties of greens that

Shepherds in Ikaria climb hills all day, every day—a probable contributor to their overall health.

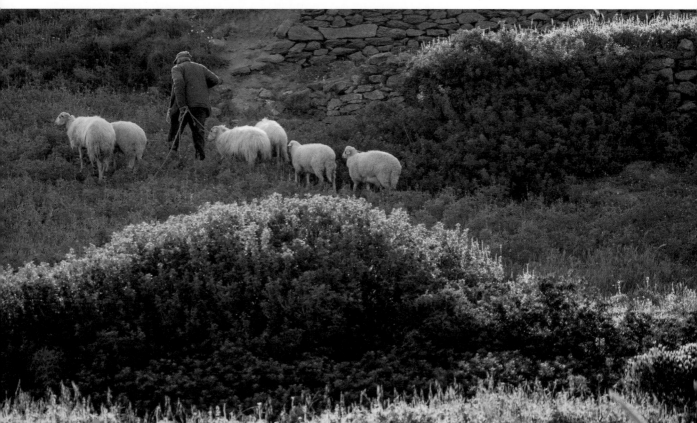

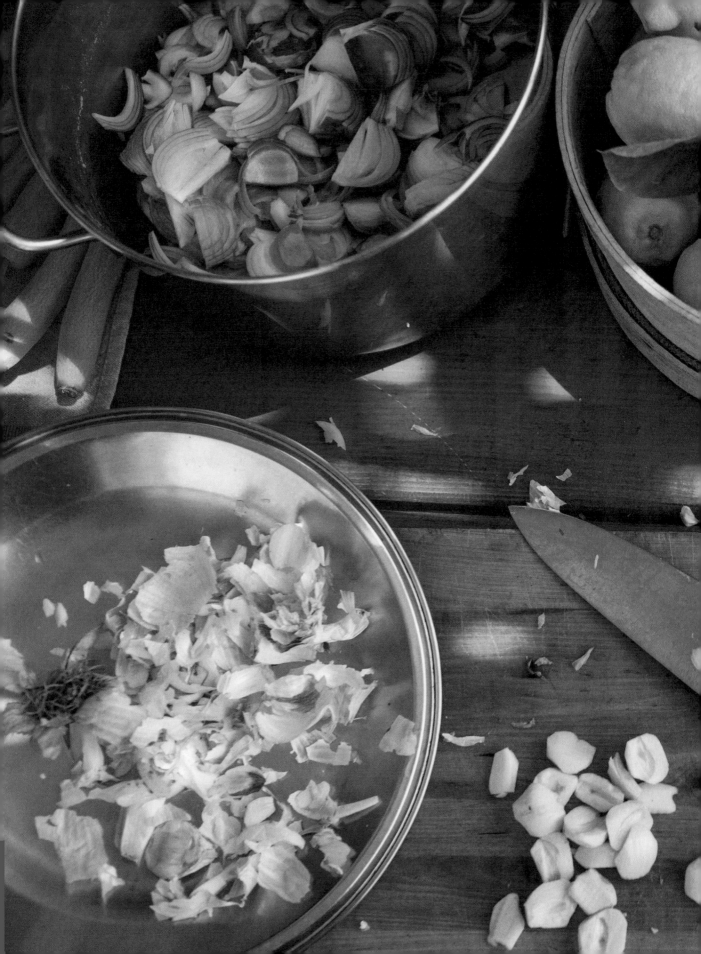

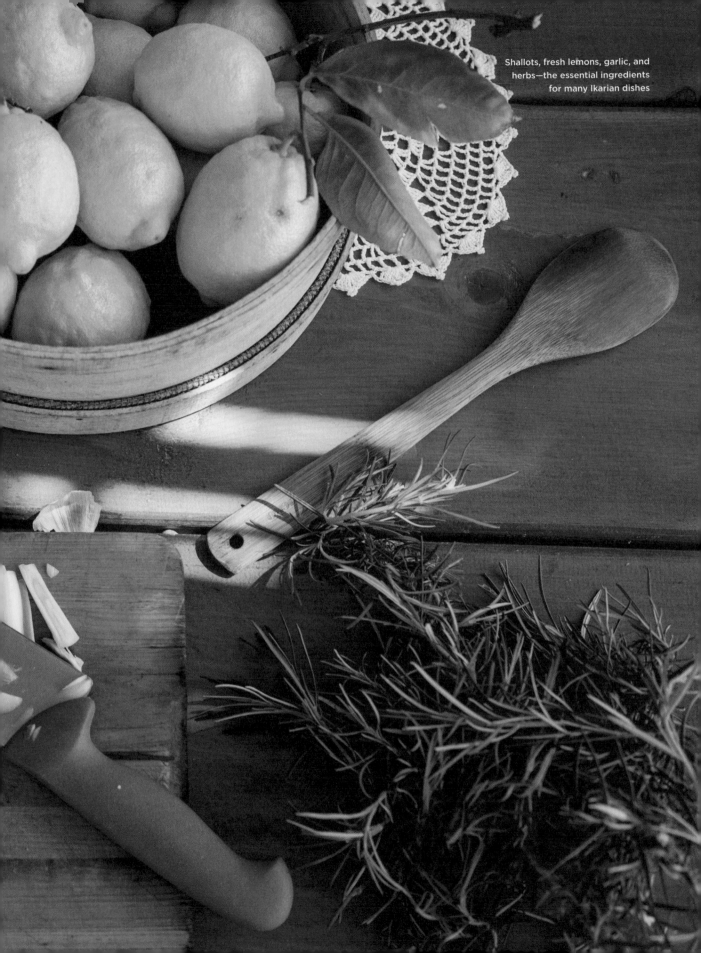

Shallots, fresh lemons, garlic, and herbs—the essential ingredients for many Ikarian dishes

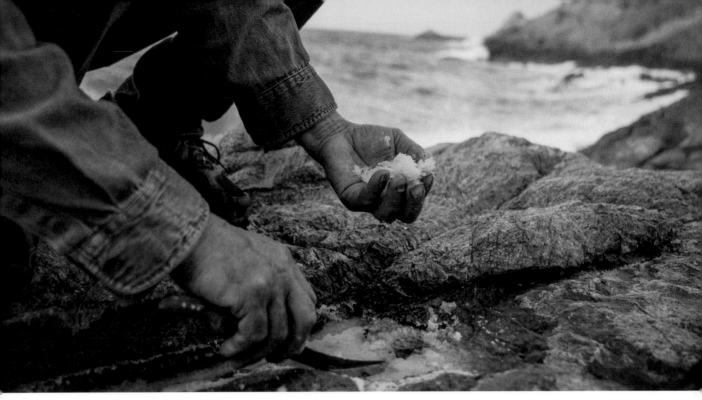

In Ikaria, this is how many people gather salt—fresh from the sea, as it gets trapped in rocks.

grow wild throughout the island. Visit and you'll see women on the side of the road with a knife in one hand and a sack in the other, brimming with fennel fronds, parsley, samphire, wild dandelion, and chicory. Most look like the types of plants Americans would likely choose to whack. But these rich greens contain 10 times the antioxidants of red wine and make for delicious bites when boiled and baked into pies or added to salad.

And then there are the herbs: endemic oregano, thyme, rosemary, sage, and mint. These add a delightful, pungent flavor to foods; dried or fresh and infused in hot water, they offer a readily available and free daily beverage in the form of herbal tea. Used as medicines, they give your mind and digestive system a boost (rosemary), reduce stress (oregano), and relieve cold symptoms (sage). Most interestingly, when I sent samples of these herbs to the University of Athens for testing, I discovered that they are all anti-inflammatory and diuretic (which lowers blood pressure). The daily dosing of these herbs over a lifetime could explain the island's low rates of both heart disease and dementia. Moreover, some studies show that sage and rosemary specifically may trigger genes that help protect against dementia.

ON GEORGE AND ELENI KARIMALIS'S rolling vineyard located splendidly high above the Aegean, I watched Eleni, a kinetic culinary genius, prepare a few of her specialties (mostly modified from her grandmother Helen's repertoire). She baked chickpeas (page 211), sweetened ever so lightly with grape syrup; baked a fennel pot pie (page 199) accented with mint; and milled dry bread, garlic, tarragon vinegar, and olive oil into a beguilingly delicious garlic spread (page 214). For dessert, she created pastries blending orange juice, olive oil, nutmeg, and flour to produce a confectioner's equivalent of Vivaldi's *Four Seasons* (honey cookies, page 227).

Eleni's grandmother taught her not to cook with olive oil, but rather to use it for finishing dishes; unheated olive oil, she said, tastes richer and fresher. Today we also know that olive oil used at too-high temperatures breaks the chains of polyunsaturated fats and makes them less healthy. Unknowingly, Eleni's grandmother was following her taste buds to healthier recipes.

For the chickpea dish, I watched Eleni "kill" onions by kneading them before baking with them; this way, they cooked easier, and caramelized into a sweet glaze. Also, baking beans—rather than stewing them—creates a browned crust that imparts a savory, almost meaty texture to the dish.

Eleni's husband, George, a severe, introspective man with bushy eyebrows and calloused hands, stood at my side during the entire demonstration. In the lulls between dishes, he offered his own time-honored advice gleaned from his ancestors:

- Make your meals special: Focus only on food and conversation
- Eat with people you love
- Drink a glass of wine with lunch and dinner
- Stop eating long before you feel full

An hour later, when Eleni served us her afternoon's production, it completely filled a colorful table. I was able to follow three of George's rules but failed the last one miserably. *

FLAVOR PROFILE

These flavor pairings form the backbone of Ikaria's most popular dishes. You can use these complementary combinations to help enhance any meal.

* * *

dill + lemon + onion

dill + mint + garlic + olive oil

basil + garlic + tomatoes

lemon + olive oil + herbs

oregano + fennel + olive oil

garlic + olive oil + red wine vinegar

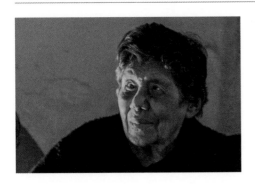

Helen Mazari, 103 YEARS OLD

Eleni's 103-year-old grandmother ate dried bread, sage tea, honey, and olives for breakfast most mornings. Like other Ikarian centenarians, her close family ties, along with a diet rich in legumes, wild greens, and herbs are key to her long, healthy life. Helen has also passed down her recipes and tradition of sharing meals with loved ones to her children and grandchildren. During our visit, she served us one of the most deliciously simple meals of our entire time in Ikaria: a simple soup of orzo and freshly picked tomatoes (page 194).

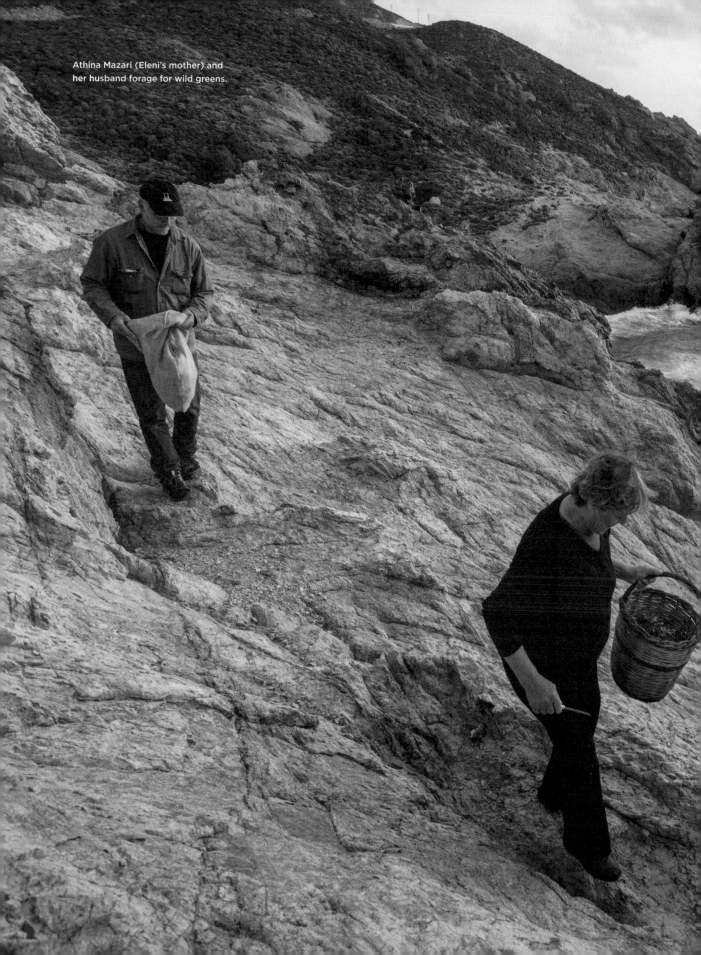

Athina Mazari (Eleni's mother) and her husband forage for wild greens.

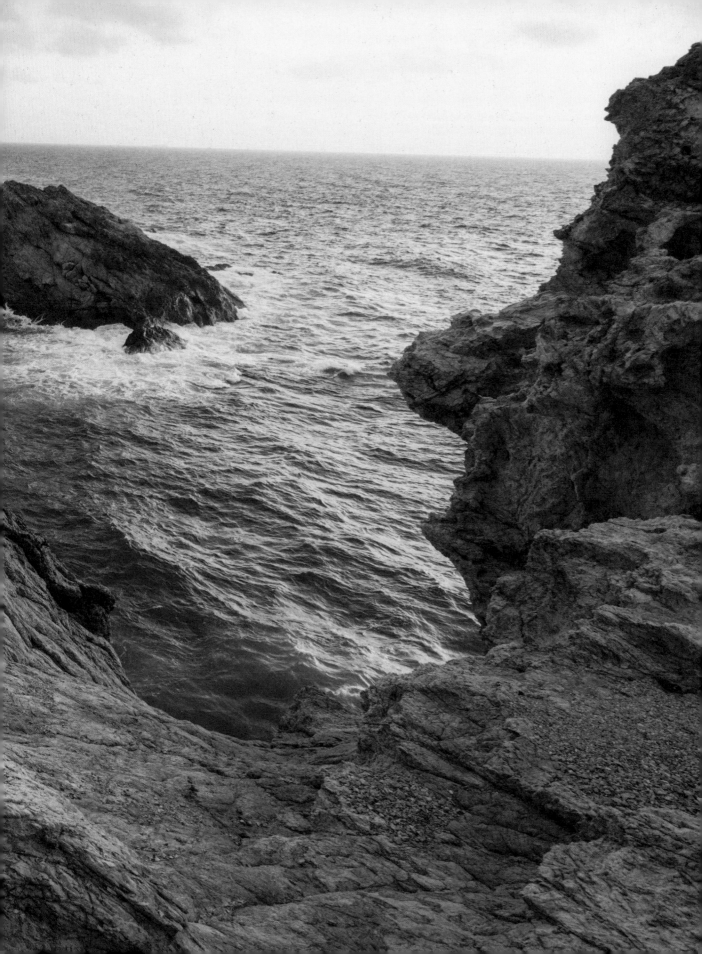

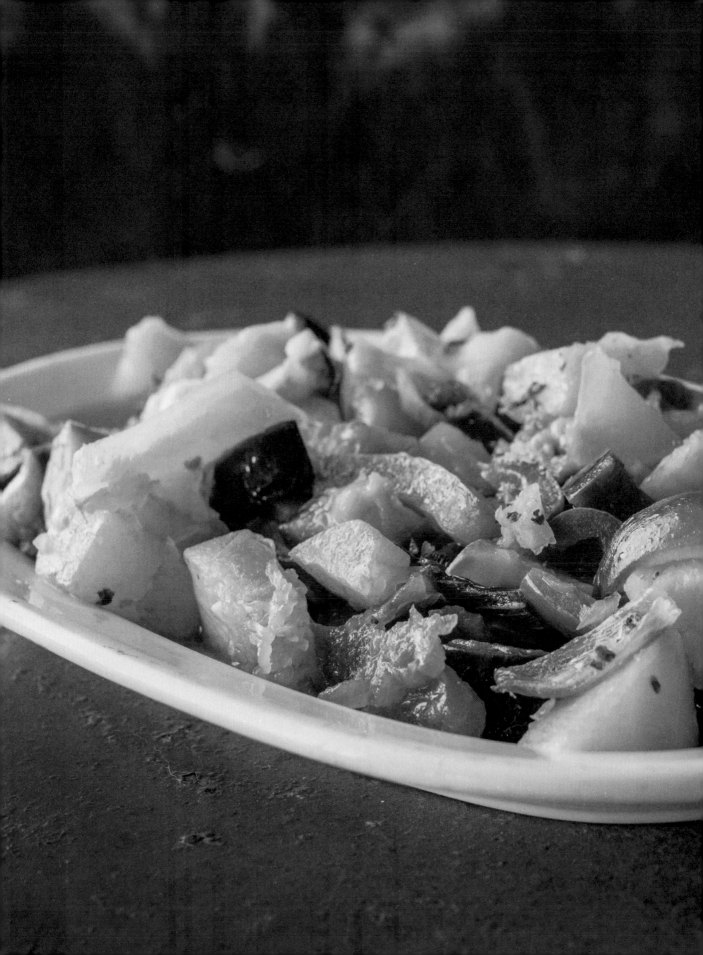

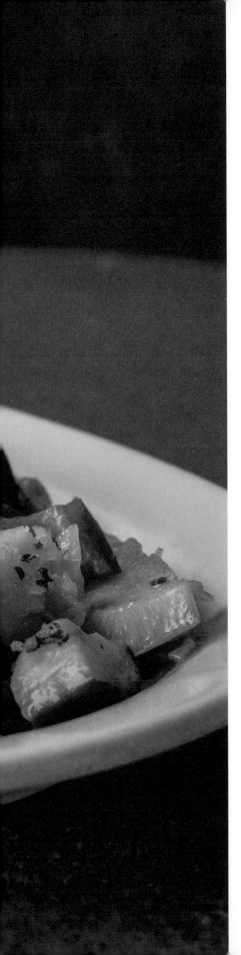

Springtime Soufiko

TOTAL COOK TIME: 30 MINUTES | MAKES 4 SERVINGS

A uniquely Ikarian dish, *soufiko*—a vegetable stew that varies depending on what's in season—is the perfect example of garden-to-table cooking. This springtime version makes great use of warmer weather veggies like bell peppers and sun-ripened tomatoes. Unlike the winter *soufiko,* which is baked in the oven, this dish is cooked quickly on the stovetop.

2 medium zucchinis, cubed

2 Italian eggplants, cubed

½ butternut squash, peeled and cubed

1 green pepper, seeded and chopped

1 red onion, thinly sliced

1 bunch green onion, cut into 1-inch strips with tops removed

1 large tomato, chopped

4 garlic cloves, minced

½ cup extra-virgin olive oil

½ cup red wine (dry and medium-bodied work well)

1 teaspoon salt

In a pot, cook all vegetables and garlic together over medium-high heat, reducing heat to simmer when liquid begins to bubble.

Cook vegetables in their own juices, about 5 minutes.

Once the vegetables have cooked, add olive oil, red wine, and salt. Stir, reduce heat to low, and continue to cook over low heat for 10-15 minutes, or until vegetables are soft.

Remove from heat and serve with a hearty sourdough bread.

Tomato Pasta Soup

TOTAL COOK TIME: 30 MINUTES | MAKES 4 SERVINGS

My Ikarian guide Eleni's 103-year-old grandmother taught me this easy soup recipe, which she called *kritharaki*. She whipped it up quickly, and it satisfied me as much as a meal that takes 20 times longer to prepare. Made with tiny, torpedo-shaped orzo, a Greek variation on risotto, this is peasant food at its best—healthy, hearty, and simple.

4 cups water

2 cups vegetable broth

1 fresh vine-ripened tomato, chopped (or one 15-ounce can fire-roasted chopped tomatoes)

1 cup roasted tomato sauce, either fresh or store-bought

2 tablespoons extra-virgin olive oil

1 pound orzo or similar short-cut pasta

1 teaspoon salt

Salt and pepper (optional)

In a large soup pot, bring water and broth to boil.

Add tomatoes, tomato sauce, olive oil, orzo, and 1 teaspoon salt. Stir to combine.

Reduce heat to low and bring pot to a simmer. Cook until you see very small bubbles and broth is thickened, about 20 minutes. Stir occasionally so orzo doesn't stick to bottom of pan.

Add salt and pepper to taste.

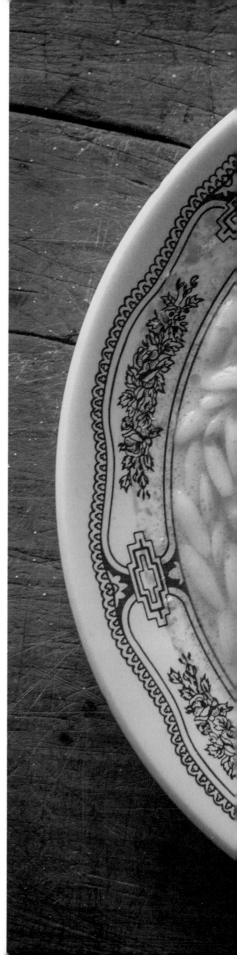

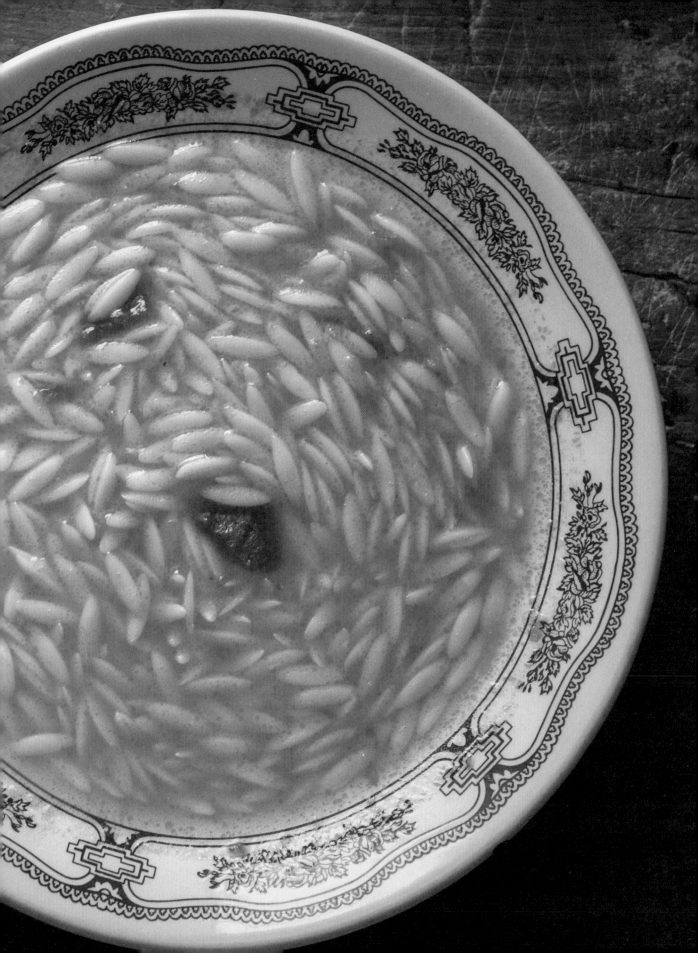

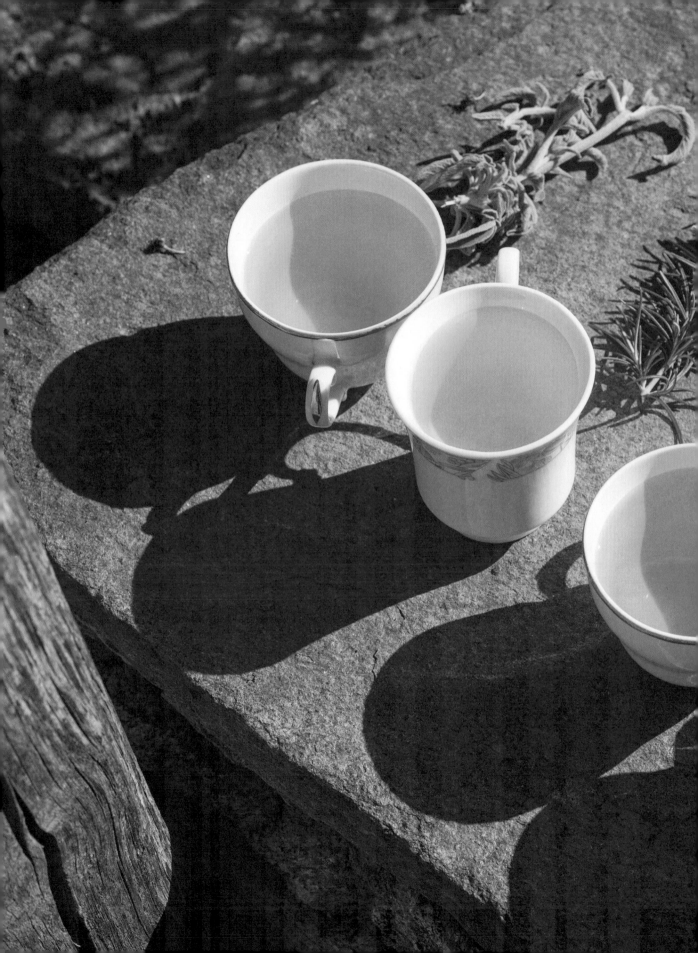

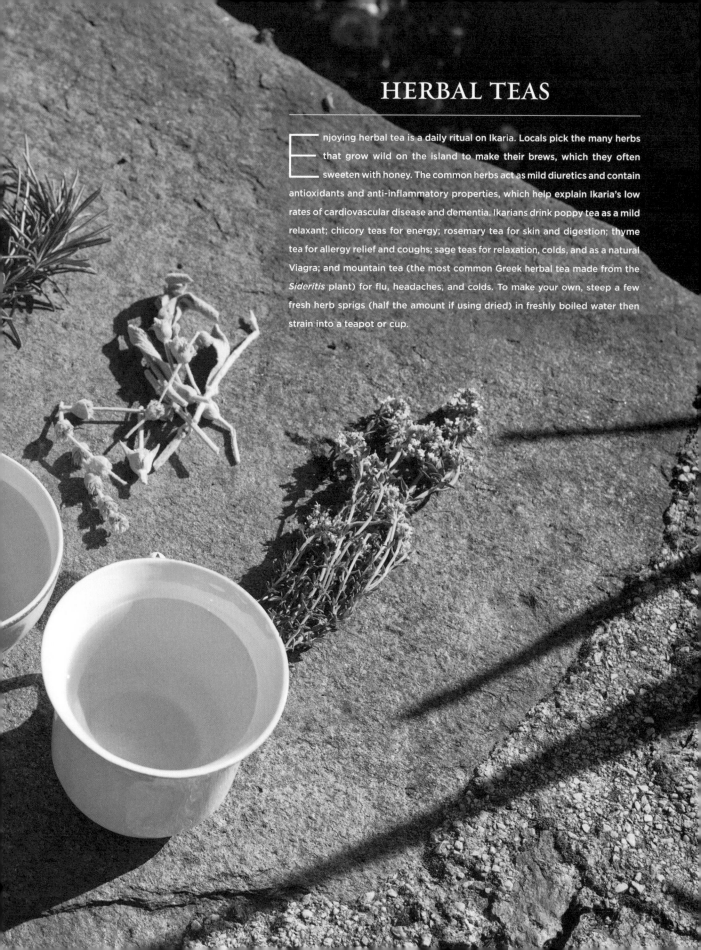

HERBAL TEAS

Enjoying herbal tea is a daily ritual on Ikaria. Locals pick the many herbs that grow wild on the island to make their brews, which they often sweeten with honey. The common herbs act as mild diuretics and contain antioxidants and anti-inflammatory properties, which help explain Ikaria's low rates of cardiovascular disease and dementia. Ikarians drink poppy tea as a mild relaxant; chicory teas for energy; rosemary tea for skin and digestion; thyme tea for allergy relief and coughs; sage teas for relaxation, colds, and as a natural Viagra; and mountain tea (the most common Greek herbal tea made from the *Sideritis* plant) for flu, headaches, and colds. To make your own, steep a few fresh herb sprigs (half the amount if using dried) in freshly boiled water then strain into a teapot or cup.

Seasonal Ikarian Stews

Ikarians use ingredients that are in season and available in their gardens to cook. Both of these one-pot meals make a fantastic and comforting dinner with the addition of some good-quality bread.

SPRING IKARIAN STEW

TOTAL COOK TIME: 30 MINUTES | MAKES 3 SERVINGS

1 sweet onion (like Vidalia), sliced

1 medium carrot, peeled and thinly sliced into rounds

1 tablespoon extra-virgin olive oil

1½ cups water

1 cup vegetable broth

12 to 16 ounces artichoke hearts (halves or quarters), drained

1 large potato, scrubbed and cut into medium dice with skin on

1 leek, chopped

1 pound baby peas, fresh or frozen

Small bunch fennel fronds,* chopped

Salt and pepper (optional)

In a soup pot, sauté onion and carrot in olive oil over medium-high heat for 3 to 4 minutes, or until onion is lightly browned.

Add water and broth to the pot and bring to a boil.

Add artichokes, potato, and leek; cook for 10 more minutes. Then add peas and fennel fronds and cook for another 10 minutes, stirring occasionally.

Remove from heat and add salt and pepper to taste. Serve with crusty bread.

*Fennel tops have a delicate anise flavor and can be used as an herb. In this recipe, you can use chopped fresh dill if you don't have fennel.

SUMMER IKARIAN STEW

TOTAL COOK TIME: 70 MINUTES | MAKES 8 SERVINGS

1 pound fresh black-eyed peas (or four 15-ounce cans, drained)

1 medium bunch collard greens, with stems removed and coarsely chopped

1 red onion, chopped

2 bunches green onion, chopped with whites removed

2 potatoes, peeled and cubed

6 sun-dried tomatoes, drained and chopped

Salt and pepper (optional)

In a pot, cover black-eyed peas with water and bring to boil. Lower heat to reduce to a simmer and cook for 30 minutes.

After black-eyed peas are cooked but still firm, add all other ingredients. Cook over medium heat for about 30 minutes.

Remove from heat and add salt and pepper to taste. Serve hot with crusty bread.

Fennel Pot Pie (next page)

TOTAL COOK TIME: 1 HOUR | MAKES 6 SERVINGS

In Ikaria, families make pies with phyllo dough using whatever vegetables are available on a weekly basis. Wild sea fennel coats Ikaria from April through June and is used locally in pies, fritters, and rice dishes. Its licorice aroma adds a refreshing quality to dishes that is unmistakably Ikarian. Wild fennel is also prized for its many health-promoting properties: It is rich in iron, iodine, calcium, vitamin K, potassium, vitamin C, fiber, and many other nutrients. Fennel fronds, which most American cooks throw away, are used in Ikarian cooking to add a light licorice flavor to dishes.

4 small onions, minced

2-3 bunches scallions, chopped

6 leeks, thinly sliced

6 medium carrots, peeled and grated

Handful fresh oregano, chopped

Handful fresh mint, chopped

Pinch of salt

1 pound fennel fronds, chopped

¾ cup extra-virgin olive oil

1 pound store-bought frozen phyllo dough or homemade*

Preheat oven to 375 degrees.

In a large pan over very low heat, sauté onions, scallions, leeks, carrots, herbs, and salt for about 10 minutes, stirring constantly until soft. (Do not use oil to sauté.)

Add fennel fronds and oil; cook until soft.

Coat a 10-inch round baking dish with oil.

Place 3-4 layers of phyllo dough in dish, leaving some hanging over the edge. Brush lightly with olive oil between layers.

Top the phyllo dough with the fennel and vegetable filling, spreading evenly on top.

Top the filling with 4 layers of phyllo, brushing lightly with olive oil between layers.

Trim any excess phyllo.

Brush the top layer of phyllo with olive oil and use a sharp knife to score the top so steam can escape. Bake for about 40 minutes or until dough is golden and crisp.

Remove from the oven and let cool before cutting to serve.

*To make your phyllo dough: Sift 4 cups flour and 1 teaspoon salt into a large mixing bowl. Add 1 cup room temperature water and ¼ cup olive oil. Mix until soft dough forms, and knead for 10 minutes. After dough is smooth, cover with plastic wrap and let rest at room temperature for one hour. Divide dough into 10 equal portions and roll into smooth balls. Shape them into cubes. On a floured surface, roll into 12-inch squares with a rolling pin. Repeat the process with the remaining dough cubes.

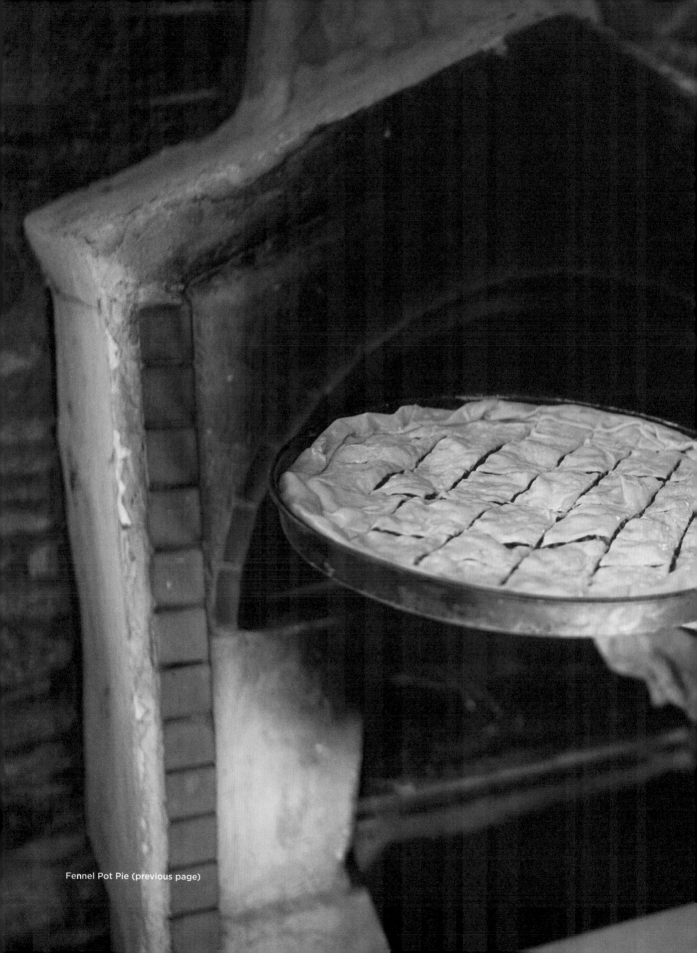

Fennel Pot Pie (previous page)

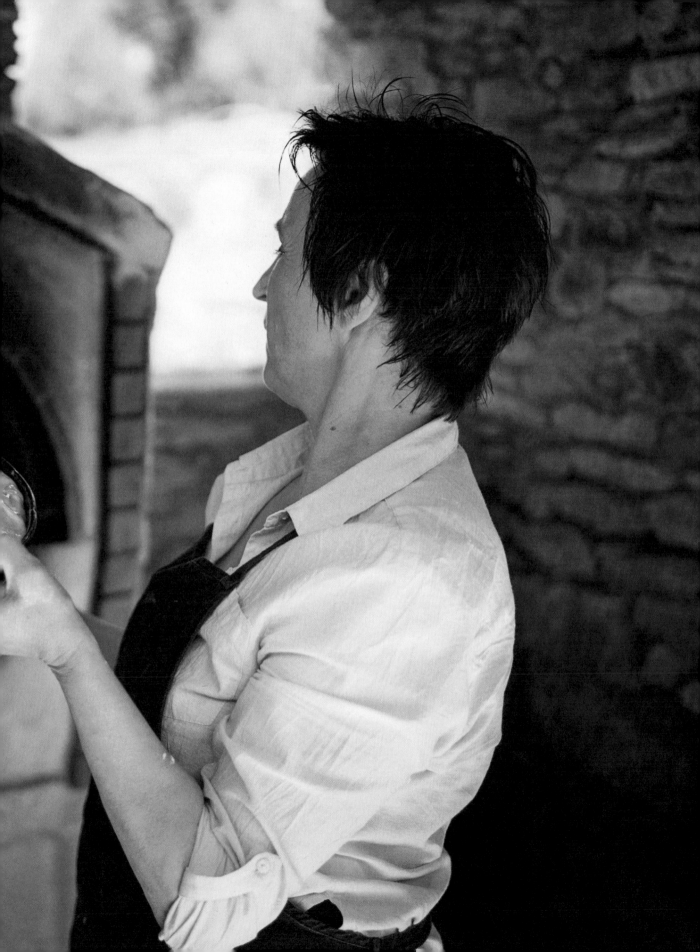

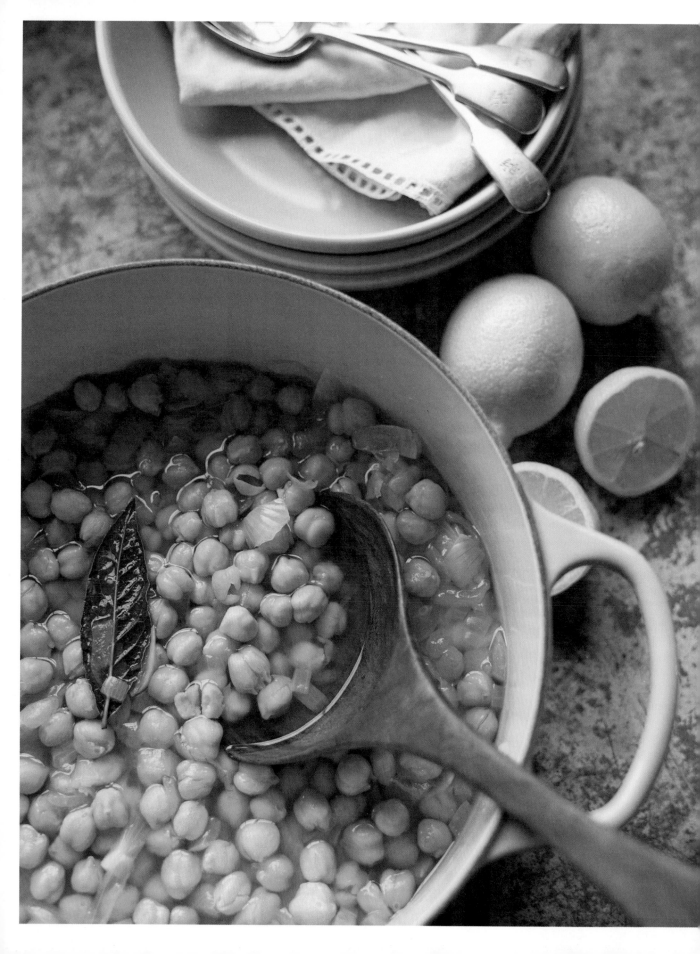

Chickpea Soup With Lemon and Herbs

TOTAL COOK TIME: READY IN 2 HOURS 20 MINUTES; 45 MINUTES IF USING CANNED CHICKPEAS |

MAKES 6 SERVINGS

Greeks and Ikarians especially have mastered the art of blending lemon, olive oil, and herbs. This simple soup is a warming alternative to chicken soup in the winter and provides yet another way to creatively render and incorporate beans into your daily diet. Chickpea soup is one of the most classic comfort foods in Ikaria; you'll find it in almost every home and tavern.

1 pound dried chickpeas, soaked overnight, rinsed, and peeled (or four 15-ounce cans low-sodium chickpeas, drained)

1 medium onion, coarsely chopped

1 garlic clove, minced

1 bay leaf

½ cup extra-virgin olive oil, plus more for serving

Salt and pepper (optional)

Juice of three lemons, for serving

Place chickpeas in a pot with just enough water to cover; bring to a boil. Remove from heat, drain, rinse, and put into a clean pot.

Add onion, garlic, bay leaf, and olive oil, and enough water to cover the ingredients. Stir to combine.

If using dried chickpeas, bring to a boil; then simmer for about 2 hours, or until chickpeas are soft.

If using canned, bring to a boil, then simmer for 30 minutes; add a few tablespoons of water at a time to thin the soup as needed.

Remove from heat and discard bay leaf. Add salt and pepper to taste.

Serve with generous drizzles of lemon juice and olive oil.

Winter Potato Salad

TOTAL COOK TIME: 25 MINUTES | MAKES 6 SERVINGS

I last visited Ikaria in the springtime; as a result, we were able to eat the last of the winter vegetables, as well as the freshest new spring crop. The Ikarians possess a unique talent for blending herbs with humble ingredients; this salad in particular combines the heartiness of potatoes (prominent in Ikaria's variant of the Mediterranean diet) with the aromatic qualities of fresh dill and greens. In an earlier era, when women were in the field and didn't have time to cook, this was a fast and easy meal to prepare.

8 cups water

2 pounds potatoes, peeled and cut into quarters or eighths, depending on their size (waxy potatoes like Yukon gold or red potatoes work best)

½ cup chopped fresh dill

½ cup extra-virgin olive oil

3 to 5 tablespoons red wine vinegar

Salt and pepper (optional)

2 cups arugula, chopped

2 cups spinach, chopped

1 large sweet onion (like Vidalia), thinly sliced

1 small head green leaf or romaine lettuce, chopped

1 small radish, sliced (optional, for garnish)

Bring 8 cups of water in saucepan to boil.

Add potatoes and cook uncovered until tender, about 12 minutes. Test by piercing potatoes with a fork—if they pierce easily, they are ready. Drain potatoes and let cool.

In a small bowl, combine dill, olive oil, and vinegar; season with salt and pepper to taste. Whisk until well combined.

In a large serving bowl, combine potatoes with dressing and toss well.

Just before serving, add remaining ingredients through lettuce and toss to combine. Garnish with radish, if using.

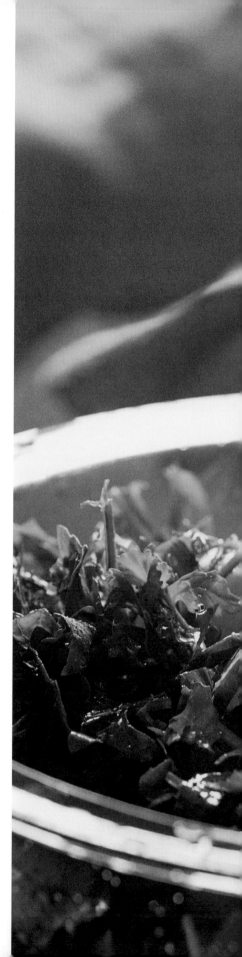

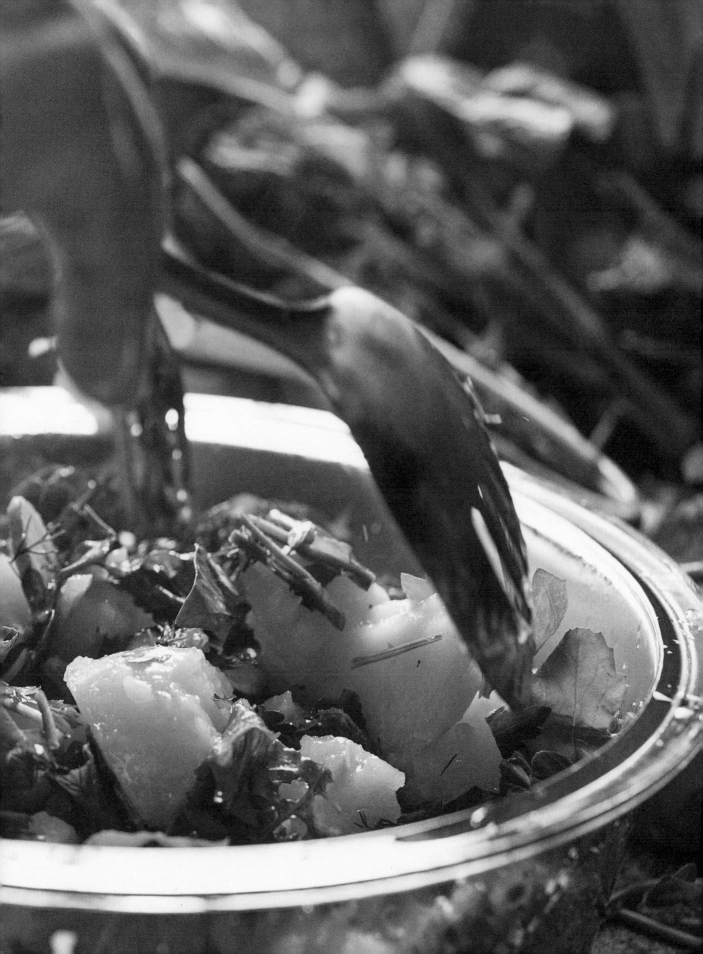

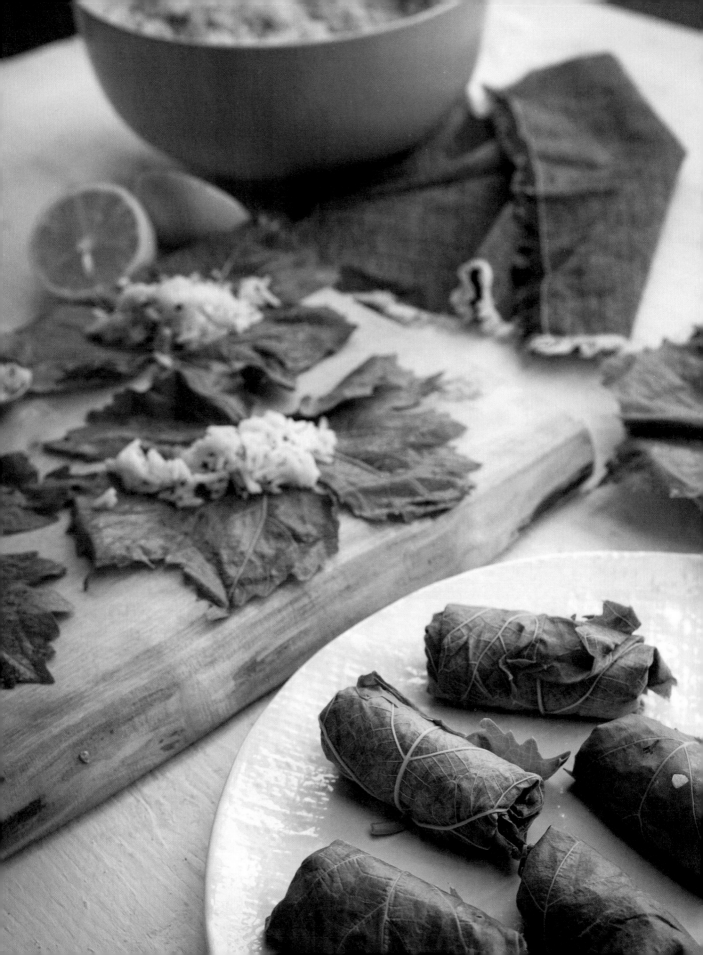

Stuffed Grape Leaves (Dolmades)

TOTAL COOK TIME: 2 HOURS | MAKES 6 SERVINGS

These gorgeous Greek morsels—one of the country's most celebrated dishes—take a little time to put together. But the end result is worth it: irresistible bundles stuffed with a mixture of rice, fresh herbs, and lemon. Rice, once extremely hard to come by, was considered a luxury item in Greece until around the 1960s—especially in Ikaria, whose humble local economy explains its more austere version of the traditional Greek diet. As a result, Ikarians traditionally stuffed their *dolmades,* whether made with grape leaves, cabbage, or collard leaves, with corn instead of rice. These can be a main dish with good crusty bread and fresh tomatoes, or a side or appetizer to a larger meal.

⅓ cup extra-virgin olive oil, divided

1 cup uncooked long-grain white rice

½ large onion, finely chopped

¼ cup chopped fresh dill

¼ cup chopped fresh mint leaves

4 cups good-quality low-sodium vegetable broth, divided

¼ to ⅓ cup fresh lemon juice, divided

30 grape leaves,* drained and rinsed

In a large pan, sauté at medium heat 2 tablespoons olive oil, rice, onion, dill, and mint for about 6-7 minutes.

Stir in half of the broth and bring to a boil. Once boiling, immediately reduce heat and simmer for 10-15 minutes, or until rice is almost cooked through.

Add 2 tablespoons of lemon juice, stir, and remove from heat.

On a clean surface, place one grape leaf with the stem facing up and the shiny side down.

Place 1 heaping teaspoon of the rice mixture at the stem end of the leaf.

Fold both sides of the leaf toward the center; then roll up from the stem to the top.

Place rolled grape leaf into a large pot, seam side down.

Repeat this process until your rice mixture or leaves are gone, placing the stuffed leaves right next to each other with no space in between—this keeps them from opening during cooking.

Sprinkle rolled grape leaves with remaining lemon juice and olive oil.

Pour the rest of the broth to just cover the grape leaves; cover pot and cook on medium heat. Lower heat as necessary to keep pot at a low simmer. Make sure not to boil, which will make the grape leaves burst.

Simmer for about 50 minutes. Remove from heat and let cool without cover for 15-20 minutes before serving.

*You can find grape leaves at specialty markets or online retailers.

Black-Eyed Pea Salad With Mint and Onions

TOTAL COOK TIME: 1 HOUR IF USING DRIED BEANS; 10 MINUTES WITH CANNED BEANS | MAKES 8 SERVINGS

This recipe represents one of my fondest revelations from cooking on Ikaria. I would never have thought to pair beans with vinegar and mint, but the result was a symphony of new and magical flavors. The vinegar not only adds the healthful digestion and immunity-boosting effects of fermentation and probiotics but also helps maintain the texture of the beans so they don't disintegrate as leftovers. Ikarians use red wine vinegar, but you can also use white or rice wine vinegar.

1 pound black-eyed peas (or four 15-ounce cans, drained)

3 green onions, tops removed and coarsely chopped

1 carrot, peeled and grated

3 tablespoons red wine vinegar

1 cup mint, chopped

½ red onion, chopped

1 cup greens like spinach, baby kale, or sweet dandelion, chopped

¼ cup extra-virgin olive oil

Salt and pepper (optional)

Dill (optional for garnish)

If using dried black-eyed peas, place them in a pot and cover with water. Bring to a boil; then reduce to a simmer and cover with a lid, tilting lid slightly to let some steam escape.

Cook for an hour, or until peas are tender.

While black-eyed peas are still hot and steaming, mix all the ingredients together in a large bowl, tossing to combine. Add salt and pepper to taste.

If using canned black-eyed peas, just drain, rinse, and heat on stovetop over medium heat with all other ingredients until warmed through (5-6 minutes).

Garnish with dill, if using.

Serve warm or cold.

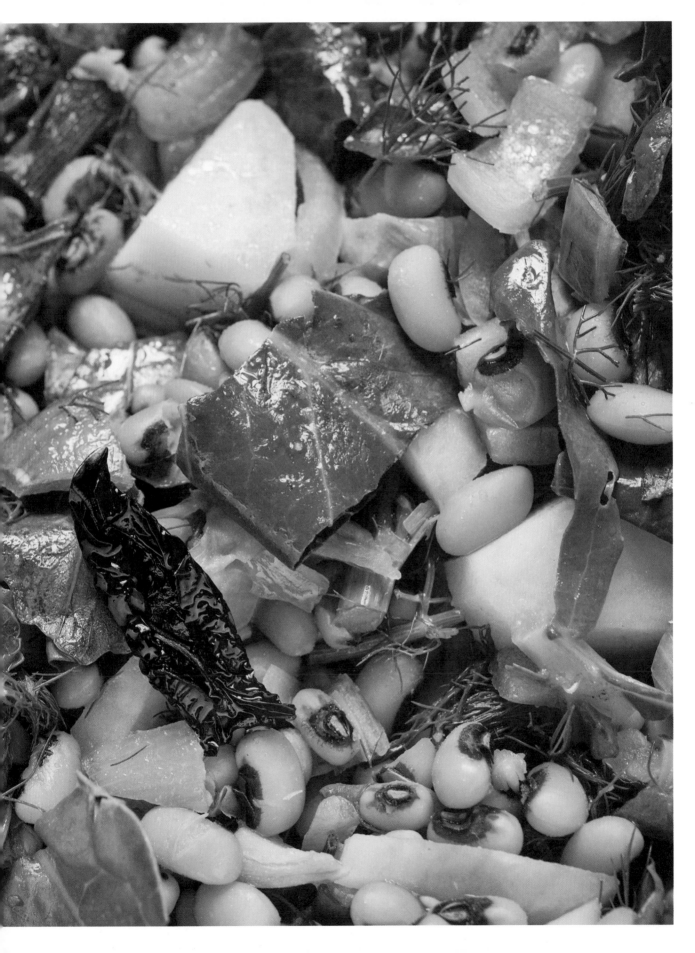

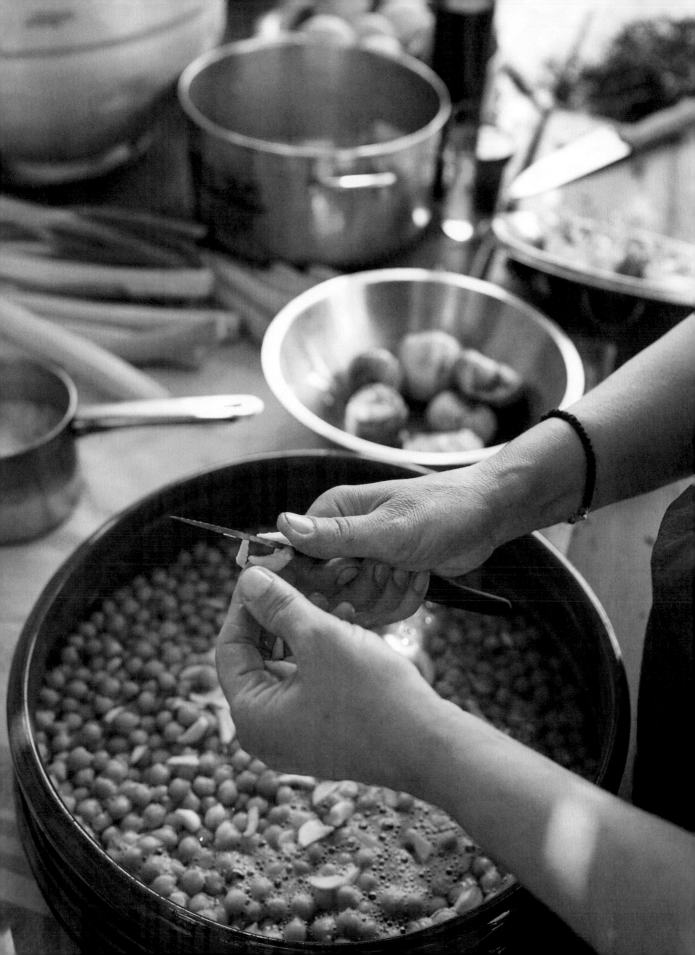

Baked Rosemary Chickpeas

TOTAL COOK TIME: 1 HOUR 50 MINUTES IF USING DRIED BEANS | MAKES 6 SERVINGS

Low in fat and packed with fiber and protein, beans and pulses (a term for edible legumes including lentils and chickpeas) are the cornerstone of every blue zones diet in the world. Historically, Ikarians have found plenty of ingenious ways to prepare beans—including slow cooking, which browns the beans and caramelizes onions, giving a rich, slightly sweet element to this hearty recipe. With a little patience, this rustic dish is easy for anyone to make, and the payoff is phenomenal: the elevation of everyday ingredients into an incredible crowd-pleaser.

1 pound dried chickpeas soaked in water and salt overnight with skins on (or four 15-ounce cans, drained)

1 bulb garlic, core removed

½ cup fresh rosemary leaves, stems removed

5 small red onions, thinly sliced

3 tablespoons extra-virgin olive oil, plus more for serving

¼ cup grape syrup*

Juice of 2 lemons, plus zest

Salt and pepper (optional)

Preheat oven to 450 degrees.

If using dried chickpeas: Drain chickpeas from soaking water; boil in new water for about 20 minutes until soft. Drain and then transfer chickpeas to a clay pot or heavy baking dish.

If using canned chickpeas, start here: Bring 6 cups water to a boil. Pour boiling water over chickpeas so the beans are just covered.

Add garlic and rosemary leaves; stir to distribute.

Using your hands, massage onions with extra-virgin olive oil until slightly softened.

Add onions and grape syrup to the chickpeas, mix to combine.

Cover the pot with foil and bake for one hour; remove cover and bake for another 30 minutes uncovered. Stir from time to time if onions are burning.

When finished, top with drizzle of olive oil, freshly squeezed lemon juice, and lemon zest. Season with salt and pepper to taste.

*Grape syrup is a condiment made from grapes cooked down into a thick syrup. It is common in Greece and other Mediterranean countries. Thick and sweet without added sugar, it's used on pancakes and bread, as well as in baking. It's often available in Italian or gourmet markets, or at online retailers; if you can't find it, substitute with 2 tablespoons brown sugar, maple syrup, or honey.

WILD, LOCAL, AND
SUN-DRIED

karia's garden-to-table cooking is seasoned with high-quality, super-local ingredients such as their world-famous honey. Ikarians pick fresh herbs and vegetables from their gardens and forage wild greens and herbs from the island's rocky landscape. They sun dry herbs to enjoy in meals and medicinal teas. Wild greens and plants often contain a higher and wider variety of plant nutrients than commercially cultivated crops—and the hunt provides seekers with an opportunity for natural movement.

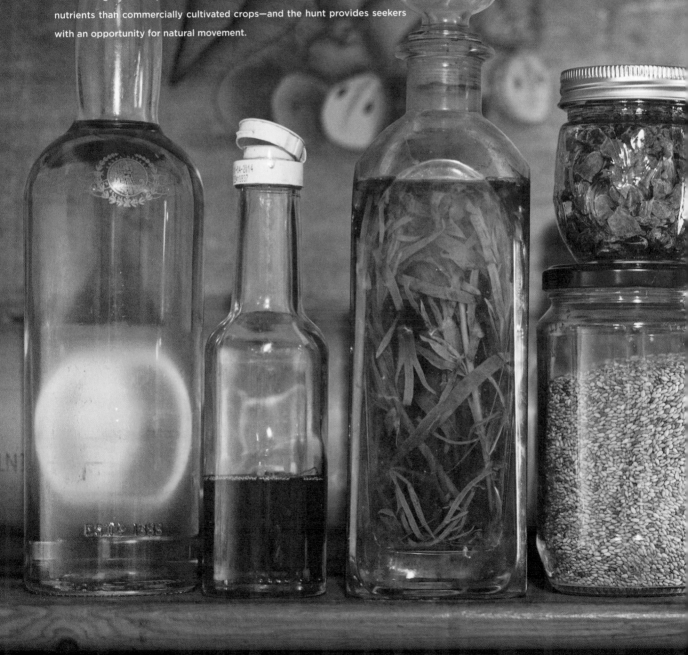

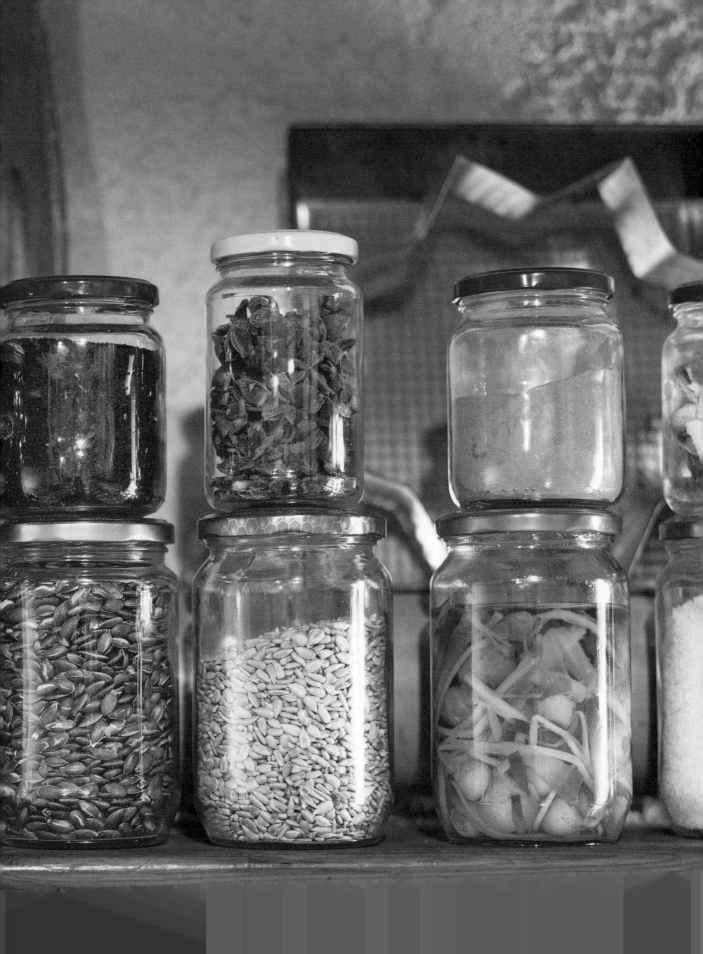

Ingenious Garlic Spread

TOTAL PREP TIME: 5 MINUTES | MAKES 4 SERVINGS

Instead of throwing away stale bread, the thrifty cooks of Ikaria put it to work in this surprisingly simple and flavorful recipe called *skordalia*. The result is a puree that can stand alone as a side dish or be used as a dip for fresh vegetables.

4 pieces of dry bread, cubed, soaked in water; or about 2 cups bread crumbs, soaked in water

½ cup extra-virgin olive oil

2 garlic cloves, minced

2 teaspoons tarragon vinegar*

Salt (optional)

Olives (optional)

Put all ingredients except salt and olives in a food processor or high-power blender and blend to consistency of hummus.

Add salt to taste before serving. Top with olives, if desired.

*Tarragon is a bittersweet herb that has a licorice/anise-like flavor and aroma. If you can't find tarragon-infused vinegar, you can substitute with white wine vinegar.

Ikaria's Longevity Wild Greens

TOTAL PREP TIME: 15 MINUTES | MAKES 6 SERVINGS

Ikarians still forage for wild foods, searching the hills, roadsides, and fields for the best of the season, including fiddlehead ferns, wild asparagus, nettles, fennel, wild dandelion, and other edible greens and herbs. *Horta* is the catch-all phrase used to signify all greens gathered in the mountains, fields, and gardens of Ikaria. They're prepared simply and eaten daily; you can adapt this cooking method with your preferred greens.

8 cups leafy greens, such as dandelion greens, Swiss chard, mustard greens, collards, kale, escaroles, beet greens, or turnip greens, roughly chopped (and stemmed, if applicable)

⅓ cup extra-virgin olive oil

3 tablespoons fresh lemon juice

Salt and pepper (optional)

Rinse greens in running water.

Fill a clean sink or a very large bowl with cold water. Submerge and agitate greens in bowl to remove any grit or sand. Let float for 10 minutes, and then remove greens from bowl, leaving water and sediment behind.

Bring a large pot of water to boil. Add greens and blanch them for 1 minute. They will become bright in color. Drain greens in colander.

Transfer to a serving platter. Drizzle with olive oil and lemon juice and season with salt and pepper to taste.

Spiced Beans

TOTAL COOK TIME: 2 HOURS IF USING DRIED BEANS; 35 MINUTES IF USING CANNED BEANS | MAKES 6 SERVINGS

Another ingenious Ikarian creation, this sublimely flavorful dish combines mint, chili peppers, and garlic to bring out the island's North African and Middle Eastern influences. Ikaria is at the crossroads of East and West, and this history is often reflected on the dinner table.

1 pound fresh beans (giant, lima, or navy) soaked in water overnight (or three 15-ounce cans, drained)

1 large tomato, quartered

1 large onion, finely chopped

1 pound butternut squash, peeled and cut into 2-inch cubes

2 garlic cloves, chopped

1 cup celery, chopped

5 mint leaves

4 chili peppers,* soaked in oil and chopped

½ cup bean broth (from cooked beans) or vegetable broth

½ cup extra-virgin olive oil

Salt and pepper (optional)

If using dried beans, bring to a boil in water, and simmer until almost cooked through. (Giant beans will need to simmer for 60-80 minutes, lima beans for 20 minutes, navy beans for about 50 minutes.) Drain when done, reserving water for broth. If using canned beans, skip this step.

Preheat oven to 350 degrees.

In a 9 x 13 casserole dish (make sure it's deep enough that you won't have overflow), mix beans and remaining ingredients—except salt and pepper—together and spread evenly in dish.

Bake, uncovered, for around 20 minutes, or until all veggies are cooked and soft.

Add salt and pepper to taste before serving.

*You might be able to find Italian Calabrian chili peppers in oil at your local grocery. If not, you can substitute with 2 tablespoons of harissa—a spicy Middle Eastern chili garlic sauce—or other preserved chili peppers. You can also omit them entirely if you prefer less spice.

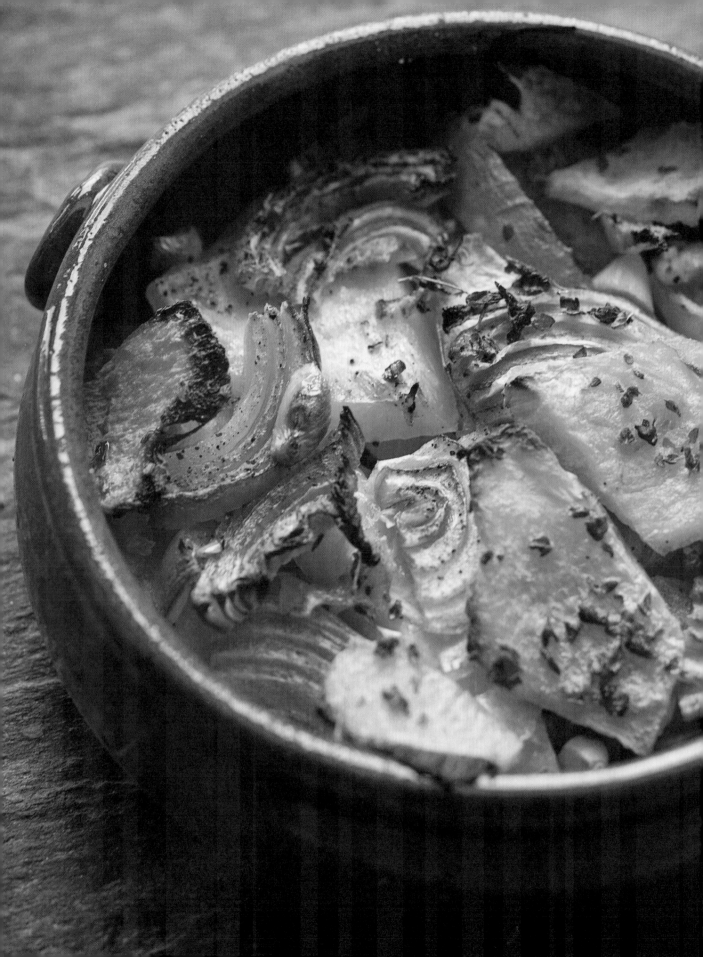

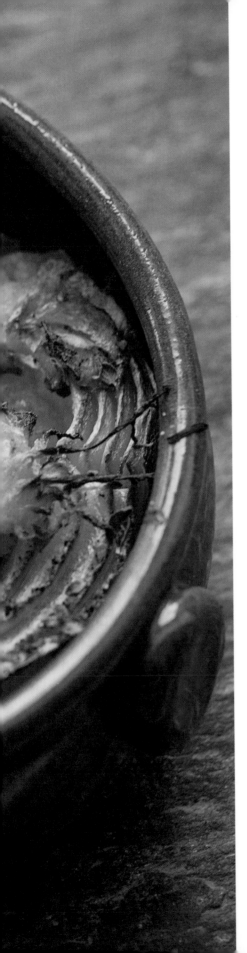

Ikarian Winter Ratatouille

TOTAL COOK TIME: 40 MINUTES | MAKES 8 SERVINGS

This Ikarian version of ratatouille takes advantage of local humble vegetables that are easy to find almost everywhere and transforms them into a satisfying, delicious stew with the island's unique flavor profile. The result is a chunky, hearty, and consummately filling one-pot meal that will satisfy vegetarians and meat eaters alike.

3 medium zucchini, cut into medium dice

2 potatoes (Yukon gold work well), cut into medium dice

2 medium tomatoes, chopped

1 onion, halved and sliced

1 green bell pepper, seeded and chopped

3 to 4 cloves garlic, chopped

⅓ cup extra-virgin olive oil, plus more for serving

1 tablespoon dried oregano, plus more for serving

Salt and pepper (optional)

Preheat oven to 350 degrees.

In a baking dish, mix all ingredients—except salt and pepper—together with your hands, making sure everything is well combined.

Cover dish with foil and bake for 15 minutes. Remove cover and bake for an additional 10 minutes.

Season with salt and pepper to taste. Drizzle with more olive oil and sprinkle with additional oregano to serve.

Serve hot or cold.

Lentil Salad
With Garlic and Herbs

TOTAL COOK TIME: 45 MINUTES │ MAKES 8 SERVINGS

Most Ikarians are Greek Orthodox, and their religion calls for them to fast on Wednesdays and Fridays. This means no meat, fish, eggs, or dairy—but beans are just fine. In Thea's kitchen, Fridays are lentil days, and Ikarians have a prescribed method for preparing them. To start, they don't have the habit of sautéing only aromatics (garlic and onion) first. Instead, they cook all the ingredients together, so the oil doesn't burn. It turns out that science is validating Ikarian cooking wisdom: After olive oil hits the smoking point (at around 320 degrees), it starts to give off fumes and the oil decomposes to negatively affect the food's flavor. This cooked lentil salad, which can be an entrée or a side dish, is simple to make and tastes even better the next day. Enjoy this as a meal with feta, good bread, and olives.

1 pound dried lentils

2 bay leaves

2 cloves garlic, minced

1 medium white onion, chopped

1 carrot, peeled and grated

2 tablespoons extra-virgin
   olive oil

Salt and pepper (optional)

White wine vinegar, for serving

Rinse the lentils, then pour into a large soup pot with bay leaves. Cover with water and bring to a boil. Reduce heat to low and simmer for 25 minutes, or until the lentils are tender and done. Remove bay leaves and drain.

In a pan, sauté cooked lentils, garlic, onion, and carrot together in olive oil over medium heat for 10 minutes, until the vegetables are cooked through.

Remove from heat and add salt and pepper to taste. Top with a splash of vinegar before serving.

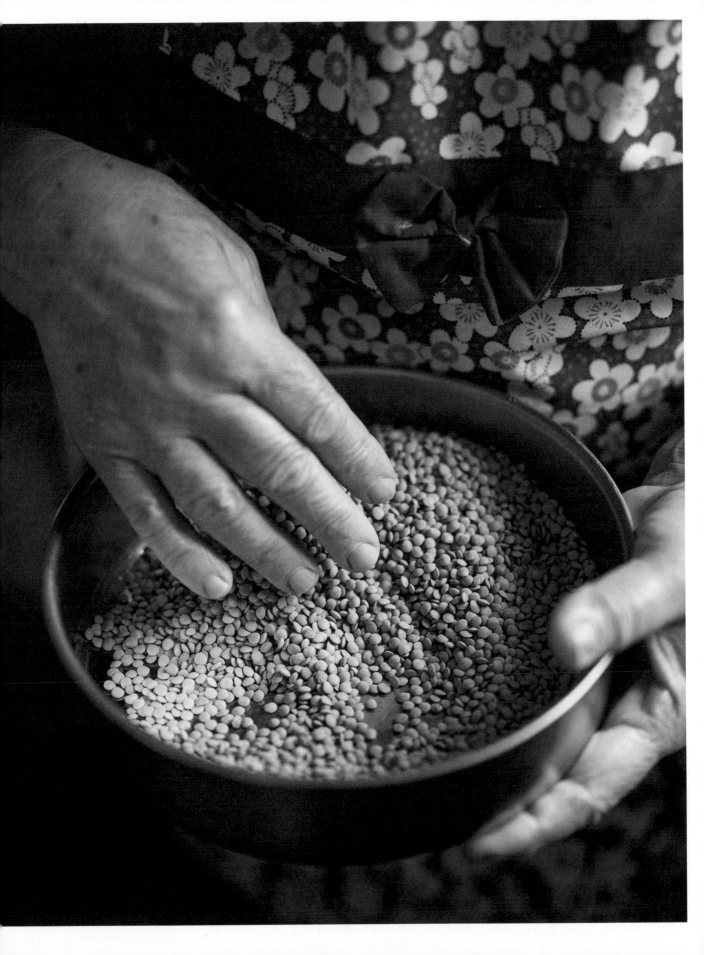

PLANTS, WINE, AND PEOPLE

With a rugged landscape, bright turquoise ocean views, and fields of vines and olive groves, Ikaria looks very similar to many other Greek islands. But Ikarians live much longer than other Greeks—and they live better, with much lower rates of heart disease, cancer, dementia, and depression. Because of their isolated locale, their traditional rhythms of village life, regular natural movement, and afternoon naps have been mostly unaffected by westernized customs and habits. Their food is also key in their longevity: They eat a distinct version of the Mediterranean diet that is heavier on beans, legumes, potatoes, honey, wild greens and herbs, fruit, and whole grains yet lighter on meat and fish than the diet of other Greeks.

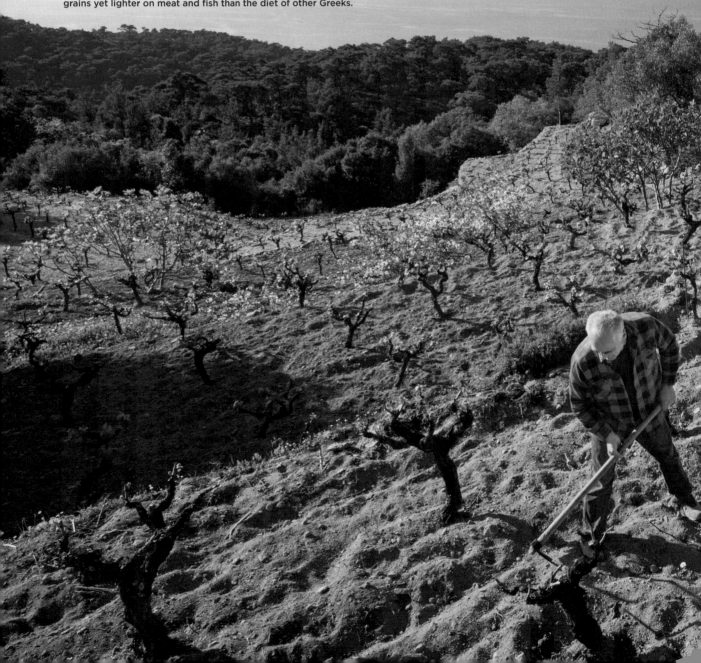

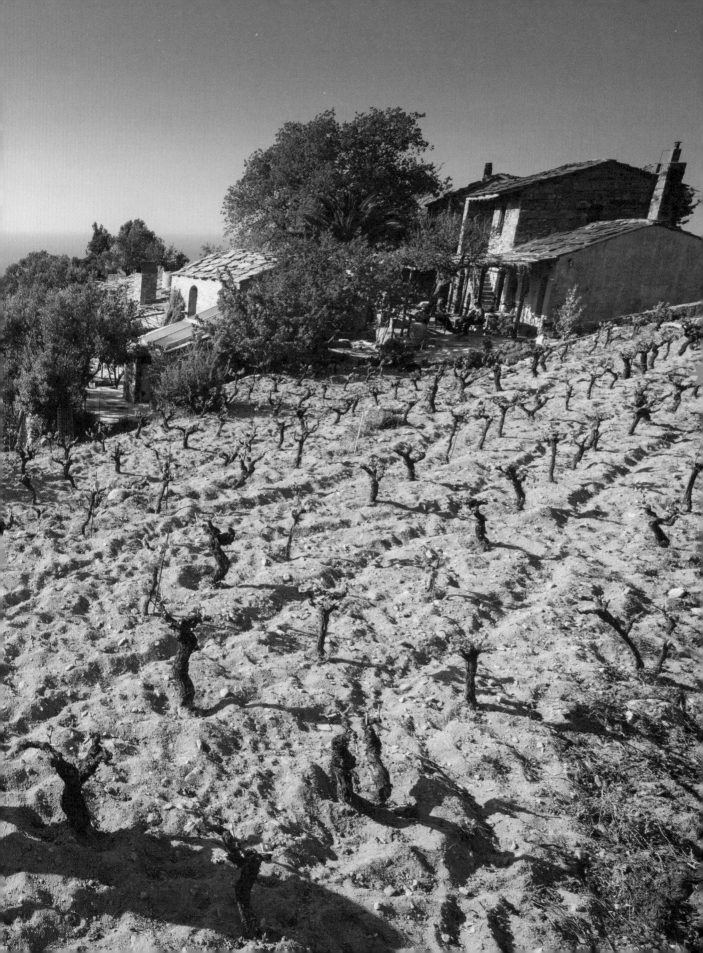

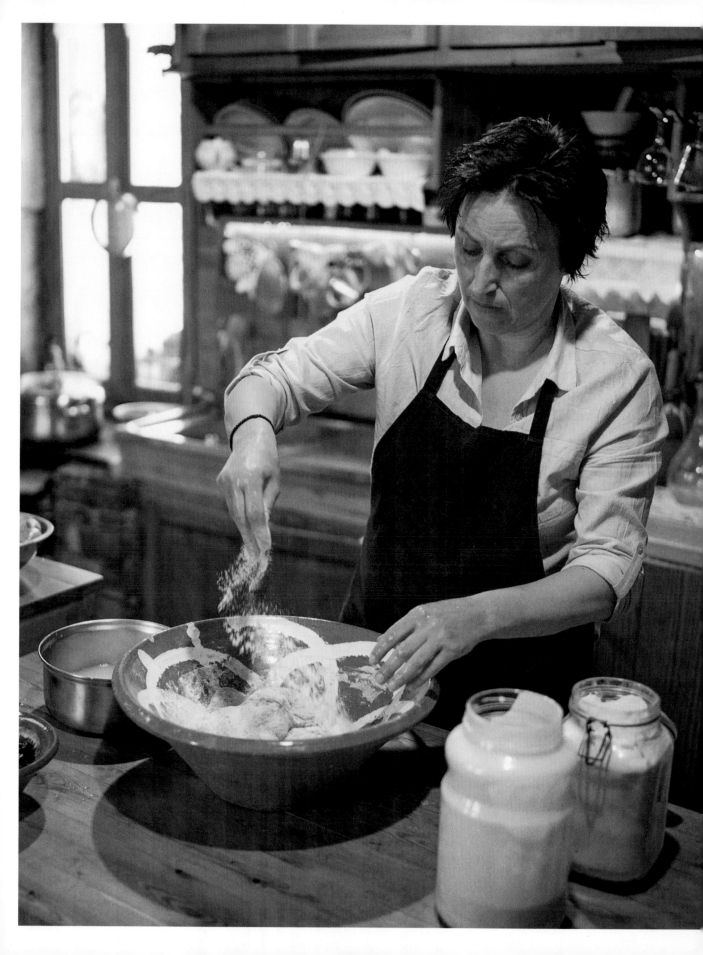

Eleni's Sourdough Bread

TOTAL COOK TIME: 4 HOURS | MAKES 6 SERVINGS

I learned this recipe from Eleni, an energetic, fast-talking 70-something-year-old with strong arms and a youthful face. As she was beating and kneading the dough, I could see that her exercise routine and level of fitness didn't come from spending hours in the gym.

Like Sardinia's sourdough bread, Ikaria's signature loaf harnesses the digestive power of wild yeast to break up simple sugars, eliminate much gluten, and produce a bread that will make your entire meal healthier. Studies show that true sourdough bread actually lowers the glycemic load of a meal, which is to say it slows the absorption of sugars into the blood. More importantly, this bread tastes delicious, so you'll want to eat it every day.

2 cups sourdough starter,*
   store-bought or homemade

1 cup room temperature water

3⅓ cups (1 pound) whole wheat
   flour

2¾ cups (1 pound) semolina flour

Pinch of salt and pepper

Sesame seeds (optional)

In a very large bowl, mix starter and water together.

In another bowl, combine flours with salt and pepper.

Add the flour mixture, 1 cup at a time, to the water mixture, and stir thoroughly with each addition. Use your hands and continue to add flour until well combined.

Knead the dough for at least 20 minutes.

Plop dough into a low, round 20-inch pan and cover with olive oil; top with sesame seeds, if using.

Cut a small cross in the middle of the dough; then cover with a towel and let rise for 2 hours.

Bake in the oven for 20 minutes at 250 degrees, then 20 minutes at 200 degrees, and another 20 minutes at 180 agrees. This makes for a perfect loaf inside and out.

*Baking with a sourdough starter (or wild yeast, a mixture of flour and water that's fermented) captures beneficial lactic acid bacteria and results in a healthier, tastier bread than if you were to use premade yeasts. The easiest way to make sourdough is to ask another baker for some starter. If that's not possible, make your own:

In a large glass jar with a lot of room, mix together 2 cups whole-wheat flour and 1½ cups water until it forms a thick liquid. Cover with cheesecloth or a paper towel and secure; keep on your kitchen counter away from direct sunlight. After 2 days, the starter will begin to rise and air bubbles will appear.

Scoop out three-quarters of the mixture and throw away. Add 1 cup whole-wheat flour and ½ cup water to the remaining mixture. Mix well. Cover again and set for 24 hours. Some foam will develop at the top when the starter is active and ready. Store it in the refrigerator.

You should feed your culture once a week if it's refrigerated by adding 1 cup flour and ½ cup water. Mix and let sit for an hour or two at room temperature before refrigerating again.

Hummus With Parsley

TOTAL PREP TIME: 10 MINUTES | MAKES 6 SERVINGS

Chickpeas are the foundation of the Ikarian diet and have been since Neolithic times. Over the centuries, Ikarian cooks have found hundreds of unique ways to transform beans, chickpeas, lentils, and split peas into tasty dishes.

A key ingredient to the blue zones diet is our belief that beans add healthy years to life. In this regard, hummus is the perfect food. Ikarians make this variation lighter than what you'd typically find at stores or in restaurants by leaving out tahini and making up the flavor with parsley and red wine vinegar. While islanders always make theirs with dried chickpeas, grown locally, it's perfectly OK to use canned beans as a timesaver.

1 pound dried chickpeas, soaked overnight and cooked until soft (or three 15-ounce cans, drained)

2 to 3 cloves garlic

½ cup extra-virgin olive oil, plus more for serving

2 tablespoons red wine vinegar

¼ cup parsley, chopped

Salt (optional)

Put cooked chickpeas and garlic in a food processor or high-powered blender and blend until roughly pureed.

Drizzle with olive oil and vinegar.

Sprinkle with parsley and salt to taste. Serve with raw vegetables, pita, or good, crusty bread for dipping.

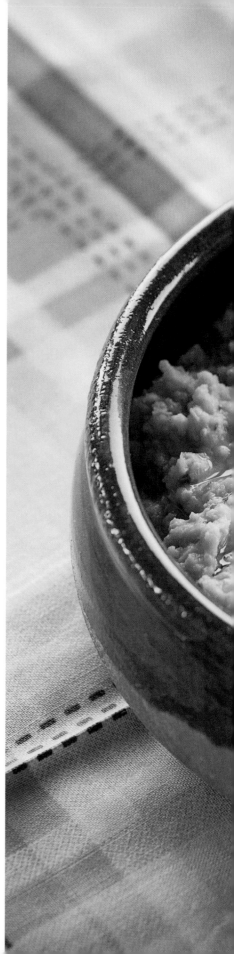

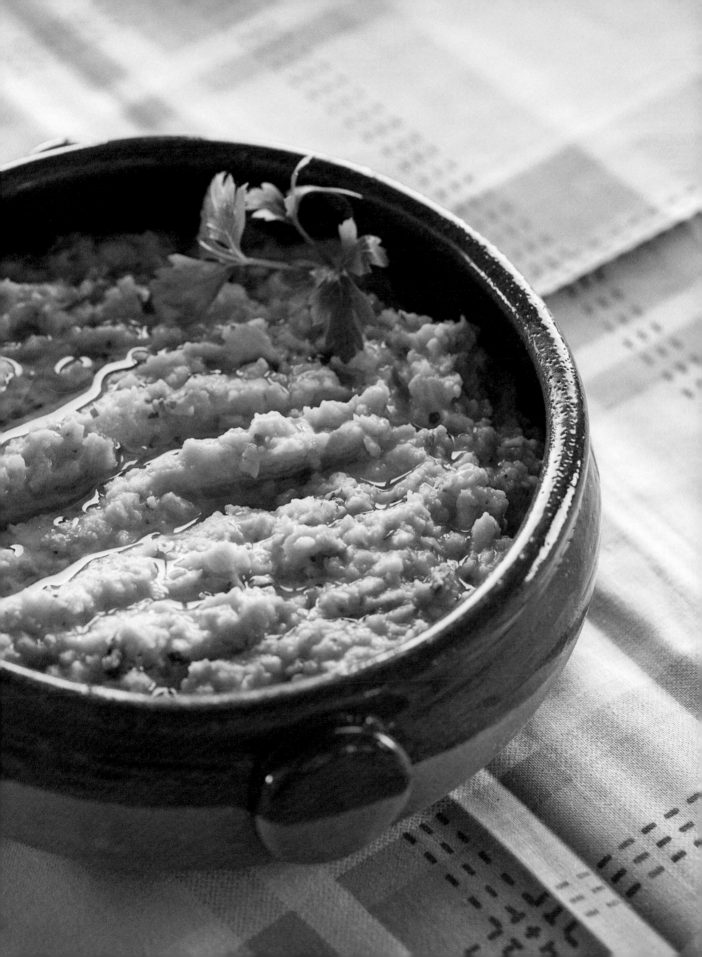

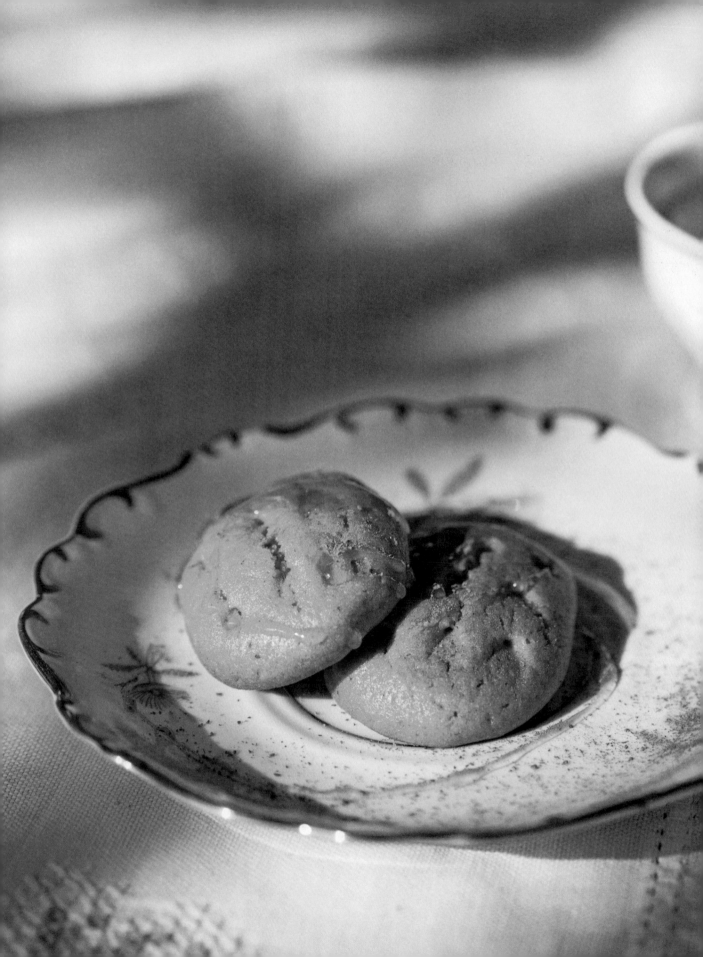

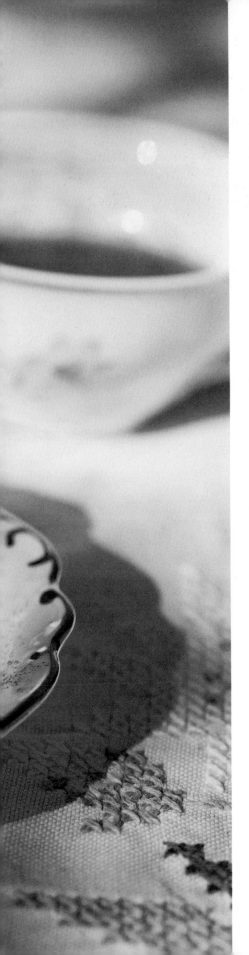

Honey Cookies (Finikia)

TOTAL COOK TIME: 70 MINUTES | MAKES 24 COOKIES

I learned how to prepare this delicious treat from Eleni Karimalis, who showed me how to make traditional Ikarian specialties based on her grandmother's recipes in the scenic kitchen overlook of her rolling vineyard. It's rare to find a delicious cookie that doesn't use eggs or dairy, but this one won't disappoint. The result is a healthier, yet every bit as satisfying, dessert. It combines the tang of orange juice, the richness of nuts, and the sweet spiciness of cinnamon and honey. Ikarian wild honey is distinctive in its taste and its anti-inflammatory and antibacterial properties.

¾ cup orange juice

¾ cup honey, plus more for drizzling

Juice from ½ lemon

1 tablespoon lemon zest

1 teaspoon vanilla

1½ ounces cognac or rum

¾ cup extra-virgin olive oil

1 teaspoon baking soda

1 teaspoon baking powder

3½ cups all-purpose flour

Pinch of cloves

2 teaspoons cinnamon

1 teaspoon nutmeg

Preheat oven to 325 degrees.

In a large bowl, whisk together orange juice, honey, lemon juice, lemon zest, vanilla, and cognac or rum. Gradually drizzle in olive oil, whisking to combine.

In a separate bowl, combine baking soda, baking powder, flour, cloves, cinnamon, and nutmeg.

Slowly add dry ingredient mixture to wet ingredients and stir until just combined. Do not overmix or knead, as the dough will become tough.

Let rest for 30 minutes at room temperature.

Roll dough into walnut-size balls and score with a fork. Place balls on a baking sheet, about an inch apart from each other.

Bake for 14-18 minutes, or until golden.

Drizzle with honey, if desired.

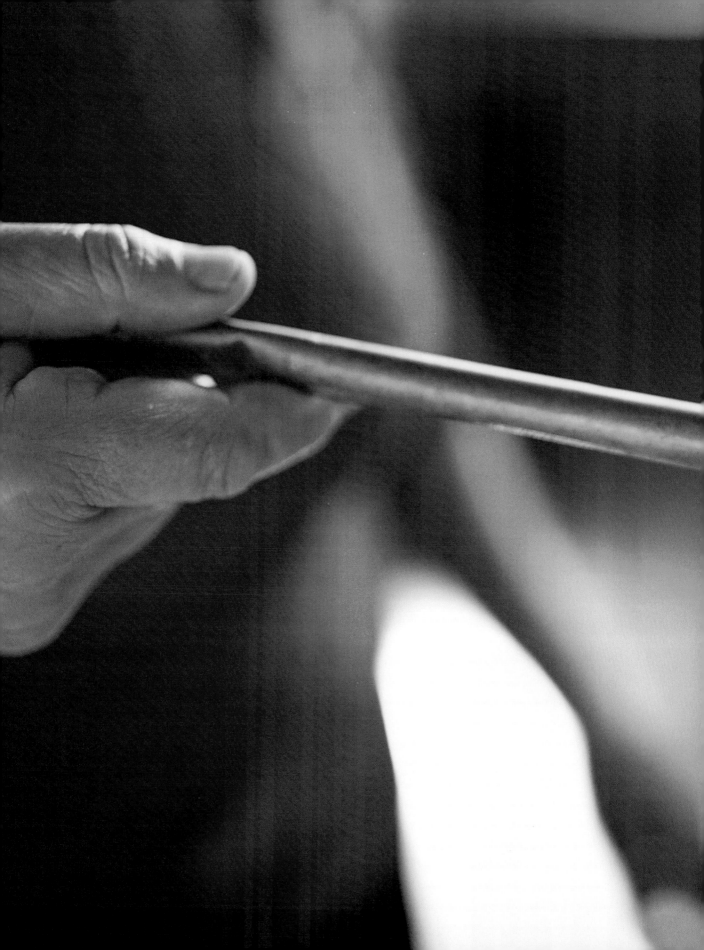

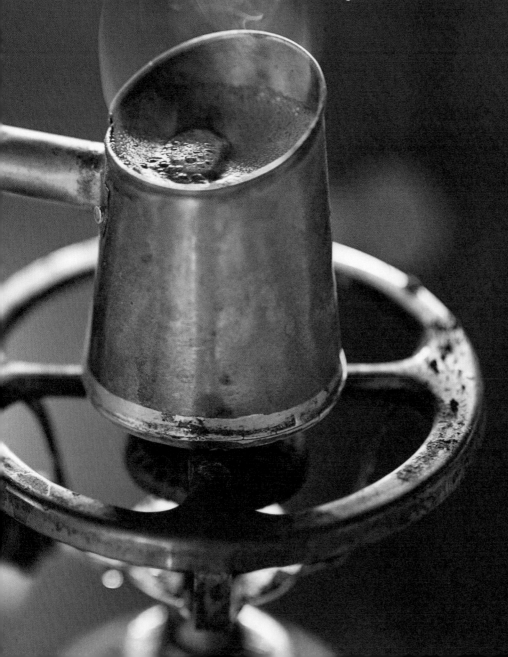

IKARIAN COFFEE

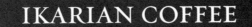

karians savor their coffee with family and friends, at the table or in social café settings. Brews from their island contain more protective antioxidants and polyphenols than your average cup of joe. Made in a small pot called a *briki,* it's a daily treat, and boiling the grounds extracts more of the healthful chemical compounds in the coffee. This preparation, also popular in Turkey and the Middle East, creates a foam and rich creaminess to the coffee. To prepare this at home, add 2 cups cold water and 2 teaspoons Greek coffee to a *briki* or saucepan. Stir until grounds dissolve and slowly bring mixture to a boil. When you see foam, remove from heat. Evenly divide the foam between two cups; then pour the coffee over it. Wait for grounds to settle to the bottom of the cup before drinking.

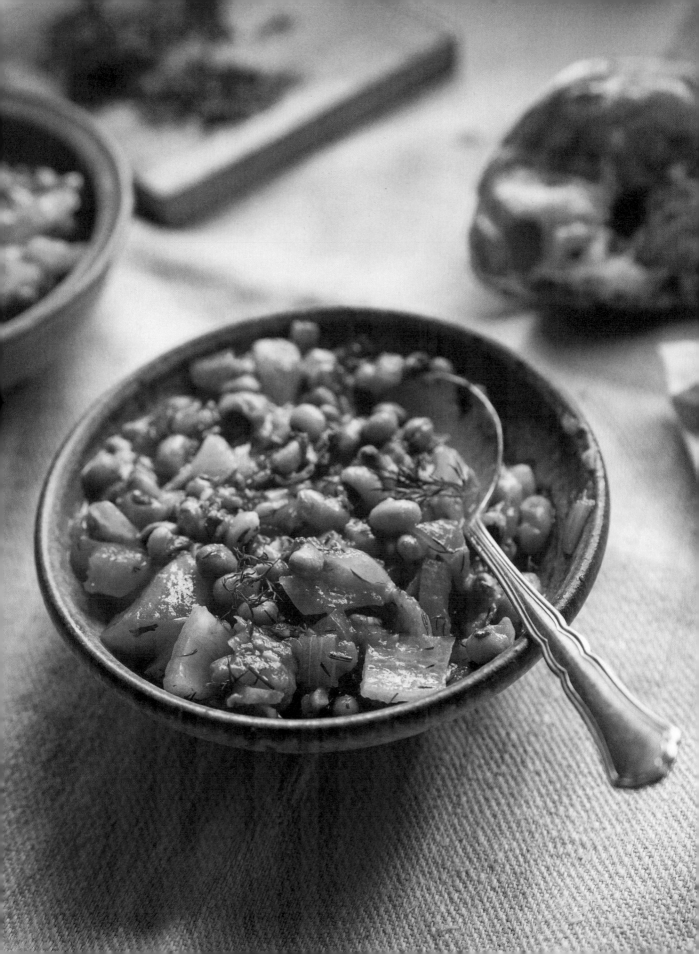

Ikarian Longevity Stew

TOTAL COOK TIME: 80 MINUTES | MAKES 4 SERVINGS

When I asked Dr. Antonia Trichopoulou, a Mediterranean diet expert, how I could get the small American city of Albert Lea, Minnesota—famous for meatpacking—to eat more vegetables, I knew I had come to the right person. We were sitting at Thea's Guesthouse, in front of one of her amazing spreads of Ikarian cuisine. Dr. Trichopoulou paused for a moment and then gestured to the food and said, "Feed them."

I had my marching orders, so I searched for a recipe that people would like. Several months later, I invited the entire city of Albert Lea to dinner. More than 2,200 people showed up as chefs demonstrated how to make this Ikarian stew in two enormous boiling cauldrons. For these people, vegetables were typically the orange flecks you see in Hamburger Helper. I was nervous to serve them a 100 percent plant-based meal. Less than an hour later, the two pots were completely empty and the city had taken its first step to changing its diet for the better.

After just one year, participants added an estimated 2.9 years to their average life span, while health care claims for city workers dropped 49 percent. This city experiment was the pilot for what is now Blue Zones Project, which has expanded to 47 communities across the United States.

Here's the exact recipe, which also happens to be one of our reader favorites.

1 cup dried black-eyed peas (or 8-ounce can, drained)

½ cup extra-virgin olive oil, divided

1 large red onion, finely chopped

4 garlic cloves, finely chopped

1 fennel bulb, chopped

1 large, firm ripe tomato, finely chopped

2 teaspoons tomato paste, diluted in ¼ cup water

2 bay leaves

1 bunch dill, finely chopped

Salt (optional)

If using dried black-eyed peas: Cover with water and bring to a boil for 1 minute. Remove from heat, cover, and let stand for an hour. Drain and rinse. (If using canned black-eyed peas, skip this step.)

In a large pot, heat half the olive oil over medium heat and cook the onion, garlic, and fennel, stirring occasionally, until soft, about 12 minutes.

Add the black-eyed peas and toss to coat with oil. Add the tomato, tomato paste, and enough water to cover the beans by about an inch. Add the bay leaves.

Bring pot to a boil, reduce heat, and simmer until the black-eyed peas are about halfway cooked (if using dried peas). Check after 40 minutes, but it may take over an hour. If using canned, skip to next step after 10 minutes.

Add the chopped dill and season with salt to taste. Continue cooking until the black-eyed peas are tender, about 20 minutes.

Remove from heat and pick out and discard the bay leaves. Pour in remaining olive oil, stir, and serve.

* By Dan Buettner

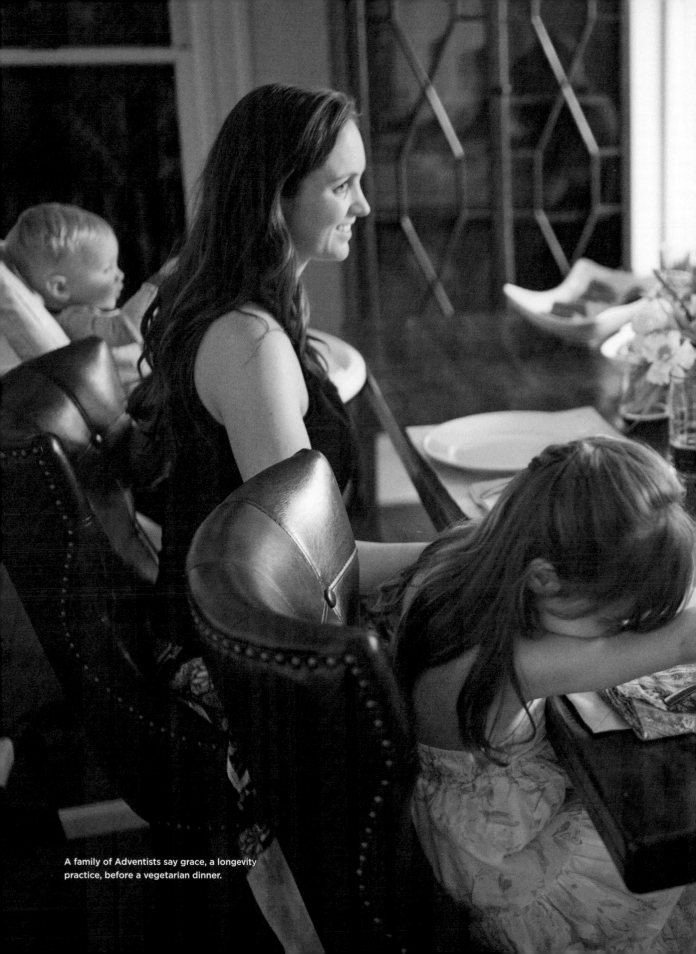

A family of Adventists say grace, a longevity practice, before a vegetarian dinner.

CHAPTER FIVE

Loma Linda

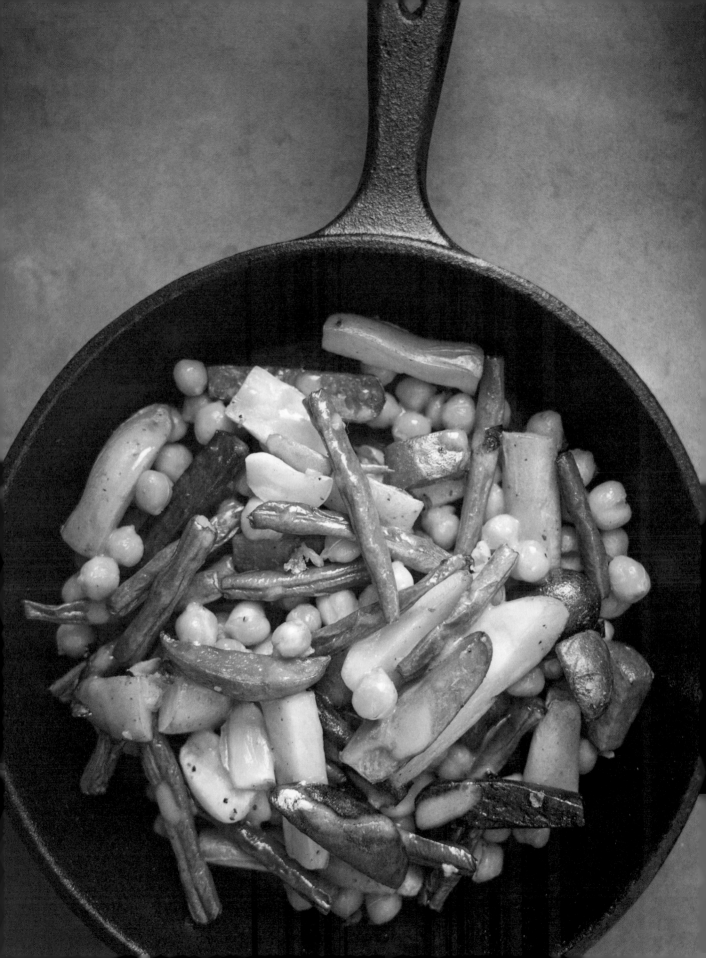

Loma Linda, California

Over the years, we've turned to doctors, scientists, and celebrities for diet advice. But here's a source we've largely overlooked: the Bible. In Genesis 1:29, God actually offers the diet for the Garden of Eden: *I have given you every plant that bears herb bearing seed . . . and every tree, in the which is the fruit of tree yielding seed; to you it shall be for meat.* • In the late 19th century, a housewife named Ellen White latched onto these Bible passages, along with a few others.

With austerity, clairvoyance, and a penchant for visions, White went on to found what would become the Seventh-day Adventist Church. She also articulated a diet that has helped produce the longest lived Americans.

In her *Councils on Food and Diet,* White offers 400 pages of Bible-inspired dietary instruction, which she sums up as follows: "Grains, fruits, nuts, and vegetables constitute the diet chosen for us by our Creator. These foods, prepared in as simple and natural a manner as possible, are the most healthful and nourishing. They impart a strength, a power of endurance, and a vigor of intellect, that are not afforded by a more complex and stimulating diet."

White warned against cooking with grease, spices, and salt and recommended whole grain over white flour. She also warned against sugar ("clouds the brain and brings peevishness into the disposition") and pickles. She endorsed potatoes as long as you don't fry them and extolled the virtues of beans and nuts.

In retrospect, White was remarkably prescient. Her recommendations are not far from the dietary guidelines of the American Cancer Society and

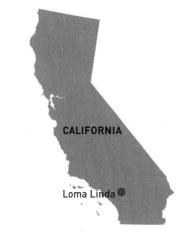

CALIFORNIA

Loma Linda

A skillet filled with roasted potatoes and green beans with a mustard drizzle (page 257)

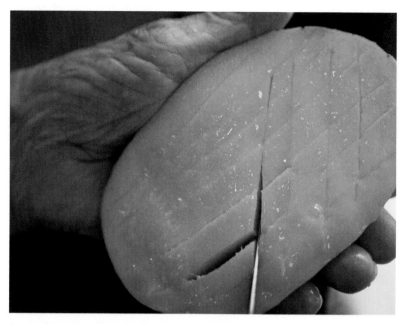

A man slices into a ripe and salted mango—a great snack idea.

the American Heart Association and are almost identical to Harvard University's Healthy Eating Plate recommendations.

White also seems to have foreseen the fouled water, salmonella, and animal cruelty as well as the risks associated with antibiotic overuse by the dairy and poultry industries. She wrote: "Let the people be taught how to prepare food without the use of milk or butter. Tell them that the time will soon come when there will be no safety in using eggs, milk, cream, or butter, because disease in animals is increasing in proportion to the increase of wickedness among men."

Today some 25 million Seventh-day Adventists—conservative Methodist Christians—have taken this dietary direction seriously and largely follow White's teachings. Strict vegetarian Adventists live nearly a decade longer than their U.S. counterparts, suffering a fraction of the rate of heart disease, diabetes, and certain cancers. They also weigh about 20 pounds less than their meat-eating counterparts. According to the Adventist Health Studies, which have followed more than 100,000 Adventists for more than 30 years, the longest-lived among them are pescatarians (vegan or vegetarian plus one small portion of fish daily). In other words, they eat a blue zones diet.

I MET ELLSWORTH WAREHAM in the early 2000s, when he was in his early 90s and still performing heart surgery. He passed away at 104 years old in December of 2018. When I met him, he credited much of his century-long vitality to a plant-based diet. He ate twice a day: A huge, 10 a.m. brunch of fruits, grain cereal, soy milk, and nuts—and a 4 p.m. dinner of pasta or rice dishes with a huge salad and vegetables. He once told me that he loved to eat, so keeping to only two meals a day helped keep him fit and trim. He also drank two glasses of water every morning and continued to drink water throughout the day. A renowned pioneer of open-heart surgery who practiced cardiology until the age of 97, Wareham became a vegan after he noticed that meat eaters' arteries were plaque filled and that plant eaters' arteries were clean and supple. When I last saw him last year, at age 103, he spotted me on the street, jumped out of a van, and gave me a hug.

Recently, I learned about cooking Adventist dishes from 90-year-old Dorothy Nelson, a culinary descendant of Ellen White. She greeted David McClain and me in her brightly lit Loma Linda townhouse wearing running

A young Adventist helps her family prepare for dinner while washing greens in the kitchen.

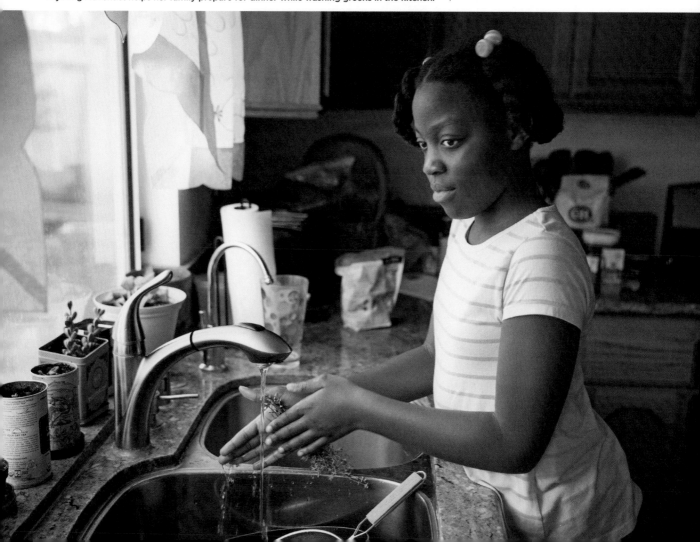

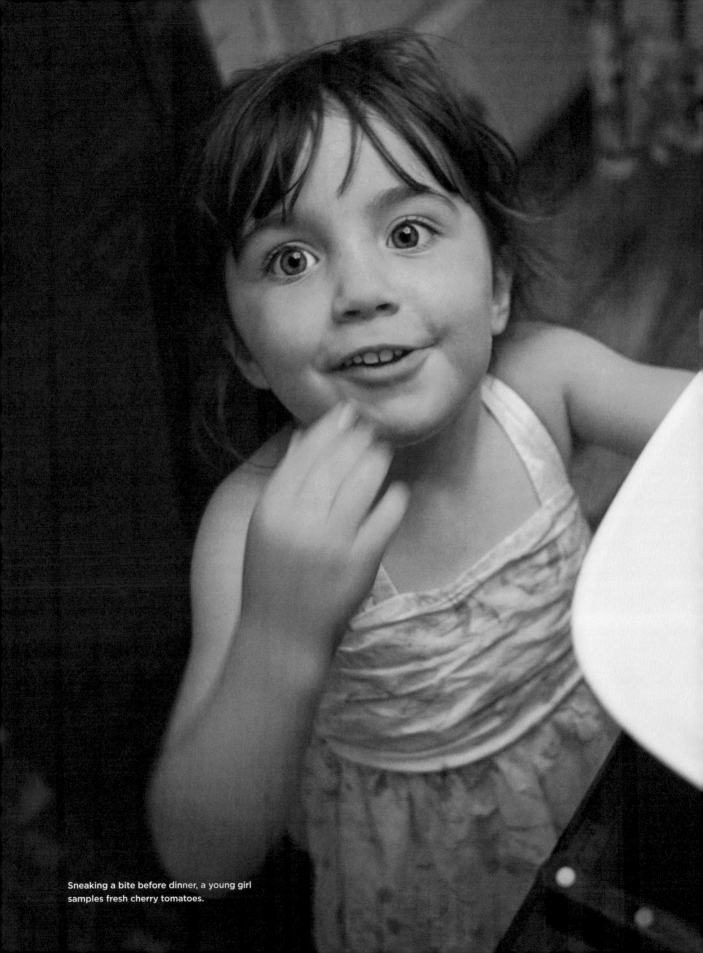

Sneaking a bite before dinner, a young girl samples fresh cherry tomatoes.

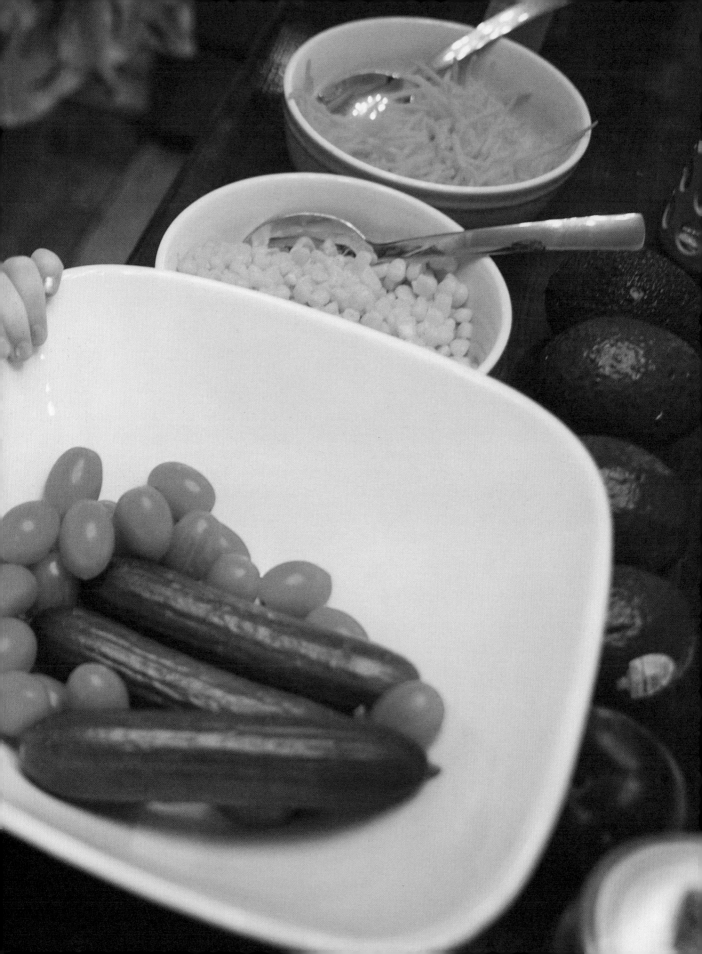

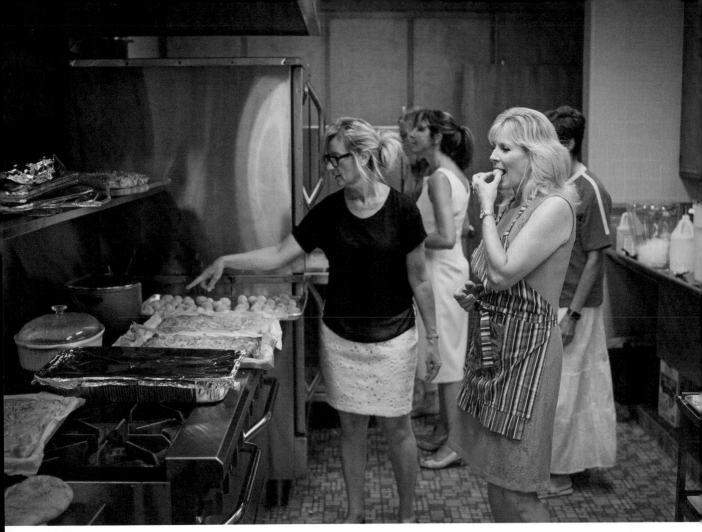

A group of women prepare food for a potluck in the church kitchen in Loma Linda. Vegetarian potlucks are a fixture in Adventists' social lives.

sneakers, a bright red T-shirt, and schoolgirl bangs cut just above crystalline blue eyes. A former pilot who once crash-landed in the Arctic and miraculously survived, today she limits her adventures to her garden.

For lunch, she cooked us black beans and rice, steamed garden cabbage and cauliflower, and browned a slice of tofu in sesame oil. After combining all the ingredients in a bowl, she added the sliced tofu, sesame seeds, and Bragg Liquid Aminos (non-fermented type of soy sauce) and served everything in huge, steaming bowls around her kitchen table. We dug in. The result was a savory, delicious compost pile of complex carbs, protein, and antioxidants: a panoply of micronutrients that filled our stomachs with fewer calories than a small bag of French fries. (You can find a few different grain bowl variations on page 262.)

"I've never tasted meat," she bragged adding that she has perfect blood pressure, has a resting heart rate of 60, and walks three miles a day. "I owe my health to God and a vegetarian diet," she told me. Then, she added three more rules for eating to 100:

• **Minimize the microwave:** "People cook food to death and destroy the nutrients. They should be lightly steaming them and eating them as close to the way they were grown."

• **Breakfast like a king, lunch like a prince, and dinner like a pauper:** Dorothy eats a savory breakfast; her favorite is brown rice and lentils with minced carrot, onion, basil, and marjoram and sprinkled with Bragg's. She lunches at about 2 p.m.—usually her last meal of the day—on a huge salad or steamed vegetables. If she eats dinner, it's usually just a piece of fruit.

• **Sweets as treats:** Dorothy allows herself sweets occasionally, and they are always, *always* homemade. The oatmeal breakfast cookies, on page 251, are based on her "power ball" recipe: a nutrient-heavy, consummately satisfying dessert that would also make a great workout snack.

The Adventist diet may not look like the most exotic cuisine in the world. But when you stop napalming taste buds with fat, sugar, and salt, nuanced flavors emerge from food and textures become more pronounced. So, the Asian-Influenced Heavenly Grain Bowl, with chickpeas, slivered nuts, avocado, and radishes (page 262), or the Perfect Slow Cooker Beans, with black-eyed peas, red wine vinegar, and mint (page 268), become a symphony of subtle delights. Moreover, eating this way has manifestly produced the longest lived Americans. And, if Ellen White is right, you'll not only last longer, you'll also be stronger, faster, and smarter along the way. ✳

FLAVOR PROFILE

These flavor pairings are the foundation of the most popular Adventist dishes. You can use these delectable combinations to help enhance any recipe.

✳ ✳ ✳

oats + nuts

oats + nuts + honey + cinnamon

fruit + nut butter

beans + corn + tomatoes

carrots + onions + garlic + legumes/beans

onions + peppers + herbs

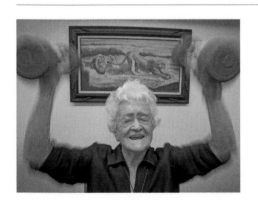

Marge Jetton, 100 YEARS OLD

For 15 years now, I've been visiting the modern Adventist community in and around Loma Linda, California. Early on, I spent several days with Marge Jetton, an energetic centenarian who woke every morning at 5:30 a.m., read her Bible, and ate precisely the same breakfast every day: steel-cut oatmeal with nuts and dates, topped with soy milk and followed by a "prune juice shooter." She'd pump iron, ride her bike, and then drive her 1994 Cadillac to the Loma Linda Senior Center to "help out the old folks." Most were in their 70s—30 years younger than Marge.

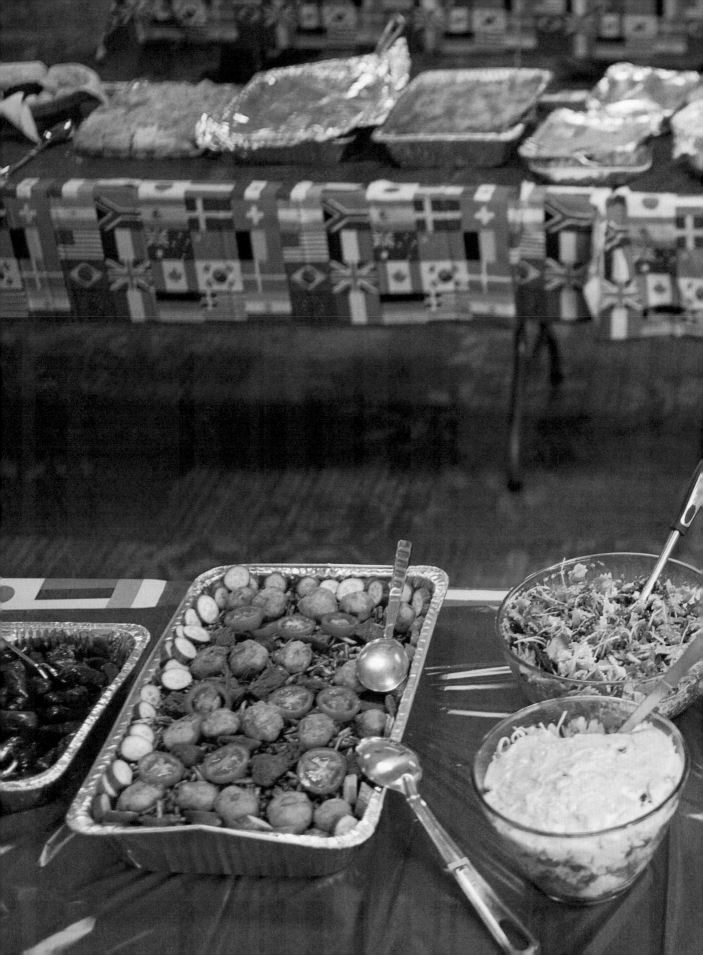

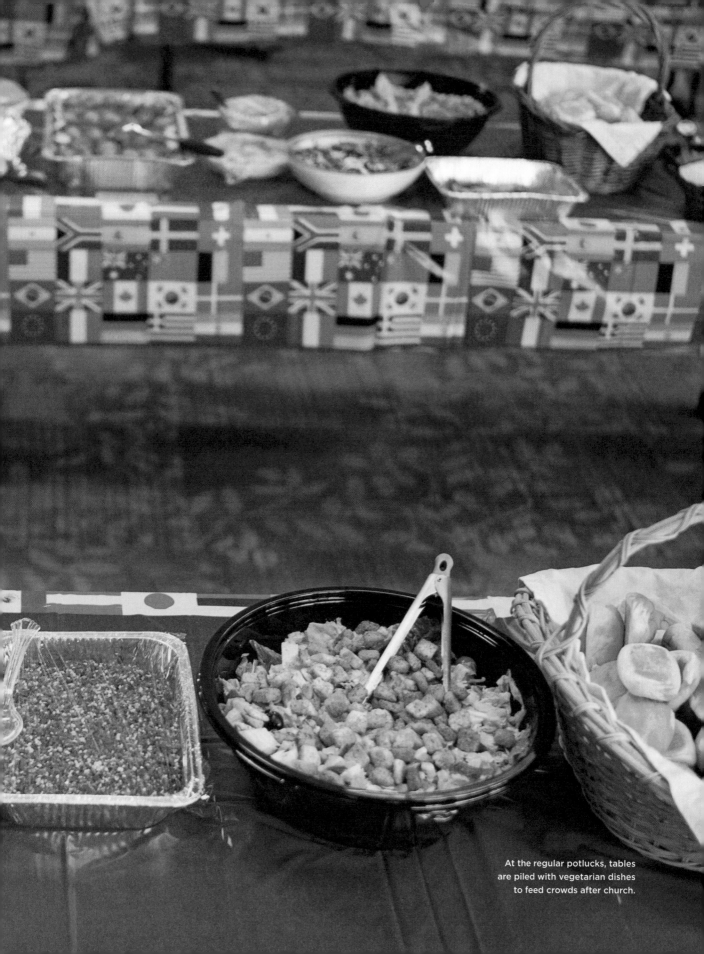

At the regular potlucks, tables are piled with vegetarian dishes to feed crowds after church.

Coconut Chia Pudding

TOTAL PREP TIME: 45 MINUTES | MAKES 6 SERVINGS

Chia seeds, a staple of the Adventist diet, which pack a punch of nutrients as well as an energy-boosting blend of omega-3 fats, fiber, protein, vitamins, and antioxidants, have recently become a popular superfood, but their origins are ancient; the Maya used them as food for runners and warriors to enhance endurance and strength. Chia seeds gel up and thicken in liquid, which makes this smooth, creamy pudding something that is healthy enough to eat for breakfast but decadent enough to enjoy as a dessert.

1 cup coconut cream

1 cup coconut milk

3 tablespoons agave nectar

½ teaspoon finely grated lemon zest

½ cup (3 ounces) chia seeds

Whisk coconut cream, coconut milk, agave nectar, and lemon zest together. Pour over chia seeds and stir well.

Cover with plastic wrap and let sit until thickened, at least 40 minutes or overnight in the refrigerator.

When ready to eat, stir well and top with fruit, nuts, and seeds, if desired.

Note: You can substitute stevia or honey for the agave, and swap in soy milk, almond milk, or rice milk for the coconut milk. If you're watching your fat intake, reduce the amount of coconut or just use a plant-based milk. If you do so, reduce the liquid to 1½ cups to maintain consistency.

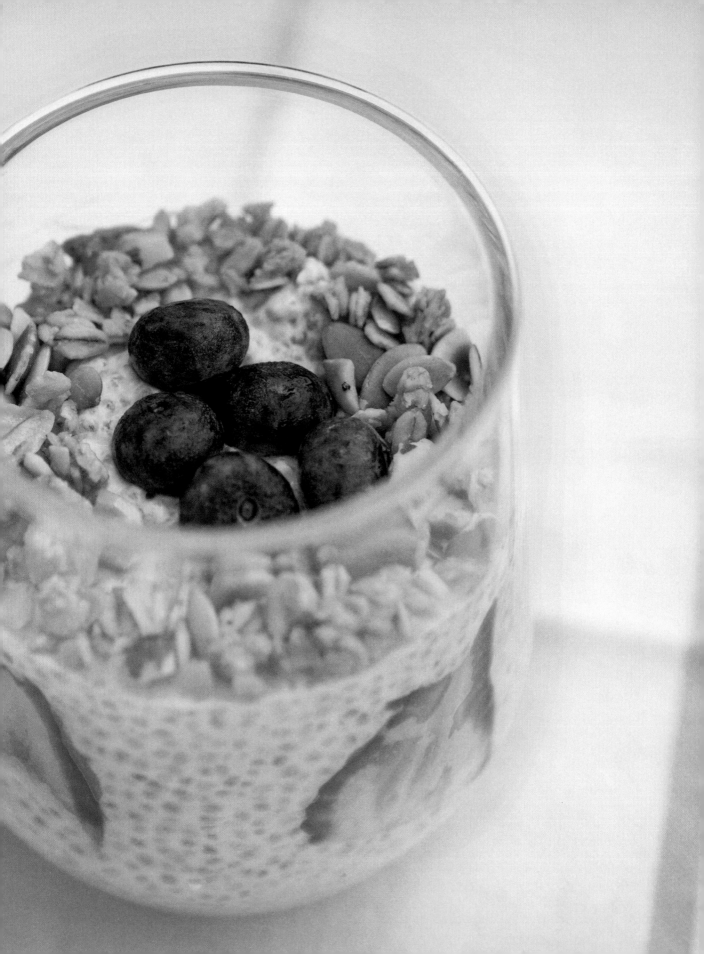

Supercharged Smoothies

TOTAL PREP TIME: 5 MINUTES | MAKES 1 SERVING

Fruits, nuts, and greens are staples in all longevity-promoting blue zones diets around the world. Combine them in these delicious smoothies to get a morning energy boost from nutrient-packed ingredients.

Research on the dietary patterns of Seventh-day Adventists reveals that front-loading calories earlier in the day is associated with a lower risk of obesity and heart conditions (which validates the age-old adage to not skip breakfast). Still, it's not always easy to put together a full meal when you're on the go—so try these filling and satisfying smoothies. Choose your favorite blend or alternate between a few to keep your breakfast feeling inspired. You can also enjoy these delicious drinks as portable snacks, light afternoon meals—and even dessert.

EVERYDAY ICY SMOOTHIE

1 frozen very ripe large banana, cut into 1-inch pieces

½ cup frozen blueberries or strawberries

Small handful frozen broccoli

½ cup vanilla almond milk

1 tablespoon almond butter

½ cup ice

2 teaspoons honey, especially if using nonripe bananas

Combine all of the ingredients in the blender and process until smooth.

ENERGY SMOOTHIE

1 banana

1 cup frozen peaches

1 cup nondairy vanilla yogurt

½ cup vanilla almond milk

1 tablespoon chia seeds

Pinch of ground cayenne to boost metabolism (optional)

Puree all ingredients in a blender until smooth.

Smoothie Bowl Option: Pour smoothie into a cereal bowl and top with ¼ cup granola and the zest of 1 orange as a garnish.

PROTEIN SMOOTHIE

¼ cup rolled oats

1 cup almond milk

3 tablespoons almond or peanut butter

1 banana

1 cup baby spinach leaves

1 tablespoon cocoa powder

1 tablespoon flax seeds

1 tablespoon agave syrup

Pinch of ground cinnamon

Pulse the oats a few times in your blender so they grind up; then add the other ingredients and puree until smooth.

Let the smoothie sit for about 3 to 5 minutes before drinking so the ground oats aren't grainy.

Smoothie Bowl Option: In a bowl, top smoothie with ¼ cup granola, 1 tablespoon shredded coconut, 1 tablespoon blueberries, and 1 tablespoon cacao nibs as a garnish.

CANTALOUPE BERRY COOLER

1 cup cantaloupe, seeded and cut
   into 1-inch cubes

½ cup frozen strawberries

½ cup frozen blueberries

1 tablespoon honey

1 cup ice

Combine all ingredients in a blender or food processor until smooth.

TROPICAL GREEN SMOOTHIE

2 cups spinach

1 ripe banana

½ cup frozen pineapple

½ cup frozen mango

3 dates, pitted

1 tablespoon almond butter

Combine all ingredients in a blender or food processor until smooth.

FROZEN MANGO LASSI

¼ cup coconut cream

¾ cup coconut milk

1 cup frozen mango

½ cup ice

Honey

Fresh mint leaves (optional as
   garnish)

Combine coconut cream, milk, mango, and ice in a blender or food processor until smooth.

Add honey to taste and blend again, adding more water or ice if necessary to reach desired consistency.

Serve with mint leaves on top, if using.

Granola Every Day, Every Way

TOTAL COOK TIME: 40 MINUTES │ MAKES 6 SERVINGS

Adventists believe in eating a hearty breakfast and a light dinner, and they often use nuts and seeds in their oatmeal and breakfast goods. Research reveals that nut eaters, on average, outlive non–nut eaters by two to three years. Nuts are also shown to reduce "bad" LDL cholesterol by 9 percent to 20 percent, regardless of the fat level or amount consumed.

This hearty granola is the perfect addition to morning oatmeal, coconut yogurt, or alone as a mid-morning snack; the variations that follow allow you to mix and match your favorite flavors, revealing just how versatile this food can be. Use it in a trail mix, in a breakfast parfait, or as a dessert topping to add a delicious boost of health to your day.

3 cups old-fashioned oats

1½ to 2 cups raw nuts like walnuts, almonds, pecans*

3 tablespoons coconut oil

½ cup honey or maple syrup

¼ teaspoon ground cinnamon

½ cup dried fruit (optional)

Chocolate chips (optional)

Preheat the oven to 300 degrees. Spray a large baking sheet with cooking spray or line with parchment paper.

In a mixing bowl, combine oats, nuts, oil, honey, and cinnamon.

Spread onto baking sheet and bake until golden brown, stirring once in a while. Bake for about 30 minutes.

Remove from oven and transfer to cooling rack and let cool. Combine with dried fruit and chocolate chips, if using.

*If using already roasted nuts, subtract 10 minutes from the cooking time.

Try These Variations

GRANOLA MEXICANA

Mix 1 cup basic granola with ½ cup chopped fresh mango, juice of 1 lime, and ¼ teaspoon chile powder.

CHAI-SPICED GRANOLA

Mix 1 cup basic granola with ¼ teaspoon ground cardamom, pinch of cloves, and 1 piece minced candied ginger.

POWER GRANOLA

Mix 1 cup basic granola with 3 tablespoons dried blueberries, 2 tablespoons cacao nibs, and 2 tablespoons shredded coconut.

GRANOLA PARFAIT

Layer ¼ cup almond-based yogurt with ¼ cup granola followed by 1 tablespoon cacao nibs, 1 tablespoon shredded coconut, and 1½ tablespoons dried blueberries. Repeat.

ICE CREAM TOPPING GRANOLA

Add a small handful of fresh in-season berries and ¼ cup basic granola on top of your favorite nondairy ice cream for a refreshing treat.

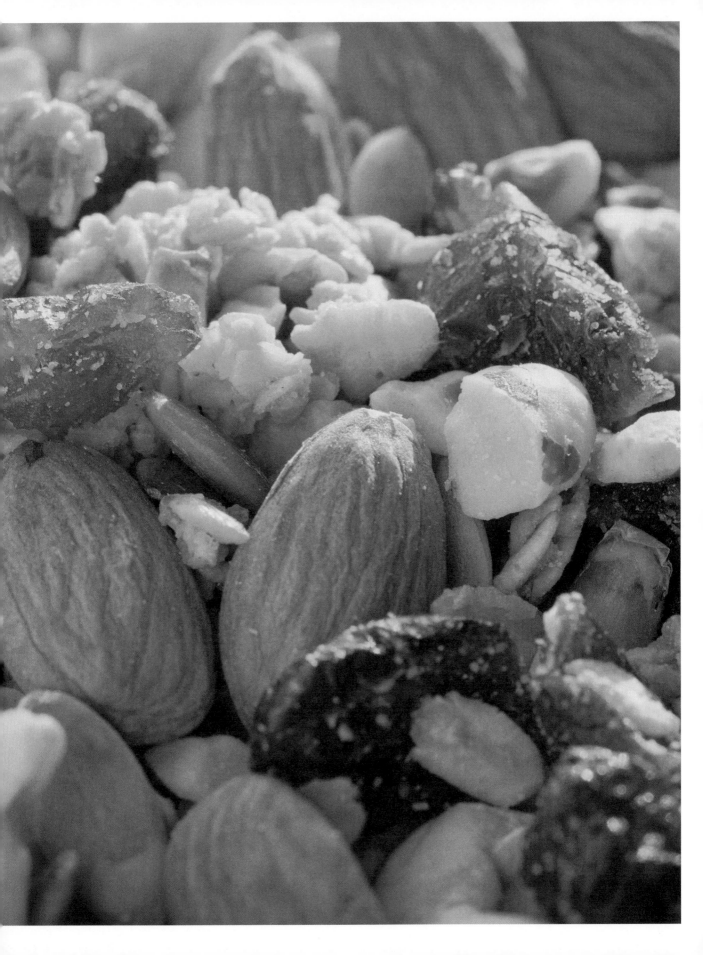

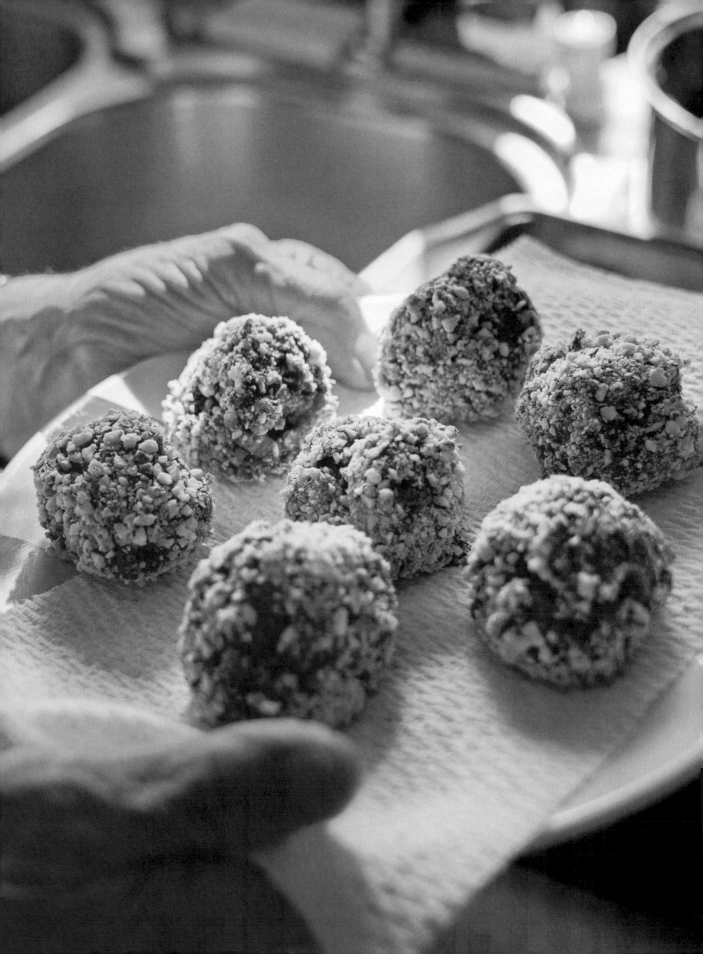

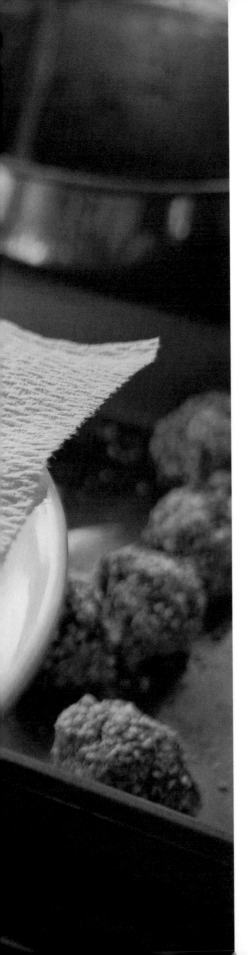

Oatmeal Breakfast Cookies

TOTAL COOK TIME: 25 MINUTES | MAKES 4 SERVINGS

Oatmeal is a dietary essential for Adventists, as both a breakfast meal and a popular ingredient in many other recipes. It provides fiber, healthy protein, complex carbohydrates, and good doses of iron and B vitamins. Because it holds up well to frying and baking, it forms the basis of many vegetarian main dishes like veggie burgers (page 278), nut loaves (page 268), and smoothies (page 246).

These quick-and-filling breakfast cookies are easy to make in advance and take on the road; they're also the perfect healthy snack or dessert. Before baking, you can flatten them into the traditional cookie shape or keep them rolled into cookie balls.

3 large ripe bananas

1¾ cups quick oats

¼ cup chocolate chips

¼ cup applesauce

Honey (optional)

Crushed nuts (optional)

Preheat oven to 350 degrees. Line a baking sheet with parchment paper or grease with cooking spray.

Mash bananas in a bowl; add oats and mix well to combine. Fold in chocolate chips and applesauce.

Use a tablespoon to measure out portions of the dough, dropping onto the baking sheet. You can shape these into balls or press and flatten each cookie with a spoon. (It will not spread out much during baking.)

Bake for about 15 minutes or until cookies are lightly browned on top.

Remove and let cool on a rack.

Roll in honey and then crushed nuts, if using, when cool enough to handle.

Longevity Smoothie Bowl

TOTAL PREP TIME: 5 MINUTES | **MAKES 2 SERVINGS**

This smoothie has all your morning protein needs packed into one, admittedly giant, bowl. It's great for a postexercise meal.

1½ cups almond milk

1 large frozen banana, cut into
  1-inch pieces*

1 cup blackberries or blueberries

½ cup chopped kale

½ cup baby spinach leaves

1 tablespoon almond butter

1 tablespoon flax seeds

¼ teaspoon turmeric

½ cup ice

1 teaspoon cinnamon, optional

Suggested Toppings:
Granola (page 248)

Fresh sliced fruit such as
  bananas, strawberries, or
  blackberries

Sliced almonds

Flax seeds

Honey

Blend smoothie ingredients until smooth, adding more milk if necessary—the consistency should be a bit thicker than a drinkable smoothie, since you will eat this with a spoon.

Pour into a bowl and add toppings.

*Be sure to use a large frozen banana or the texture of the smoothie bowl won't be thick enough.

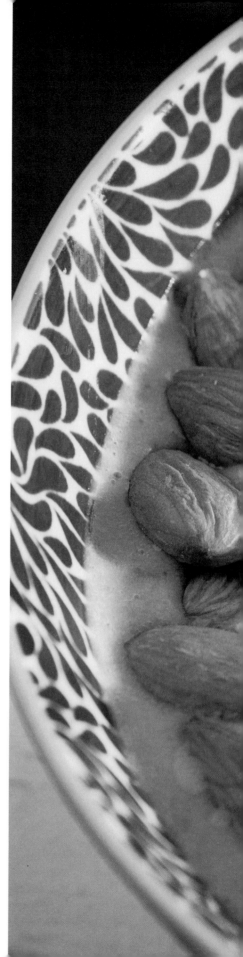

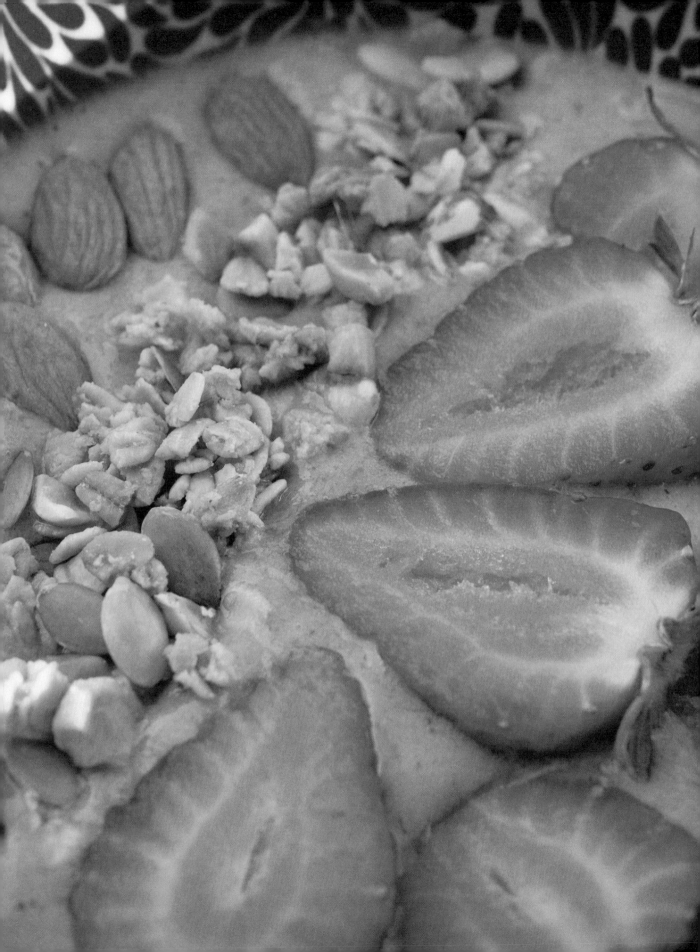

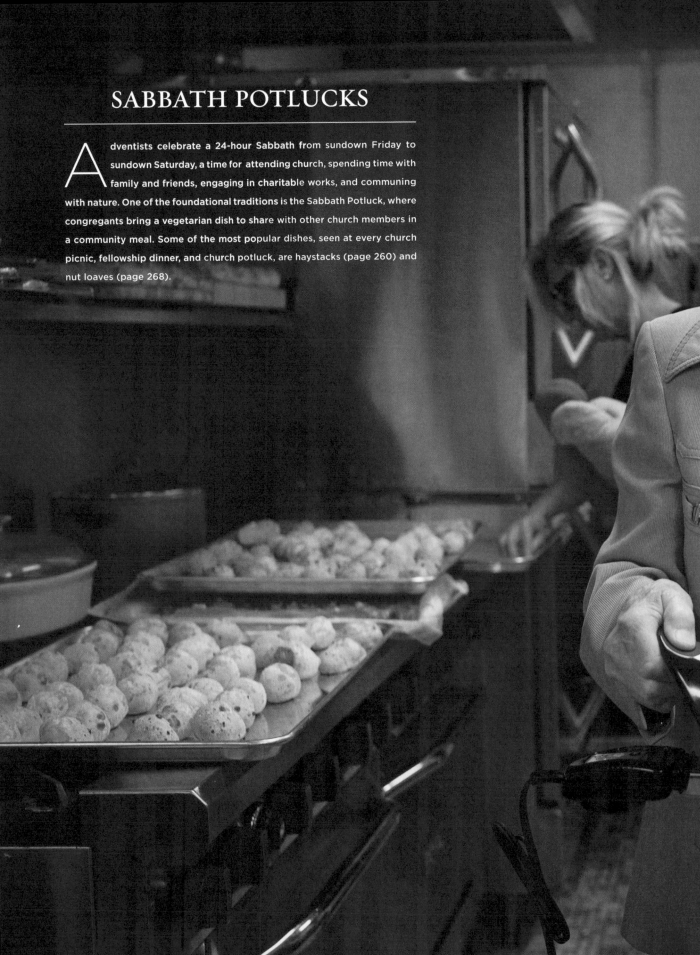

SABBATH POTLUCKS

Adventists celebrate a 24-hour Sabbath from sundown Friday to sundown Saturday, a time for attending church, spending time with family and friends, engaging in charitable works, and communing with nature. One of the foundational traditions is the Sabbath Potluck, where congregants bring a vegetarian dish to share with other church members in a community meal. Some of the most popular dishes, seen at every church picnic, fellowship dinner, and church potluck, are haystacks (page 260) and nut loaves (page 268).

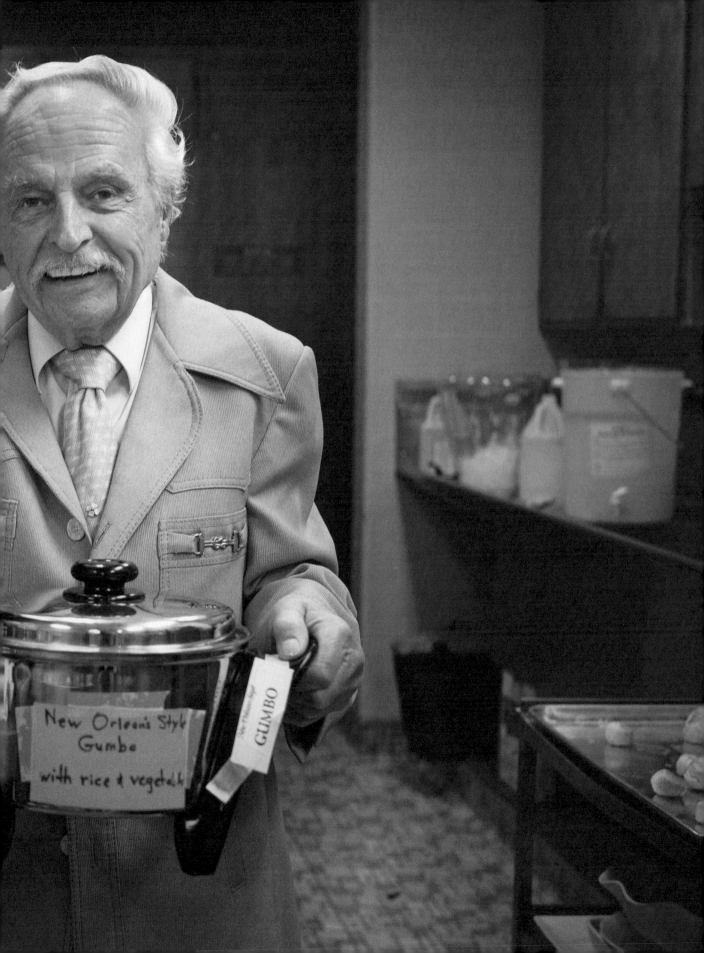

Adventist Gumbo

TOTAL COOK TIME: 45 MINUTES | MAKES 4 TO 6 SERVINGS

This aromatic gumbo uses the elements of the traditional Creole stew and is bursting with flavor. Full of greens, beans, and herbs, it's the ultimate blue zones meal. Feel free to swap the greens and beans with whatever you have on hand: Spinach, kale, turnip greens, white beans, navy beans, and black-eyed peas all work well in this dish. Since many Adventists don't eat very spicy foods—in line with traditional church teaching—this gumbo only has a mild kick. If you like yours with a little more spice, add more cayenne pepper or serve it with your favorite hot sauce.

⅓ cup extra-virgin olive oil

⅓ cup all-purpose flour

1½ large sweet onions (like Vidalia), chopped

4 garlic cloves, minced

3 bay leaves

¼ teaspoon cayenne pepper

½ teaspoon dried thyme

2 stalks celery, diced

1 red bell pepper, cored and diced

4 cups vegetable stock

⅓ cup fresh or frozen corn kernels

1½ cups cooked black-eyed peas (or one 15-ounce can, drained)

1 cup cooked brown rice

1 cup frozen cut okra

2 cups chopped spinach

¼ cup chopped fresh parsley

Salt and pepper (optional)

Make your roux: In a large soup pot, heat olive oil over medium heat. Add flour, whisking until smooth. Cook for 3 to 4 minutes, stirring often, and then turn heat down to low and cook for another 3 to 4 minutes, until roux has become golden in color.

Add onion and turn heat up to medium-low for about 5 minutes. Cook until onion is just soft.

Add garlic, bay leaves, cayenne pepper, thyme, celery, and red pepper. Cover and cook for about 5 minutes over medium heat or until vegetables are tender.

Stir in vegetable stock, turn the heat up and bring to a boil.

Add corn, black-eyed peas, rice, and okra; lower heat to a simmer and cook for about 5 minutes.

Add spinach and parsley and continue to simmer for another 5 minutes.

Remove bay leaves and add salt and pepper to taste.

Serve over rice or with a side of cornbread (page 267).

Roasted Potatoes and Green Beans With Mustard Drizzle

TOTAL COOK TIME: 45 MINUTES | MAKES 4 SERVINGS

In this deceptively simple recipe, the mustard dressing brightens all the flavors of this dish to create a spectacular one-pan meal. With beans, greens, and potatoes, it combines many of the most important staple foods from blue zones hot spots.

½ pound fingerling potatoes, halved

3 garlic cloves, sliced

3 tablespoons chopped fresh parsley or other herbs

2 to 3 tablespoons extra-virgin olive oil

½ cup cooked chickpeas (or canned, drained and rinsed), patted dry with a paper towel

½ pound green beans, washed, trimmed, and dried

For the dressing:
1 tablespoon Dijon mustard

1½ tablespoons extra-virgin olive oil

1 tablespoon white wine vinegar

2 teaspoons honey

Salt and pepper (optional)

Heat oven to 425 degrees.

In a large mixing bowl, toss potatoes with garlic, herbs, and half of olive oil.

Place in a single layer in a roasting pan and roast for 25 minutes, stirring once or twice.

When potatoes are tender and starting to brown, add the chickpeas and green beans and roast for another 10 minutes.

While that roasts, in a small bowl whisk together mustard, olive oil, vinegar, and honey to form an emulsified dressing.

Season the dressing with salt and pepper to taste.

Transfer the roasted vegetables and beans to a platter and drizzle with dressing. Serve warm.

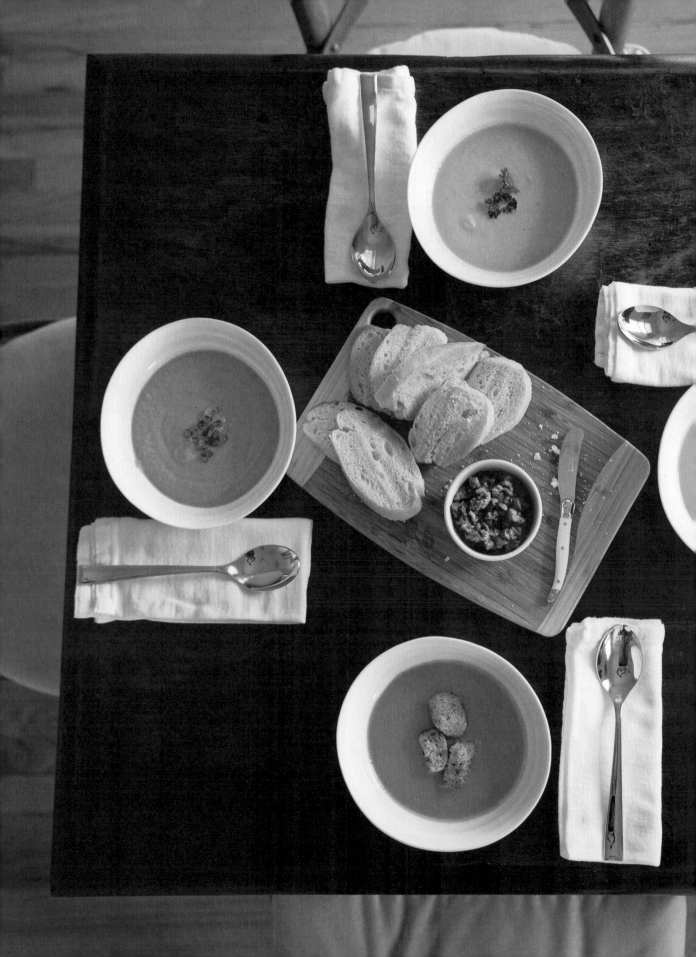

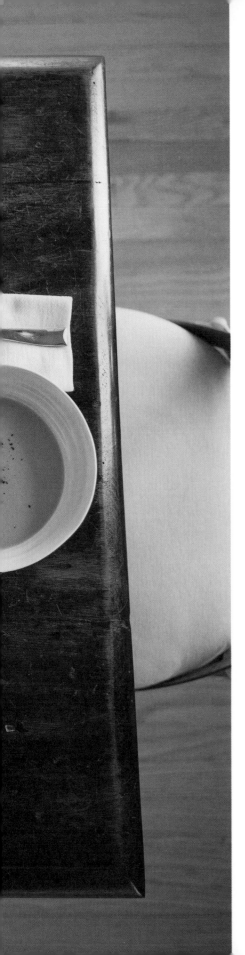

Dan's Favorite Cream Soup

TOTAL COOK TIME: 40 MINUTES | MAKES 5 SERVINGS

In just a few minutes, you can whip up this creamy, comforting soup featuring carrots, broccoli, tarragon, and onions. This dish is like a warm blanket on a cold day; try making it with different vegetables and spices to change things up.

2 tablespoons extra-virgin olive oil

2 medium onions, diced

4 stalks celery, chopped

3 carrots, peeled and chopped

3 cloves garlic, minced

Sprig of tarragon

2 bay leaves

7 cups chopped broccoli, packed

4 to 6 cups water or vegetable broth (or half water and half veggie broth)

3 to 4 tablespoons cashew cream, store-bought or home-made (page 277)

Salt and pepper (optional)

In a large soup pot over medium heat, heat olive oil and sauté onions, celery, and carrots for about 6-7 minutes.

Add garlic and herbs and sauté for another minute longer; then add broccoli and vegetable broth or water and bring to a simmer. Cook until broccoli is very tender, about 8 minutes.

Let soup cool for a few minutes, remove bay leaves, and then transfer soup to a blender, working in batches. Try not to fill blender more than halfway. Remove center of blender cap and cover with a dish towel.

Add 3 to 4 tablespoons of cashew cream and blend soup until it's pureed. If using an immersion blender, add cashew cream directly to pot and puree until smooth. Add salt and pepper to taste.

Note: You can also use this recipe as a soup base to make cream of mushroom soup, pepper cream soup, and creamy tomato soup. Just substitute mushrooms, peppers, or tomatoes for the broccoli, cooking each until tender.

Haystacks
(Adventist Taco Salad)

TOTAL COOK TIME: 15 MINUTES | MAKES 6 SERVINGS

"Haystacks" are a traditional Adventist version of a taco salad: beans, chips, salad greens, and tomatoes are assembled into a layered dish that is easy to customize. You can find it at any Adventist potluck or Friday night vespers gathering. Some people use Frito's corn chips as the base, but low-sodium tortilla chips are a healthier option. Haystack ingredients are usually served individually so that people can pick and choose what they like, assembly-line fashion: the ultimate taco bar!

2 cups lightly salted or low-sodium tortilla chips
(use blue corn chips for a nice presentation)

2 cups shredded romaine lettuce

1 avocado, chopped

1 Roma tomato, chopped

½ cup corn kernels

1 cup cooked black beans
(drained and rinsed if using canned)

1 cup good quality salsa

Suggested Toppings:
Sliced pickled jalapeños

2 to 3 green onions, sliced

Chopped cilantro, optional

Cashew cream drizzle, optional
(page 277)

½ cup meatless crumbles,
optional

If assembling as a completed dish, on a large platter spread a layer of tortilla chips.

Then add a layer of lettuce and any other chopped vegetables, followed by a layer of beans, then salsa.

Add all other toppings, then drizzle with cashew cream and a sprinkle of meatless crumbles, if desired.

Following this assembly order keeps the chips from getting soggy, allowing you to make this dish ahead of time.

Note: Feel free to get creative: Play with adding olives, cucumbers, zucchini, roasted red peppers, pepitas, or whatever other veggies you have on hand to create your own version of a haystack, adding these between the lettuce and bean layers. You can also change the flavor by changing up salsa to use as the dressing.

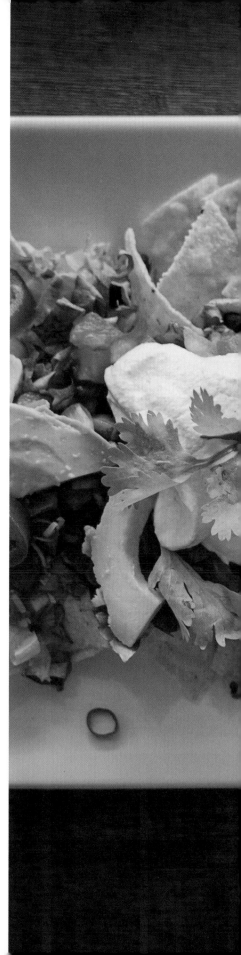

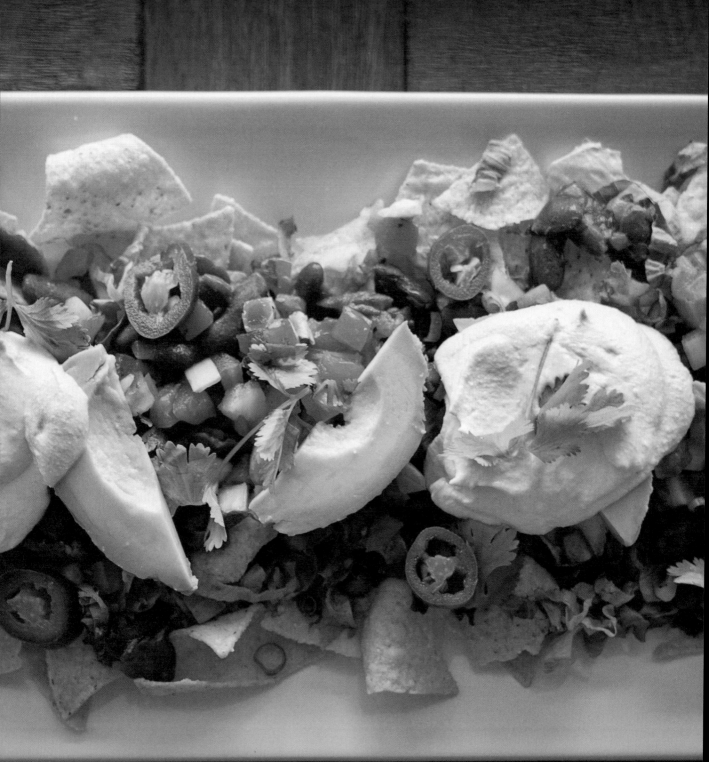

Heavenly Grain Bowls

TOTAL PREP TIME: 10 MINUTES | MAKES 4 SERVINGS

At their core, heavenly grain bowls are the perfect way to transform heart-healthy grains, beans, greens, and veggies into an easy-to-make, easy-to-store, and easy-to-eat meal. Customize your own by choosing one item from each of the categories below or follow the directions to create one of our very favorite iterations.

Grain ideas: brown rice, farro, couscous, quinoa, wheat berries, or a mixture

Veggie ideas: raw veggies and/or cooked veggies like lettuce, kale, spinach, zucchini, tomatoes

Beans or legumes: black beans, lentils, kidney beans, cannellini beans

Sauce or dressing ideas: sriracha, honey mustard, lemon vinaigrette, pesto, harissa, salsa

Crunchy toppings: crushed nuts, seeds, fried shallots

Garnishes: sliced avocado, sprouts, herbs

ASIAN-INFLUENCED HEAVENLY GRAIN BOWL

The Dressing:
¼ cup peanut butter

1 teaspoon sesame oil

¼ cup rice vinegar

3 tablespoons soy sauce

¼ cup water

1 to 2 tablespoons sriracha

The Bowl:
3 cups cooked quinoa or brown rice or a combination of both

1 avocado, peeled and chopped

1 Roma tomato, chopped

1 cup shredded lettuce or chopped spinach

½ cup cooked black beans or chickpeas

In a bowl, whisk dressing ingredients together.

Portion out grains into five bowls, then top each bowl with avocado, tomato, greens, and beans.

Drizzle each with dressing.

HEARTY BARLEY AND KALE BOWL

2 cups cooked barley

1 cup thinly sliced, loosely packed kale

½ cup cooked cannellini beans, drained and rinsed

1 carrot, peeled and cut into small dice

5 to 6 pitted Kalamata olives, sliced in half

2 cornichons, cut into small dice

3 tablespoons red wine vinegar

3 tablespoons olive oil

¼ teaspoon salt

¼ teaspoon cracked black pepper

3 to 4 basil leaves, sliced thin

1 pitted date, diced (optional)

Combine all the ingredients—except date—and let sit for at least 10 minutes before serving to allow the flavors to marry.

If you like a salty/sweet contrast, add the date; if you want something purely savory, simply omit it.

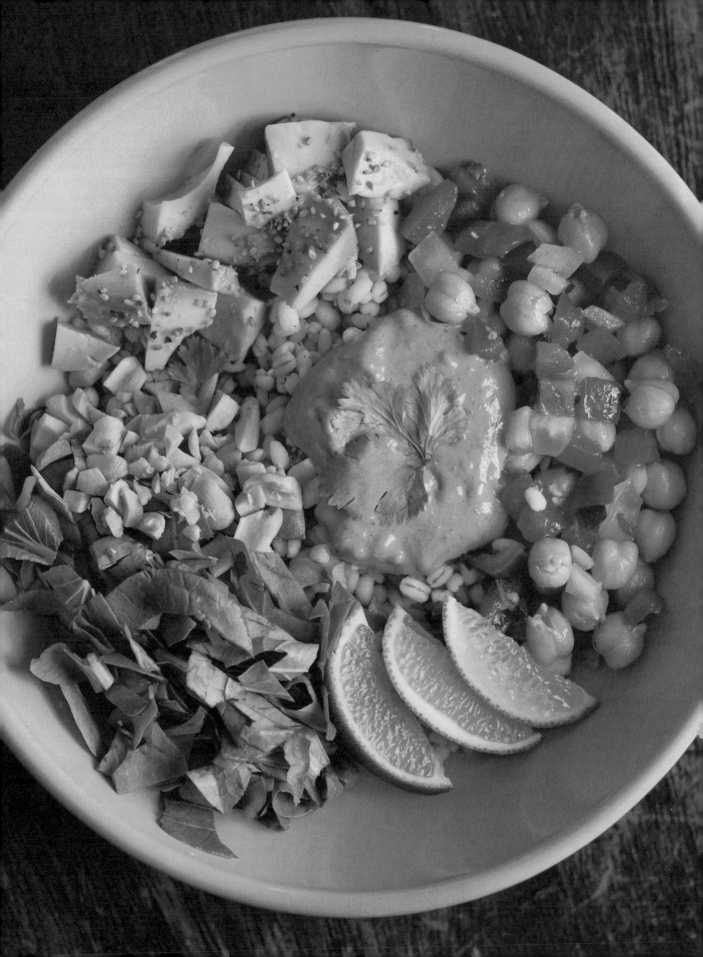

COOKING AND EATING TOGETHER

Those who follow the Adventist diet are often the healthiest and longest living Americans; studies show that Adventists in Loma Linda live a decade longer than their peers. This vegetarian eating plan emphasizes whole grains, nuts, beans, vegetables, and soy products; Adventists also generally abstain from coffee and alcohol. Beyond their everyday blue zones diets, Adventists in Loma Linda have strong family and community ties, take a full 24-hour Sabbath day to worship and to de-stress, regularly get out in nature, and often share meals with family and other Adventists.

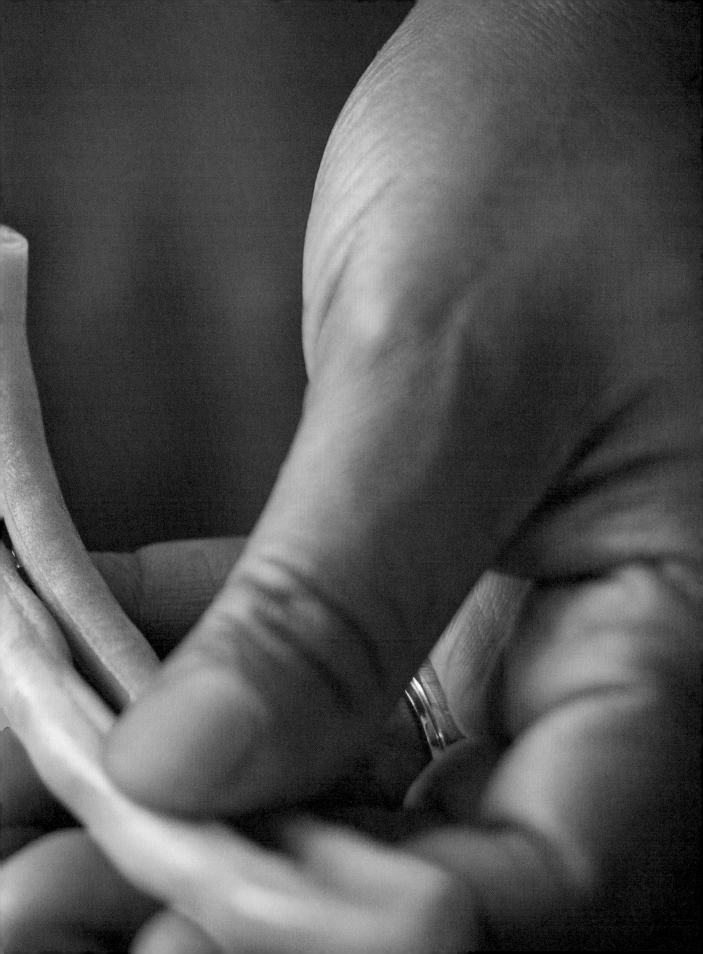

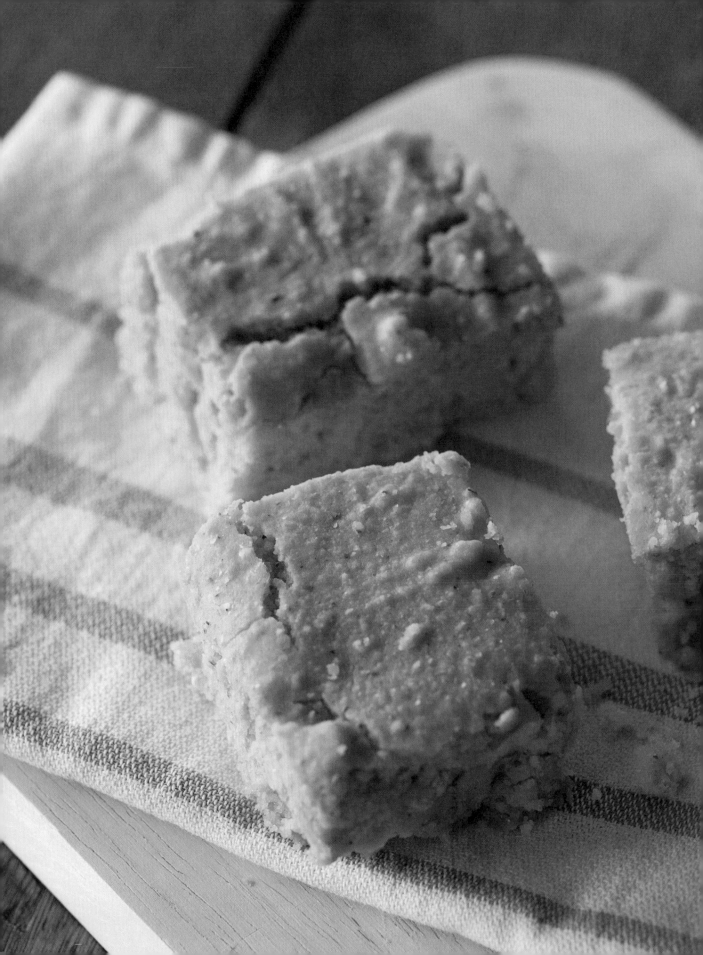

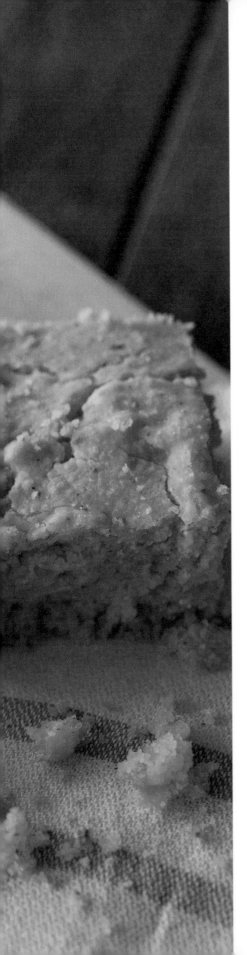

Quick Cornbread

TOTAL COOK TIME: 40 MINUTES | MAKES 12 SERVINGS

These crumbly cornbread muffins studded with corn kernels are good for breakfast, for a snack, or as a side to chili. Dress them up with jalapeño or jam or drizzle with honey.

Cornmeal, or ground dried corn, has been around for thousands of years and is the foundation of many staple foods, including polenta, tortillas, and grits. It's an excellent source of fiber, protein, vitamin A, carotenoids, complex carbohydrates, and essential minerals.

1 tablespoon flaxseed meal plus 3 tablespoons water ("flax egg")

1 cup cornmeal

1 cup unbleached all-purpose flour or spelt flour

1 tablespoon baking powder

½ teaspoon salt

¾ cup vanilla soy milk (sweetened)

¼ cup applesauce

¼ cup vegetable oil

2 tablespoons maple syrup

1 teaspoon vanilla extract

½ cup sweet corn kernels, fresh or frozen

Preheat oven to 350 degrees. Line a 9 x 13 baking pan with parchment paper, or oil a 12-cup muffin pan.

Add flaxseed meal and water to a dish and stir. Let sit for 5 minutes until thickened to create what's known as a "flax egg."

In a large bowl, mix the dry ingredients (cornmeal, flour, baking powder, salt) together.

In another large bowl, combine wet ingredients ("flax egg," soy milk, applesauce, oil, maple syrup, vanilla extract). Whisk until foamy.

Pour wet ingredients into dry ingredients and stir to combine. Add corn kernels and stir.

Pour into pan or muffin tin and bake for 30 minutes (20 minutes for muffins) or until toothpick comes out clean.

Perfect Slow Cooker Beans

TOTAL COOK TIME: 8 HOURS | MAKES 8 SERVINGS

The flavor, texture, and digestibility of these slow cooker beans are sublime! This approach is based on the way traditional Mexican cooks prepare beans—in clay, unsoaked—with seasonings and epazote for digestibility.

2 cups dried beans of choice

1 to 2 teaspoons sea salt

1 tablespoon black peppercorns

3 to 4 large garlic cloves, skin on

¼ cup diced white onion

2 bay leaves (optional)

2 chipotle peppers (optional)

2 teaspoons dried epazote* or
3 to 4 epazote sprigs (optional)

Turn empty slow cooker on low to preheat.

Meanwhile, use a sieve or colander to rinse beans in water and shake off excess liquid. Add to slow cooker.

Add sea salt, whole black peppercorns, garlic cloves, and diced onion. Add bay leaves, chipotle peppers, and epazote, if using.

Pour boiling water over the mixture until water is 2 inches above beans. Cover slow cooker and set on low for 7 to 8 hours. Remove bay leaves.

Serve beans with rice, over a salad, or in tacos.

*Epazote is an aromatic herb used in the cuisines and traditional medicines of Mexico and Guatemala; it has notes of oregano, anise, citrus, and mint. Look for it in gourmet or Latin grocers or at online retailers.

Walnut "Meat" Loaf (pages 270-71)

TOTAL COOK TIME: 95 MINUTES | MAKES 6 TO 8 SERVINGS

Like haystacks, nut loaves are Adventist staples at potlucks, picnics, and parties. Adventists make their savory loaves with a variety of nuts, grains, beans, legumes, and vegetable combinations; every family has its own version of the recipe.

1 cup whole wheat bread crumbs

1 cup seasoned bread crumbs

2 cups walnuts, finely ground

½ cup instant oats, coarsely ground in food processor

2 large onions, minced

2 celery heart stalks, minced

3 tablespoons ketchup

2 tablespoons vegetable oil

1 teaspoon poultry seasoning

1 tablespoon garlic powder

¼ cup almond or soy milk

Preheat oven to 375 degrees. Generously oil a 9 x 5 loaf pan.

In a large bowl, combine both types of bread crumbs, ground walnuts, and oats.

In a food processor, pulse onions, celery, ketchup, and 2 tablespoons oil until broken down but not completely liquefied.

Add wet ingredients to dry mixture, along with poultry seasoning, garlic powder, and milk, and mix until well moistened; add more milk if it's not moist enough.

Pour mixture into prepared pan and cover with foil. Bake for 70 minutes and remove foil. Bake for an additional 10 minutes, or until a knife or toothpick comes out clean.

Let cool 10-15 minutes before slicing. Serve with gravy or ketchup.

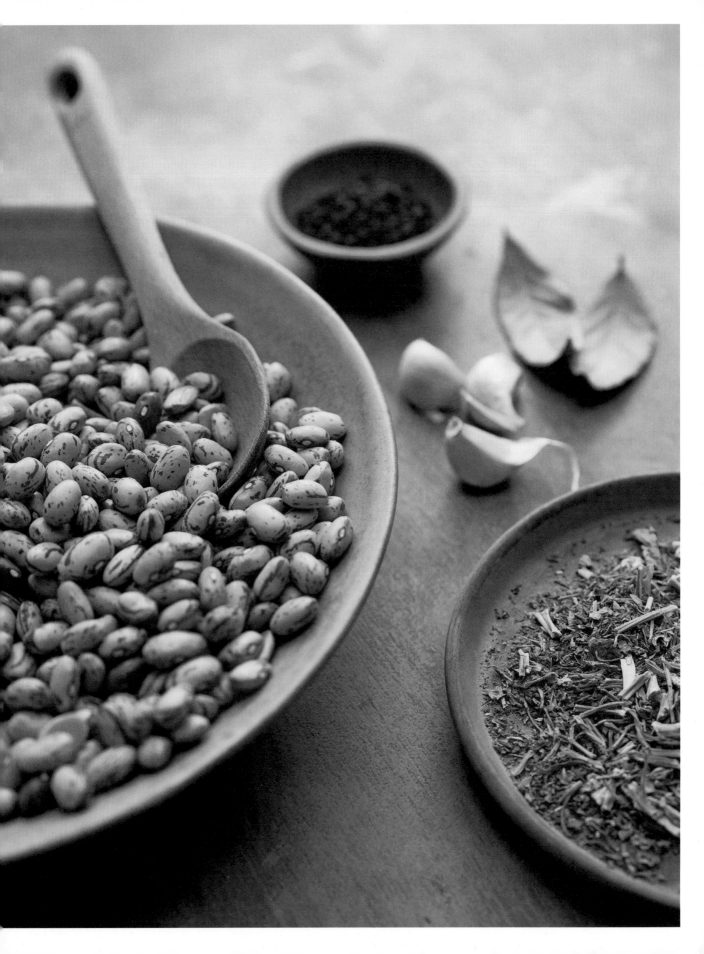

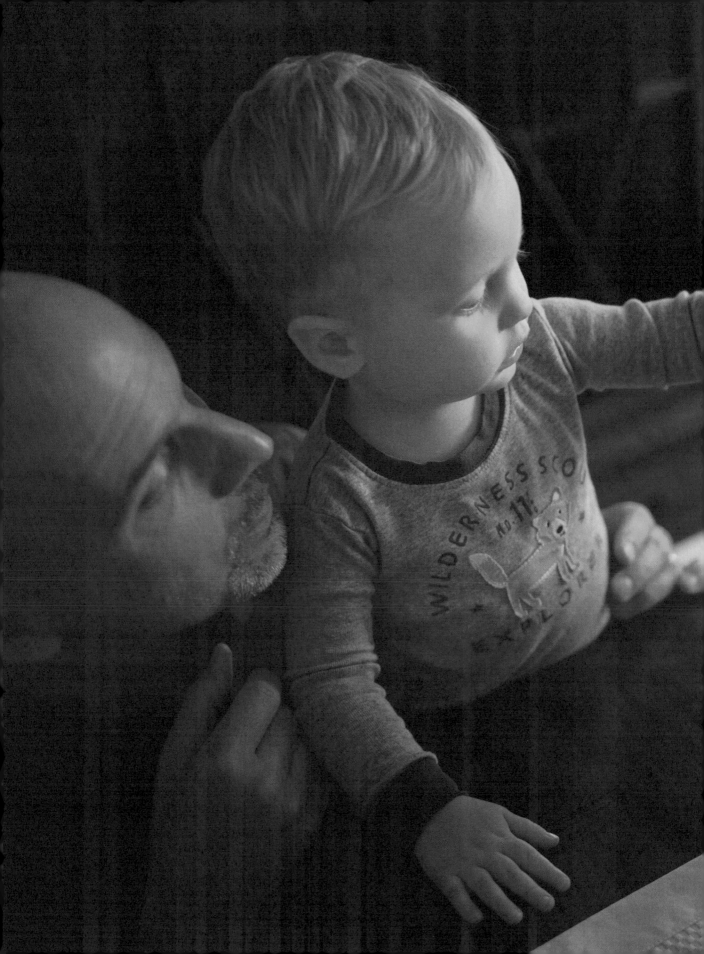

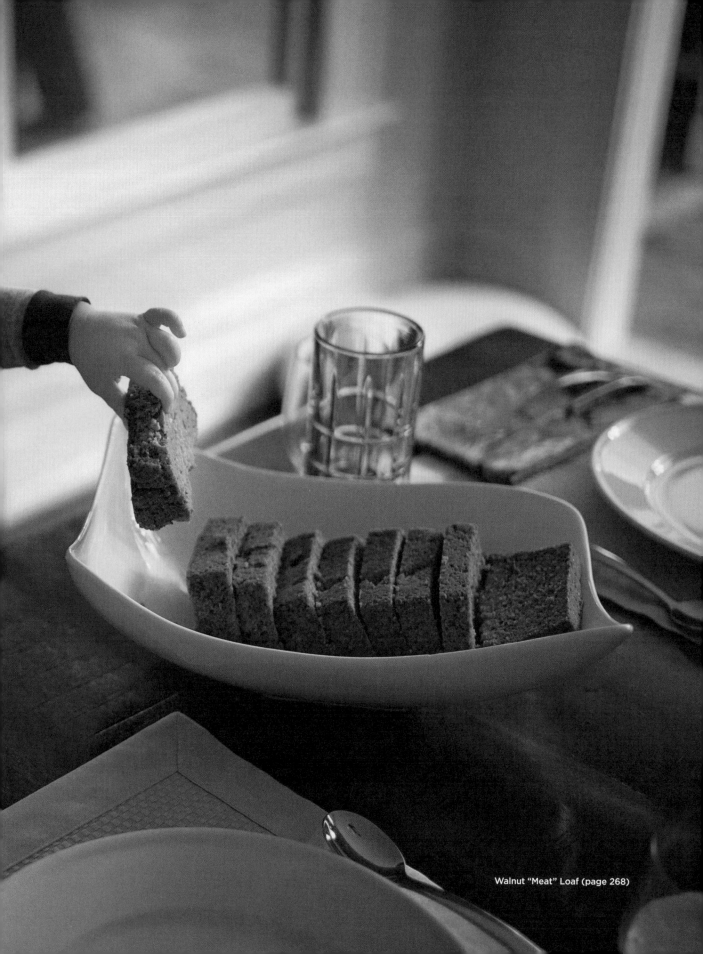

Walnut "Meat" Loaf (page 268)

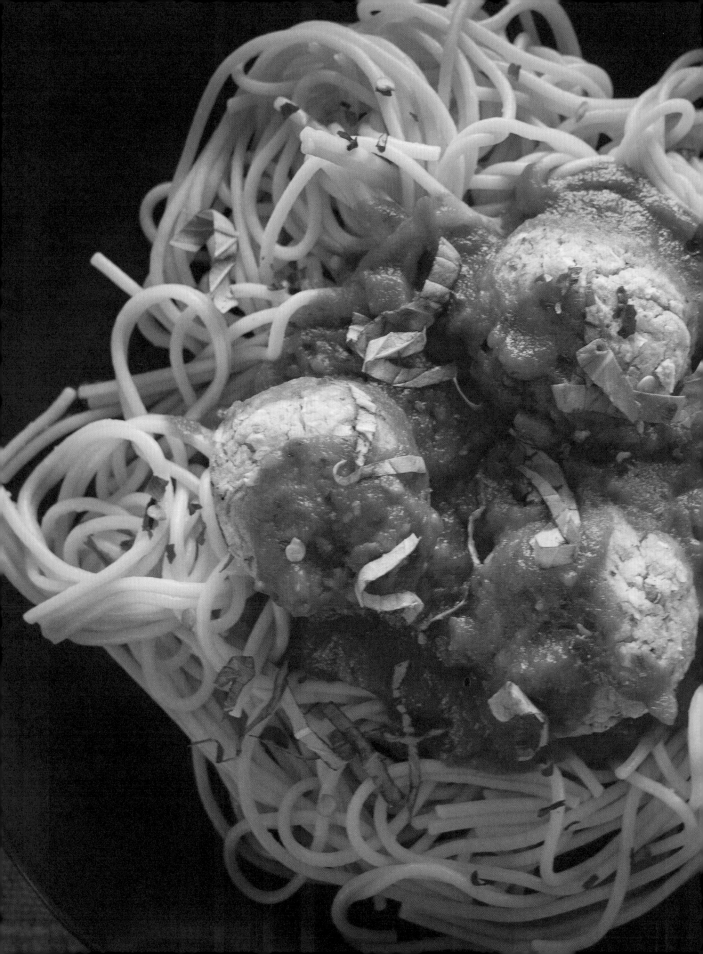

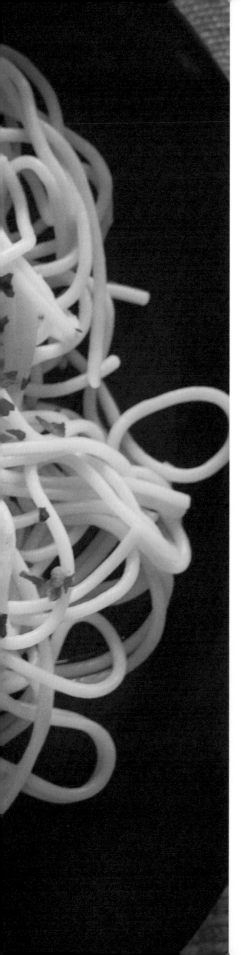

Veggie No-Meat Balls

TOTAL COOK TIME: 35 MINUTES | MAKES 4 SERVINGS

Serve these simple and savory chickpea balls over pasta or as a meatball sub in a roll. You can also make them into crumbles to use on grain bowls or in burritos in place of ground meat. However you make them, they're versatile and will freeze well.

2 cups chickpeas, drained, and liquid reserved

4 tablespoons aquafaba (chickpea liquid)

1 clove garlic, minced

½ cup panko bread crumbs, plus more if needed

½ tablespoon garlic powder

2 teaspoons onion powder

1 teaspoon salt

1 teaspoon dried oregano

½ teaspoon dried basil

¼ teaspoon pepper

½ teaspoon cumin

Preheat oven to 450 degrees.

Mash chickpeas with a potato masher in a large bowl until mostly crushed.

Stir in the remaining ingredients until combined; add more bread crumbs if mixture feels too wet and sticky. If it seems too dry, add an additional teaspoon of aquafaba at a time.

Form the chickpea mixture into balls and place onto an oiled or parchment-lined baking pan.

Bake for 20-25 minutes, turning over halfway.

Serve over whole-wheat noodles with tomato sauce (page 66).

One-Pot Lasagna Soup

TOTAL COOK TIME: 50 MINUTES | **MAKES 4 SERVINGS**

This easy-to-make soup has the comforting goodness of lasagna—but without the complicated preparation. It's also a lighter riff on the classic layered pasta dish that's made hearty with lentils and vegetables. Full of Mediterranean flavors like oregano, basil, and garlic, the aromatic broth is enhanced by red wine. (Though Adventists traditionally don't drink wine, some do use it in cooking.)

Extra-virgin olive oil, for sautéing

1 medium onion, diced

3 cups vegetable broth, or a combination of 1½ cups water and 1½ cups broth

3 garlic cloves, minced

½ cup dried brown lentils

One 28-ounce can diced tomatoes, with liquid

½ cup red wine

½ tablespoon dried oregano

½ tablespoon dried basil

¼ teaspoon ground nutmeg

½ pound lasagna noodles, broken into pieces

Salt and white pepper (optional)

Tofu ricotta* or cashew cream (page 277), for serving

Basil leaves for garnish

In a large soup pot, sauté the onion in olive oil until tender, about 6-8 minutes.

Place next four ingredients (vegetable broth, garlic, lentils, and tomatoes) into the pot. Bring it to a boil and then reduce to medium-low heat to simmer for 20 minutes.

Stir in wine, herbs, and spices and simmer for 20 more minutes.

While the broth is simmering, cook the lasagna noodles according to package directions.

Add lasagna noodles to the soup; add salt and pepper to taste.

Remove from heat and ladle into individual bowls.

Serve with a generous dollop of tofu ricotta or cashew cream and garnish with basil.

*To make tofu ricotta blend 1 pound extra-firm tofu (drained and patted dry) with 2 teaspoons garlic powder, 1 teaspoon oregano, 1 teaspoon basil, and 1 teaspoon lemon juice until combined; stream in extra-virgin olive oil until you obtain the consistency that you want. If too thick, add water, one tablespoon at a time, to thin out. Add salt and white pepper to taste.

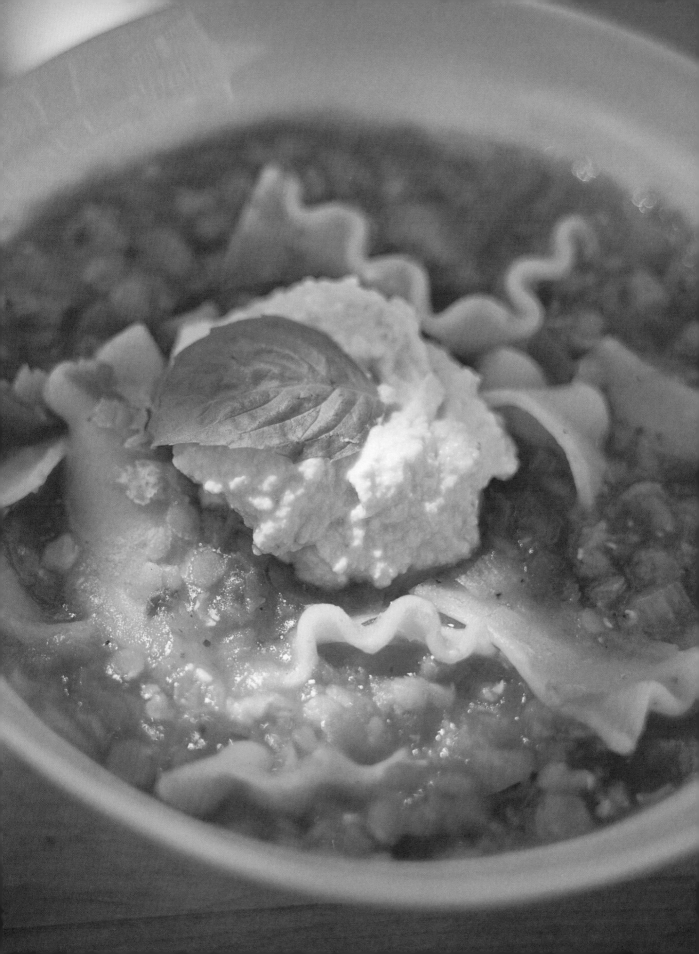

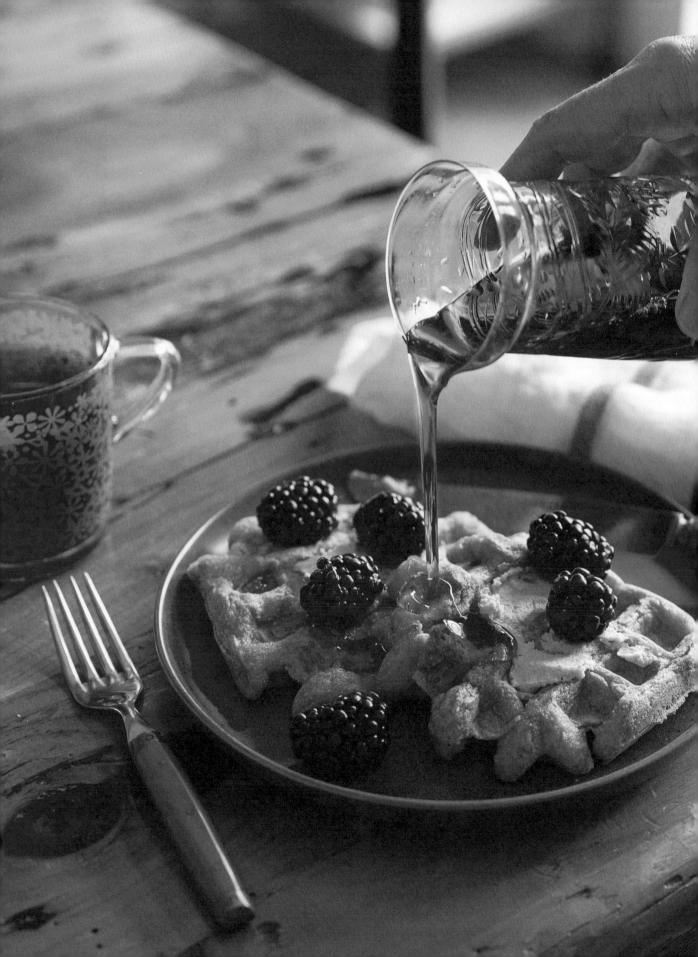

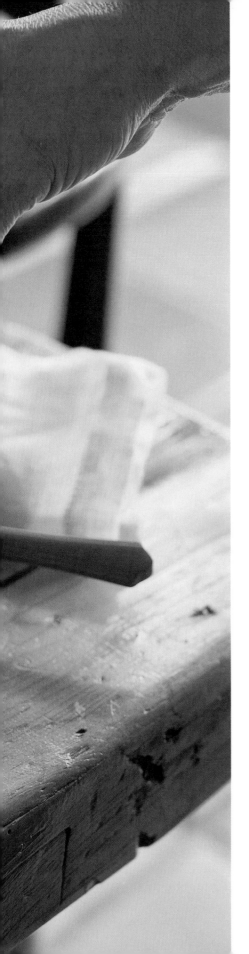

Cornmeal Waffles

TOTAL COOK TIME: 15 MINUTES | MAKES 4 SERVINGS (8 WAFFLES)

These waffles have a complex texture and a complex taste, minus the complex cooking experience. Add in the fact that they're made with whole wheat flour, heart-healthy nuts, and fresh berries and you've got a powerhouse breakfast or a fun breakfast-for-dinner meal.

The Batter:
1 cup whole wheat flour or all-purpose flour, or a combination of both

½ cup cornmeal (use blue cornmeal for a striking presentation)

½ teaspoon baking soda

⅛ teaspoon salt

2 tablespoons granulated sugar

2 tablespoons oil

¼ cup applesauce

1¼ cups almond milk

2 tablespoons diced roasted green chilies (optional)

Optional Toppings:
Cashew cream*

Maple syrup with ⅛ teaspoon salt

Blackberries

Granola (page 248)

In a large bowl, mix the dry ingredients (the first five).

Then add in the wet ingredients and chilies (if using, for a U.S. southwestern style) until thoroughly combined.

Heat a waffle iron and spray with oil.

Cook the waffles for 3 to 4 minutes.

Serve immediately with toppings of your choice.

*To make cashew cream (useful in everything from creamy soups to pasta sauces to puddings): Blend 1 cup raw cashews (soaked 3 hours or overnight in hot water and drained) with ½ cup water in a blender or food processor at high speed. Blend until completely smooth. Drizzle in extra water as needed to reach desired consistency. Try these flavor varieties:

Vegan sour cream: Mix cashew cream with a squeeze of lemon.

Cashew whipped cream: Combine with 1 teaspoon vanilla extract and 1 to 2 tablespoons maple syrup.

Vegan Alfredo sauce: Add minced garlic, blend, and stir with salt and pepper to taste.

Caesar dressing: Mix with minced garlic and nutritional yeast, lemon juice, and black pepper.

Sweet Potato Black Bean Burger

TOTAL COOK TIME: 35 MINUTES | MAKES 4 SERVINGS

This burger is a longevity powerhouse. Loaded with beans, greens, sweet potatoes, and pepitas, it's the perfect example of a blue zones–inspired twist on a classic American comfort food.

The Patty and Buns:
1½ cups rolled oats

1 cup peeled, mashed, cooked sweet potato

1 cup mashed black beans

½ teaspoon salt

2 teaspoons onion powder

1 teaspoon ground cumin

1 teaspoon smoked paprika

½ teaspoon black pepper

½ teaspoon chipotle powder, optional

Oil for cooking

4 whole wheat burger buns

The Sauce:
¼ cup toasted pepitas

¼ cup good-quality salsa verde

The Toppings:
1 avocado, sliced

½ cup loosely packed sliced kale

Pickled or thinly sliced raw red onion*

To make the patties, pulse the rolled oats in a food processor until coarsely ground and set aside.

Combine the sweet potato, black beans, salt, and spices; then incorporate the ground oats. Let this sit for about 5 minutes so flavors can marry.

Form the mixture into 4 patties. In a skillet, heat a thin layer of oil over medium heat.

Add the patties and fry on both sides until crisped, about 4 minutes per side.

To make the sauce: Puree the pepitas and salsa verde in a food processor or blender and set aside.

Build your burger: Mash the avocado and spread on the bottom bun. Then, add your patty and top with the pepita sauce. Finish off the burger with kale and red onion, then the top bun.

*To pickle red onions, submerge them in white vinegar with a generous pinch of salt for at least 6 hours.

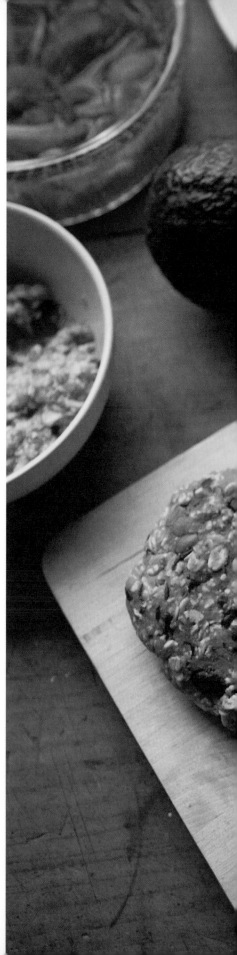

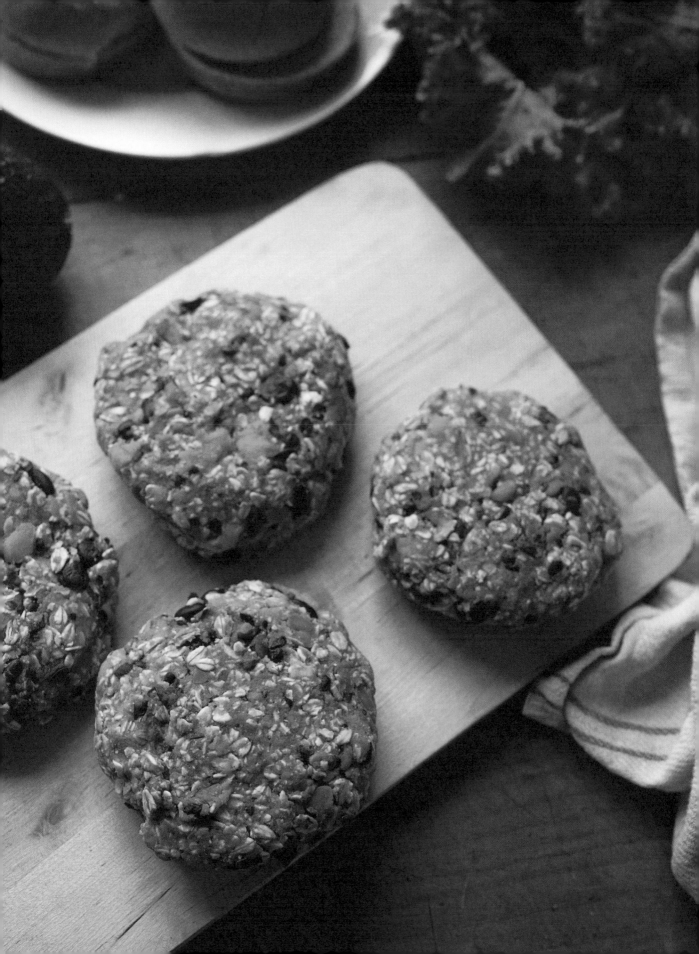

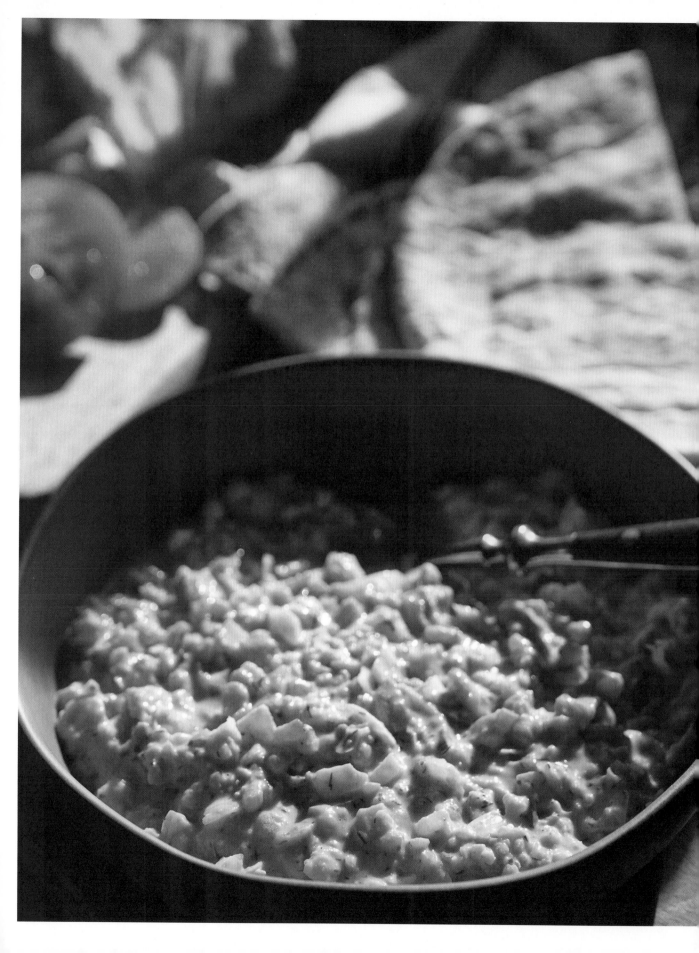

No-Tuna Tuna Salad (left)

TOTAL PREP TIME: 10 MINUTES | MAKES 2 SERVINGS

This creamy chickpea salad is a healthier take on tuna salad that hews more closely to what people eat in blue zones hot spots. Although people assume that centenarians in Sardinia, Italy, and Ikaria, Greece, eat a lot of fish, beans and legumes are the true cornerstones of their daily diet. This salad is unbelievably delicious and easy to make in bulk. You can serve it inside whole wheat sandwich bread or pita, with crackers and veggies as a dip, or on top of a green salad.

One 15-ounce can chickpeas, drained with some liquid reserved

1 tablespoon aquafaba (liquid from the canned chickpeas)

3 tablespoons vegan mayonnaise

2 teaspoons Dijon mustard

1 tablespoon maple syrup or agave nectar

¼ cup diced sweet onion

¼ cup diced celery

¼ cup relish

Salt and pepper (optional)

Kelp seasoning (optional)

Place the chickpeas in a mixing bowl and mash with a potato masher or large fork, but keep them chunky.

Add remaining ingredients and mix well to combine—add more mayo or mustard, if needed, for desired creaminess or taste.

Add salt and pepper to taste and kelp seasoning, if using.

TLT Sammy (Tempeh, Lettuce, and Tomato)

TOTAL PREP TIME: 2 HOURS | MAKES 3 SERVINGS

We love this simple, meat-free take on one of America's classic sandwiches, the BLT. Whole wheat bread, greens, and avocado make it a longevity recipe. If you don't want to make your own, you can buy already-seasoned tempeh in health food and specialty grocery stores. Tempeh, a fermented soybean cake with a nutty texture and flavor, also has the added benefits that come with fermentation.

3 tablespoons extra-virgin olive oil

5 tablespoons soy sauce or tamari

1 tablespoon balsamic vinegar

1 tablespoon maple syrup

8 ounces tempeh, cut into ⅓-inch-thick strips

6 pieces sliced hearty whole grain or sourdough bread

1 avocado, sliced (or guacamole)

Hummus, mustard, or vegan mayonnaise

1 tomato, sliced

1 cup greens like romaine, spinach, and/or sprouts

Whisk together oil, soy sauce, vinegar, and maple syrup. Pour over tempeh and marinate 1-2 hours.

In a sauté pan over medium-high heat, cook the tempeh for a couple minutes on each side, until browned. Then let cool.

Assemble your sandwich: Toast bread (if desired) and slather with smashed avocado and hummus, mustard, or mayo. Top with tomato, greens, tempeh, and another dressed slice of bread.

4-Ingredient Chocolate Mousse Pie

TOTAL COOK TIME: 35 MINUTES | MAKES 8 SERVINGS

American Seventh-day Adventists have learned to use plant foods like tofu to reinvent classic comfort-food dishes like chocolate mousse pie in a healthier way. This four-ingredient recipe doesn't require any baking, and it's fantastic enough for special occasions. This will charm even the biggest chocolate mousse lover; your guests won't know it's dairy-free unless you tell them!

1¾ cups semisweet chocolate chips

12 ounces silken tofu, drained, patted dry

½ cup vanilla almond milk

Ready-made graham cracker pie crust

Berries or chopped nuts, for topping (optional)

Melt the chocolate chips over a double boiler or in the microwave in 30-second increments.

Puree melted chocolate in a blender with tofu and almond milk until smooth, about 1 minute.

Pour the mixture into your crust and smooth with a knife. Cover and freeze until set, about 30 minutes.

Serve topped with berries or chopped nuts of your choice, if you'd like.

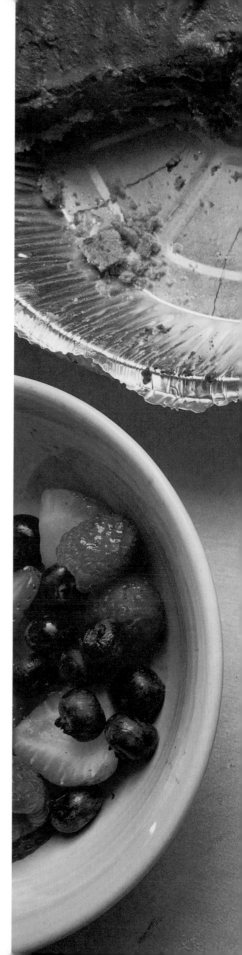

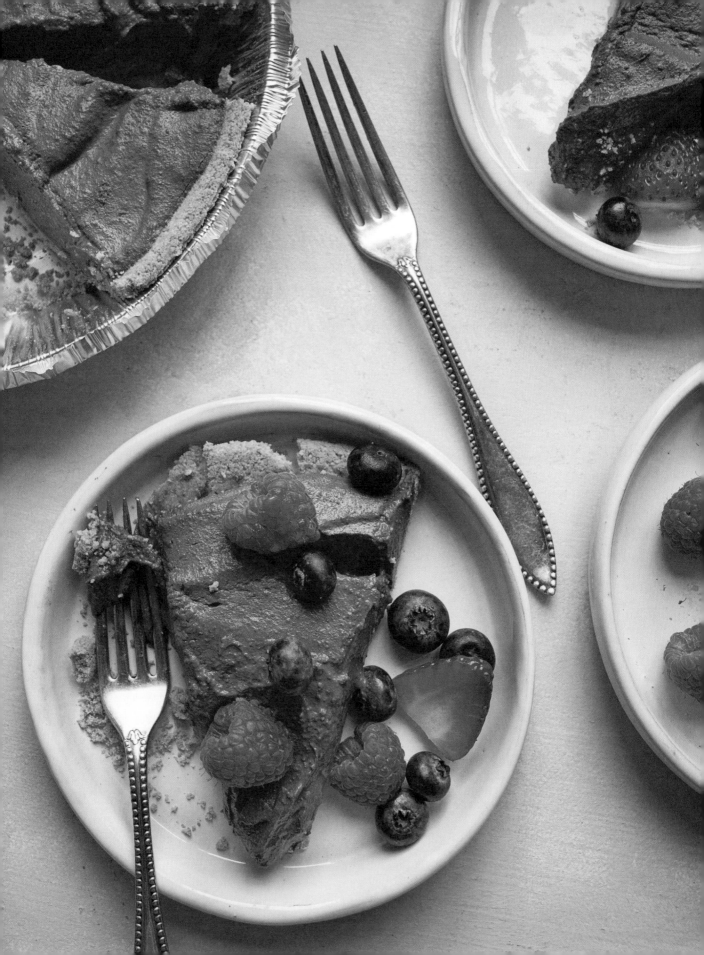

ADVENTIST STAPLES

Although health and wellness are part of the Seventh-day Adventist faith, keeping a strict plant-based diet is open to interpretation by congregants. Therefore, while most Adventists follow a vegetarian or vegan diet, every member of the church eats a little differently. Nevertheless, the Adventist staples usually remain consistent: whole grains, vegetables, legumes, fruits, nuts, and soy products, and a minimal amount of processed foods and food additives.

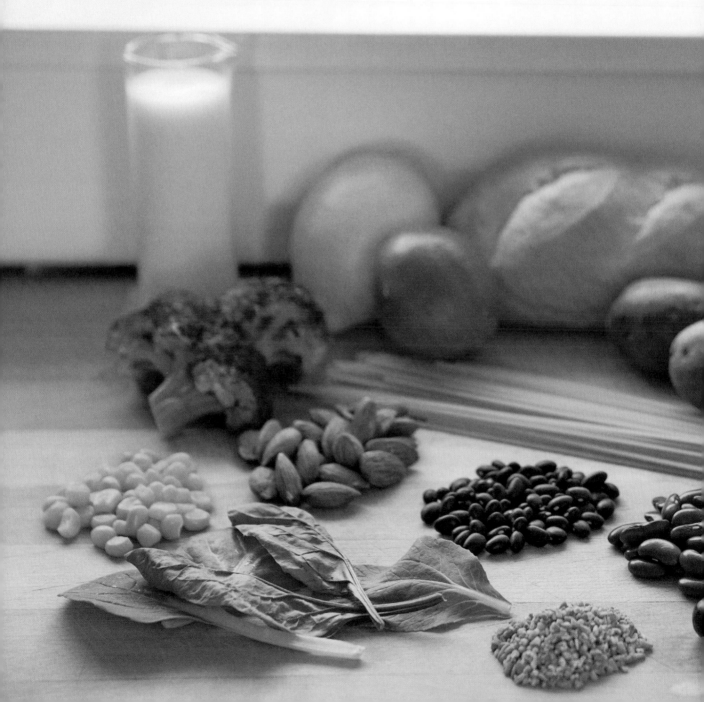

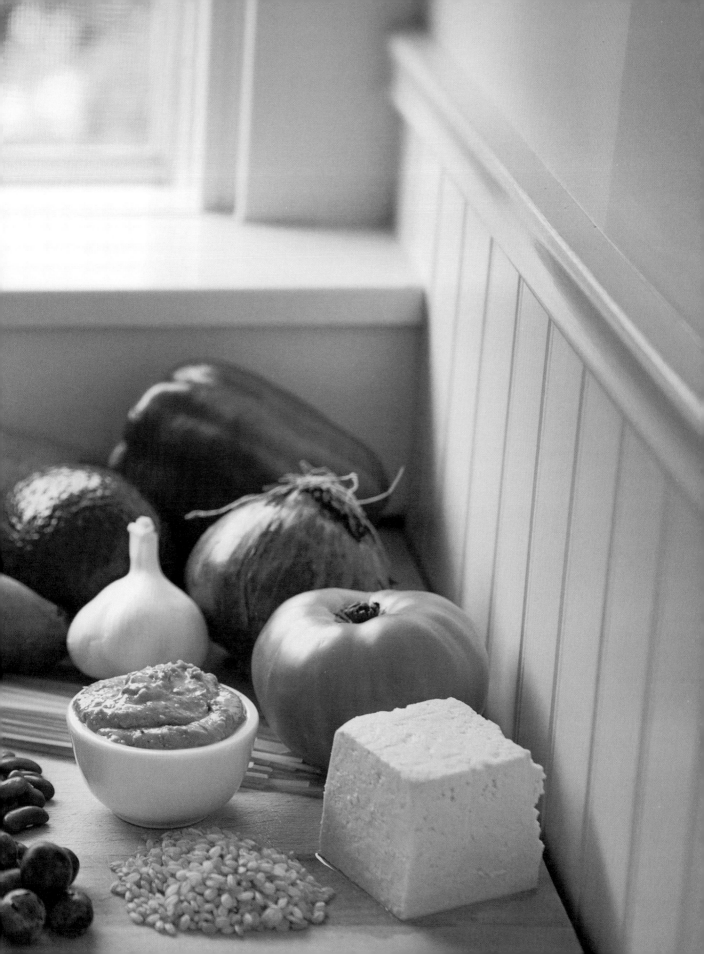

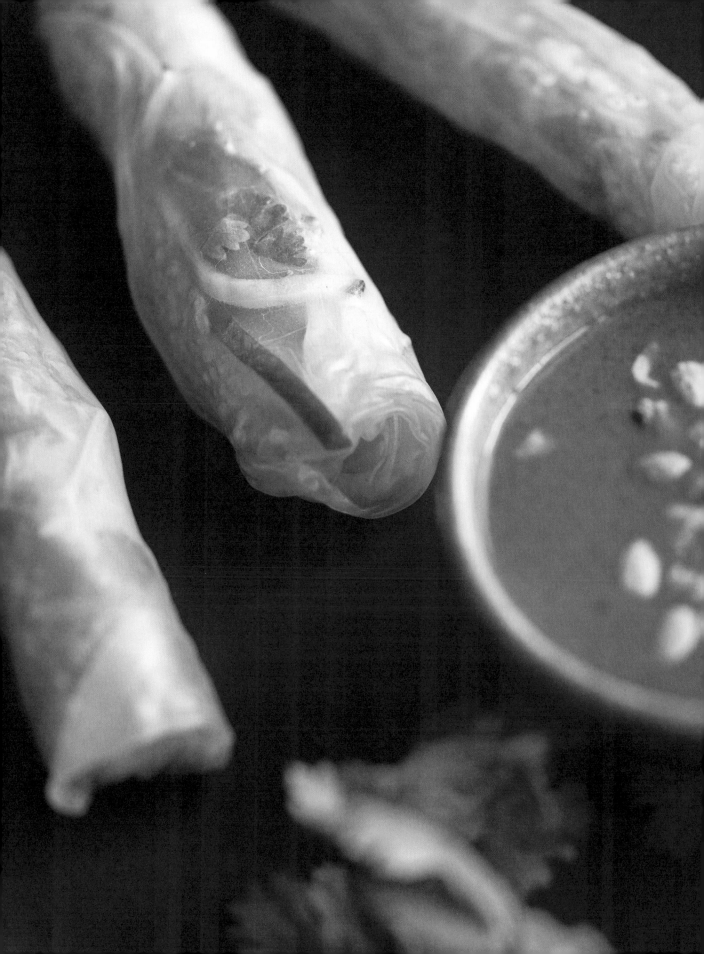

Quinoa-Stuffed Spring Rolls With Peanut Dipping Sauce

TOTAL COOK TIME: 20 MINUTES | MAKES 5 SERVINGS

These fresh no-cook spring rolls are easy to prepare but impressive when served. Feel free to also play around with the fillings—you can easily swap the quinoa for rice noodles or use Thai basil instead of cilantro.

Beaver Dam Community Hospitals is the lead sponsor for the Blue Zones Project in Dodge County, Wisconsin. Founded in 2017, the hospital system brought in the initiative to combat rising health conditions and obesity levels.

Dozens of organizations, large employers, schools, policymakers, and individuals in Dodge County have signed on to make improvements and enhancements to the health of the entire community. Beaver Dam Community Hospitals is an approved worksite, and its café, serving almost 1,000 meals per day, is also a Blue Zones–approved restaurant. It wasn't too long ago that most major hospitals in America housed fast-food chains, so serving healthy food where people need it most goes a long way in improving the health of an entire community.

Spring Rolls:
⅓ cup quinoa, rinsed

10 spring roll rice paper wrappers

1 carrot, peeled and matchstick julienned

1 cucumber, matchstick julienned

1 red pepper, matchstick julienned

Handful of cilantro (or any herb you desire)

Peanut Dipping Sauce:
¼ cup natural creamy peanut butter

1 tablespoon low-sodium soy sauce

2 teaspoons chopped garlic

1 teaspoon sriracha hot sauce (optional)

Chopped peanuts and red peper flakes (optional, for garnish)

Cook quinoa according to package directions. When done, toss to cool.

While quinoa is cooking, mix all sauce ingredients together on stove over low heat. Whisk until combined and creamy—adding water as needed to get to your desired consistency—then set aside to cool.

Pour warm water into a pan or a bowl big enough to fit the wrappers.

Working with one at a time, submerge wrapper into the water until it becomes tender but not soft. This can take anywhere from 20 to 90 seconds, depending on how old the rice papers are.

Quickly move wrapper to a dry surface and pat excess water off the wrapper.

Place a small amount of carrot, cucumber, pepper, quinoa, and cilantro in the middle of the rice paper. Do not overstuff.

Carefully roll the paper, starting from the bottom and pulling in the sides until you have rolled a tight spring roll.

Serve spring rolls with dipping sauce. Garnish with peanuts and red pepper flakes, if using.

* By Chef Kylie Peltier, Beaver Dam Community Hospitals Inc. Café, Blue Zones Project, Dodge County, Wisconsin

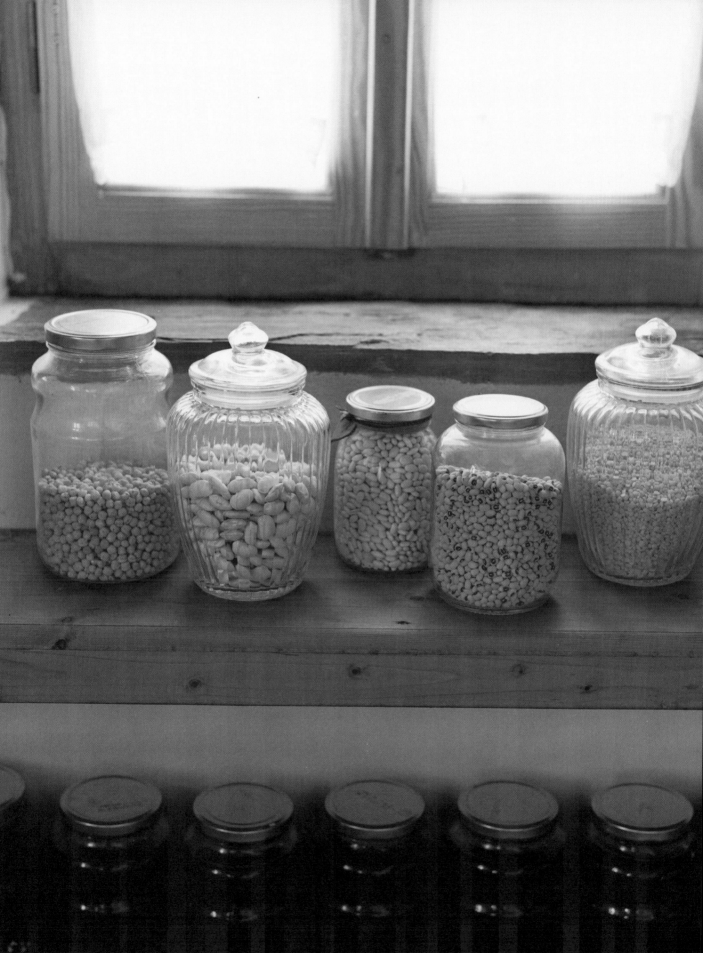

How to Cook Beans

Beans and legumes (like lentils), compared with any other food, are the most important dietary predictor of longevity. They are also affordable and probably offer the best bang for your nutritional buck than any other food out there.

As a rule, one pound of dried beans (about 2 cups) makes 5 to 6 cups of cooked beans. That means 1 cup of dried beans makes 2.5 to 3 cups of cooked beans.

THE PREP

RINSE: Rinse dried beans well, discarding any dirt or rocks.

OVERNIGHT SOAK: Put beans in a pot and cover with 2 inches of water at the top. Let soak for 8 hours or overnight. Drain beans before cooking.

QUICK SOAK: Put beans in a pot and cover with 2 inches of water at the top. Bring beans and water to boil on the stove and remove from heat. Let beans soak, covered, for 90 minutes. Drain beans before cooking.

Note: Some legumes, like lentils and split peas, do not need to be soaked. Also, if you don't have time to soak, you can still cook your beans on the stovetop or using the other methods below. You will just need to cook your beans for longer, sometimes even for double the cooking time.

HOW TO COOK

On the stovetop: In a soup pot, bring beans and water to a boil. Use 3 to 4 cups of water for each cup of beans or legumes. Generally, larger beans will need 4 cups and smaller ones will need 3. So use 3 cups water for 1 cup of lentils, soybeans, and split peas and 4 cups water for 1 cup of chickpeas and black beans. Reduce heat to medium-low to simmer. Use the guide below for how long to let beans simmer. Beans are done when they are tender and cooked through (but not mushy). Let cool in cooking liquid.

BEANS AND LEGUMES COOKING TIME ON THE STOVETOP

- **Adzuki beans:** 1 hour
- **Black beans:** 90 minutes to 2 hours
- **Black-eyed peas:** 1 hour to 90 minutes
- **Cannellini beans:** 2 to 2½ hours
- **Chickpeas:** 2 to 2½ hours
- **Fava beans:** 45 minutes
  (skins removed after soaking)
- **Great northern beans:** 90 minutes
- **Kidney beans:** 2 hours

- **Lentils, brown or green:** 25 to 30 minutes
  (no soaking required)
- **Lentils, red or yellow:** 15 to 20 minutes
- **Lima beans:** 90 minutes to 2 hours
  (no soaking required)
- **Pinto beans:** 90 minutes
- **Red beans:** 2¼ hours
- **Soybeans:** 3 hours
- **Split peas:** 45 minutes to 1 hour
  (no soaking required)

PRESSURE COOKER: Put soaked and drained beans in pressure cooker. Cover with hot or boiling water, making sure not to fill the cooker more than half full. Cook on high pressure for 2 to 18 minutes, depending on the type of beans.

SLOW COOKER: Put soaked and drained beans in slow cooker. Cover with hot or boiling water. Cook for 2 to 4 hours on high, depending on the type of beans.

Note: You can save your cooked bean liquid and use as a veggie stock.

Tip: While cooking your beans, you can add herbs to add flavor and aid in digestion. These herbs include cumin, bay leaves, fennel, and fresh epazote (available in Latin markets).

Top Longevity Ingredients From Sardinia

The typical daily diet of a Sardinian shepherd in 1943 included consumption of meat and dairy products that came almost entirely from eating milk and cheese from sheep and goats. Almost half of the daily intake consisted of grains, and a fourth came from dairy. The average wine consumption was 114 grams (4 ounces) a day. The Sardinian diet was influenced after World War II and again in the 1970s, when American foods like burgers were introduced.

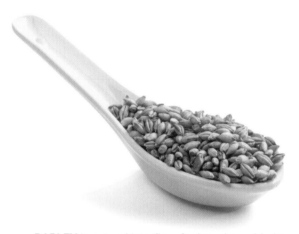

BARLEY is ground into flour for bread or added to soups. It's the food most highly associated with Sardinian men living to 100.

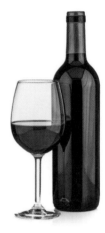

CANNONAU WINE—Sardinia's distinctive red—is made from sun-stressed Grenache grapes. Sardinians drink an average of three to four small glasses of it a day.

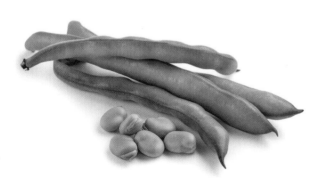

FAVA BEANS are eaten in soups and stews in Sardinia and deliver loads of protein and fiber. They are one of the foods most associated with living to 100.

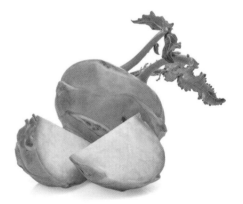

KOHLRABI contains many longevity nutrients, including copper, manganese, iron, and potassium, and it is also a rich source of fiber and calcium.

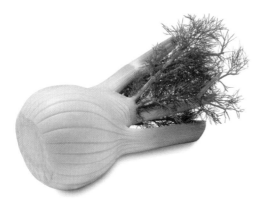

FENNEL is used as a vegetable (its bulb), an herb (its fronds), and a spice (its seeds), and is rich in fiber and vitamins A, B, and C. It's also a good diuretic, helping to maintain healthy blood pressure.

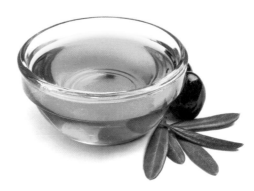

OLIVE OIL has many longevity benefits, including anti-inflammatory properties and healthy monounsaturated fats.

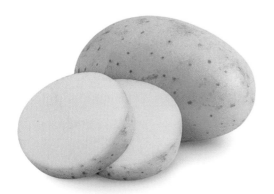

POTATOES are added to minestrone in Sardinia and help lower cholesterol and the risk of heart disease.

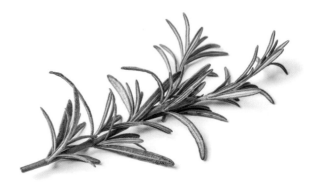

ROSEMARY, often picked fresh in Sardinian gardens, helps enhance memory, improve digestion, and prevent brain aging and cancer.

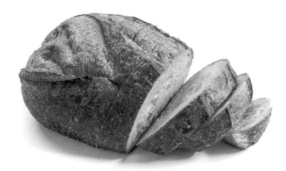

SOURDOUGH BREAD (*moddizzosu*) is made from whole wheat and live lactobacillus (instead of yeast), which gives the bread its lower glycemic index.

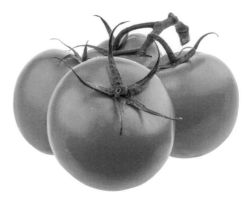

TOMATOES are a rich source of vitamin C and potassium and are used to make sauces that top Sardinian breads and pasta dishes.

Top Longevity Ingredients From Okinawa

Sweet potatoes represented two-thirds of the typical daily diet of Okinawans in 1949. Through the postwar decades, islanders continued to eat more greens as well as more yellow, orange, and red vegetables than other Japanese.

Okinawans also tended to eat more meat—primarily pork—than other Japanese, but at the same time, they ate less fish, less salt, and much less added sugar. Today, the Western influence has changed the island with fast and processed foods, and it is now one of the unhealthiest Japanese prefectures.

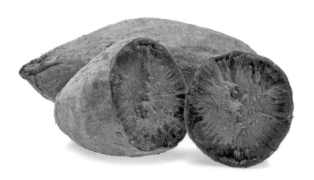

IMO is a supercharged purple sweet potato that doesn't cause blood sugar to spike as much as a regular white potato.

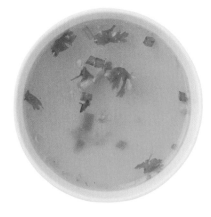

DASHI BROTH is rich in amino acids, which are fundamental to keeping your body healthy.

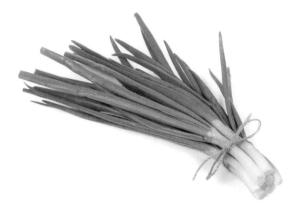

GREEN ONIONS are an excellent source of vitamin K and vitamin C and can be used top to bottom.

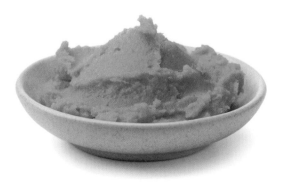

MISO is rich in various vitamins. Because it is fermented, it provides loads of beneficial gut bacteria.

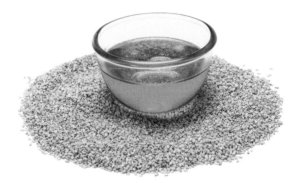

SESAME OIL is high in zinc and copper and is known to boost heart health and improve circulation.

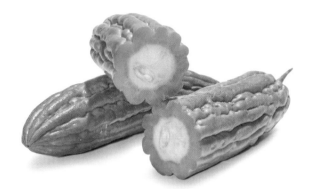

BITTER MELON, known as *goya,* is an effective antidiabetic food and helps regulate blood sugar. It is also the base of many *champuru,* or stir-fry, dishes.

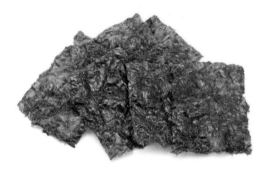

SEAWEED AND KELP in general provide a filling, low-calorie nutrient boost to the diet. They are rich in carotenoids, folate, magnesium, iron, calcium, and iodine.

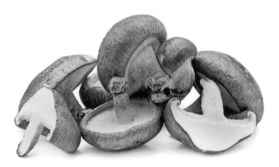

MUSHROOMS, particularly shiitake, contain more than 100 compounds with immune-protecting properties.

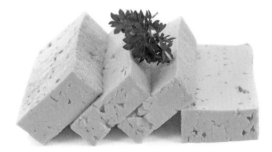

TOFU is eaten in Okinawa like bread in France. Studies show that people who eat soy products in place of meat have lower cholesterol and a lower risk of heart disease.

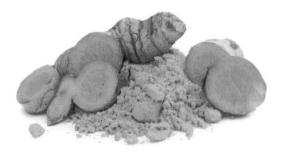

TURMERIC—ginger's golden cousin— is a powerful anticancer, antioxidant, and anti-inflammatory agent.

Top Longevity Ingredients From Nicoya

In the traditional diet of the people who live on Costa Rica's Nicoya Peninsula, about 80 percent of the daily calories come from different types of carbohydrates, including grains that add up to about 26 percent of their typical diet, with the remaining 20 percent of calories coming from various proteins and fats in about equal measure.

Black beans are eaten every day, often at every meal. The black beans they depend on contain more antioxidants than any other bean and are arguably the best in the world.

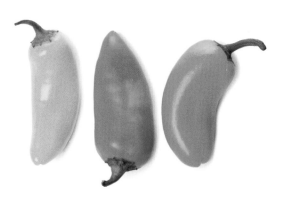

SMALL SWEET PEPPERS are rich in vitamins, especially vitamin C. There are several health benefits from eating them, including reduced risk of a number of chronic diseases.

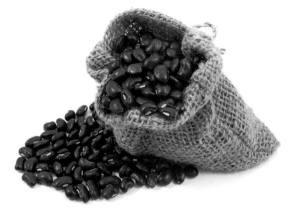

BLACK BEANS are full of fiber and protein. The soluble fiber in them helps reduce bad cholesterol. The insoluble fiber aids digestion.

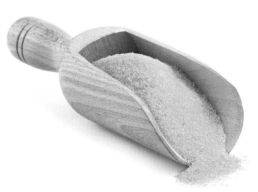

GROUND CORN, or *nixtamal,* is used to make tortillas eaten at breakfast, lunch, and dinner. It increases the body's ability to absorb calcium, iron, and minerals.

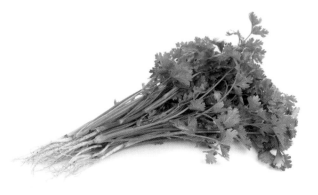

CILANTRO is an herb used in many Nicoyan dishes. It's known to help lower blood sugar levels and reduce the risk of cardiovascular diseases. It also aids digestion.

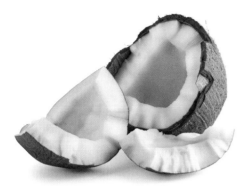

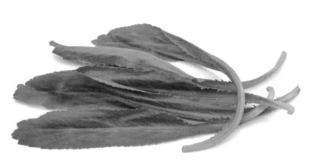

COCONUT is a good source of healthy saturated fats that actually boost fat burning. It also increases HDL cholesterol (the good kind), which is linked to a lower risk of heart disease.

CULANTRO, also known as Mexican coriander, is related to cilantro but with a much stronger flavor. It is rich in calcium, iron, and riboflavin.

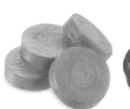
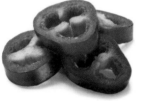

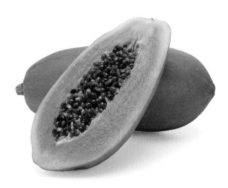

CHILERO SAUCE, probably the most popular condiment in Costa Rica, gives a probiotic boost to dishes from its vinegar and its antioxidant and antibacterial properties from its peppers.

PAPAYA TREES grow almost like weeds in Nicoya. The rich orange flesh of their fruit contains vitamins A, C, and E, plus papain, which counters inflammation.

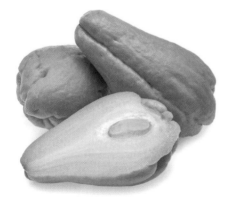

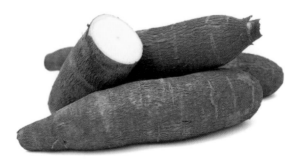

SQUASH, available in several varieties, belong to the botanical family Cucurbitaceae, known for providing high levels of useful carotenoids.

YUCA are a good source of vitamin C and antioxidants. Basically, it's a powerhouse for boosting immunity and fighting infections and viruses.

Top Longevity Ingredients From Ikaria

Older Ikarians eat a diet rich in greens and other vegetables as well as beans and fruit, which together account for 64 percent of their daily food intake—dairy products and beverages excluded. Fat accounts for a large percentage of their daily calories, but more than half the fat energy comes from olive oil, associated with positive health factors in a number of studies. Ikarians eat the purest form of the Mediterranean diet—heavier in beans and greens and lighter in fish and meat.

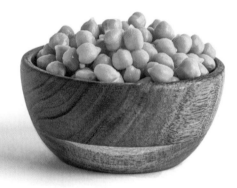

BEANS, particularly chickpeas and black-eyed peas, are eaten like a snack or added to soups and stews. Though chickpeas can be high in fat, nearly all of it is unsaturated.

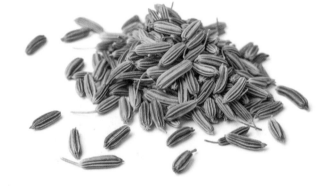

FENNEL, from bulb to seeds, is packed with nutrients, including calcium, iron, manganese, and potassium. Ikarians use it in cooking as well as in herbal teas.

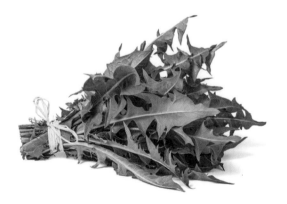

WILD GREENS like purslane, dandelion, and arugula are a great source of minerals as well as carotenoids—the colorful pigments the body converts to vitamin A.

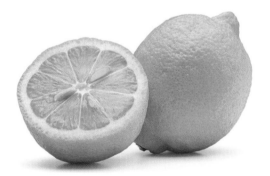

LEMONS are eaten whole, skin and all, in Ikaria. The peel may have a beneficial impact on blood glucose, helping to control or prevent diabetes.

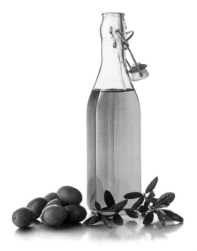

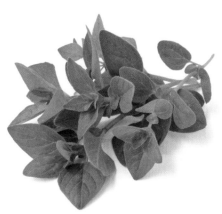

OLIVE OIL, of which Ikarians eat at least four table-spoons a day, may protect against heart disease. It's also why one study suggests Ikarians have a 50 percent lower mortality rate.

OREGANO is one of the many herbs used in Ikarian cooking. It's rich in antioxidants and compounds proved to help fight bacteria.

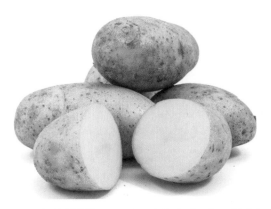

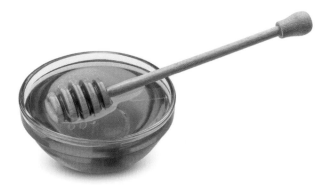

POTATOES are eaten daily in Ikaria, which is unlike other Mediterranean diets. Studies suggest potatoes can reduce blood pressure, fight diabetes, and prevent inflammation.

HONEY is used by the islanders to treat everything from colds to wounds. Besides stirring it into coffee, older Ikarians also take a spoonful in the morning and before dinner.

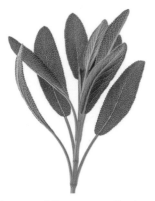

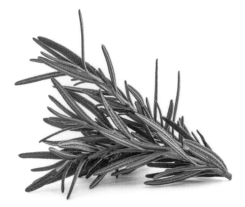

SAGE may be one of the reasons Ikarians have lower rates of Alzheimer's and dementia; it also has proper-ties that help strengthen bones.

ROSEMARY, shown to improve digestion and enhance memory, is used quite often in herbal teas throughout Ikaria.

Top Longevity Ingredients From Loma Linda

More than 50 percent of the Adventist diet comes from fruits and vegetables, according to the Adventist Health Study 2, one of the few large health studies to focus on different ethnicities and how they eat. The remainder of their diet mostly comes from legumes, soy, and grains. Adventists were decades ahead of the rest of the United States in experimenting with and using ethnic and international ingredients and flavors in their cooking.

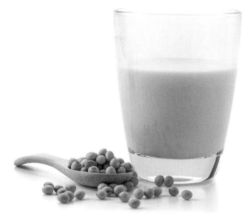

SOY MILK—not the sweetened, flavored kind—is used as an alternative to dairy. High in protein and low in fat, it contains phytoestrogens, which may protect against some types of cancer.

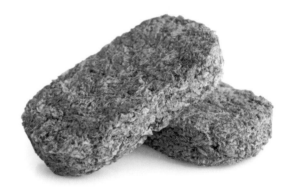

WEETABIX is a whole grain cereal mostly sold in England. Adding whole grains to your diet promotes skin and bone health, and keeps you regular, among other benefits.

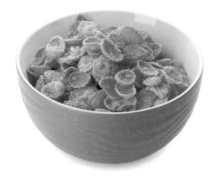

CORN FLAKES are a staple of the Adventist breakfast and are rich in vitamins and minerals like folate and thiamine.

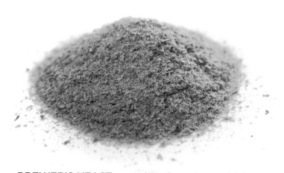

BREWER'S YEAST contains chromium, which may help control blood sugar levels and improve glucose tolerance. It also has immune-boosting properties.

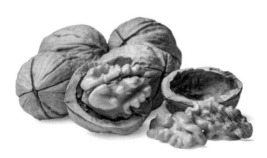

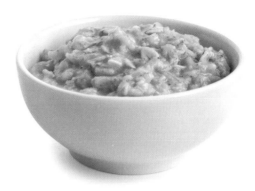

NUTS, as well as nut butters, are key to the Adventist diet. One study found that those who ate a handful of nuts at least five times a week lived two to three years longer than those who didn't eat any nuts.

OATMEAL is a staple for Adventists. Slow-cooked, it provides a balanced portion of fats, complex carbs, and plant protein, along with good doses of iron and B vitamins.

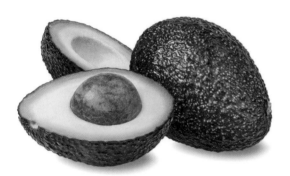

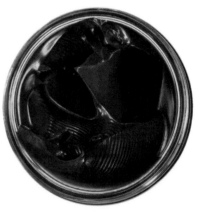

AVOCADOS are high in potassium and low in salt; they also may help reduce blood pressure and the risk of stroke. Ounce for ounce, they contain 30 percent more potassium than a banana.

VEGEMITE is an Australian spread made from brewer's yeast, salt, and vegetable extract. It is perfect for topping whole wheat toast and an excellent source of vitamins that support brain health.

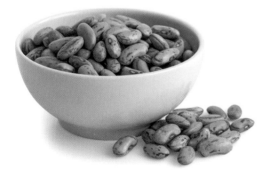

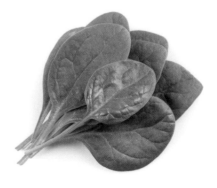

BEANS, like in all blue zones, are king. For the vegetarian Adventists, beans, lentils, and peas represent an important daily protein source.

SPINACH, or other green vegetables like broccoli, provides essential vitamins, minerals, and fiber to the Adventist diet.

Metric Conversions

The recipes in this book were developed using standard U.S. measures following U.S. government guidelines. The charts below offer equivalents for U.S. and metric measures. All conversions are approximate and have been rounded up or down to the nearest whole number.

WEIGHT CONVERSIONS

ounces	grams
½	14
¾	21
1	28
1½	43
2	57
2½	71
3	85
3½	99
4	113
4½	128
5	142
6	170
7	198
8	227
9	255
10	283
12	340
16 (1 pound)	454

VOLUME CONVERSIONS

U.S.	metric
1 teaspoon	5 milliliters
2 teaspoons	10 milliliters
1 tablespoon	15 milliliters
2 tablespoons	30 milliliters
¼ cup	59 milliliters
⅓ cup	79 milliliters
½ cup	118 milliliters
¾ cup	177 milliliters
1 cup	237 milliliters
1¼ cups	296 milliliters
1½ cups	355 milliliters
2 cups (1 pint)	473 milliliters
2½ cups	591 milliliters
3 cups	710 milliliters
4 cups (1 quart)	0.946 liter
1.06 quarts	1 liter
4 quarts (1 gallon)	3.8 liters

OVEN TEMPERATURES

Fahrenheit	Celsius	gas mark
225	105	¼
250	120	½
275	135	1
300	150	2
325	165	3
350	180	4
375	190	5
400	200	6
425	220	7
450	230	8
475	245	9

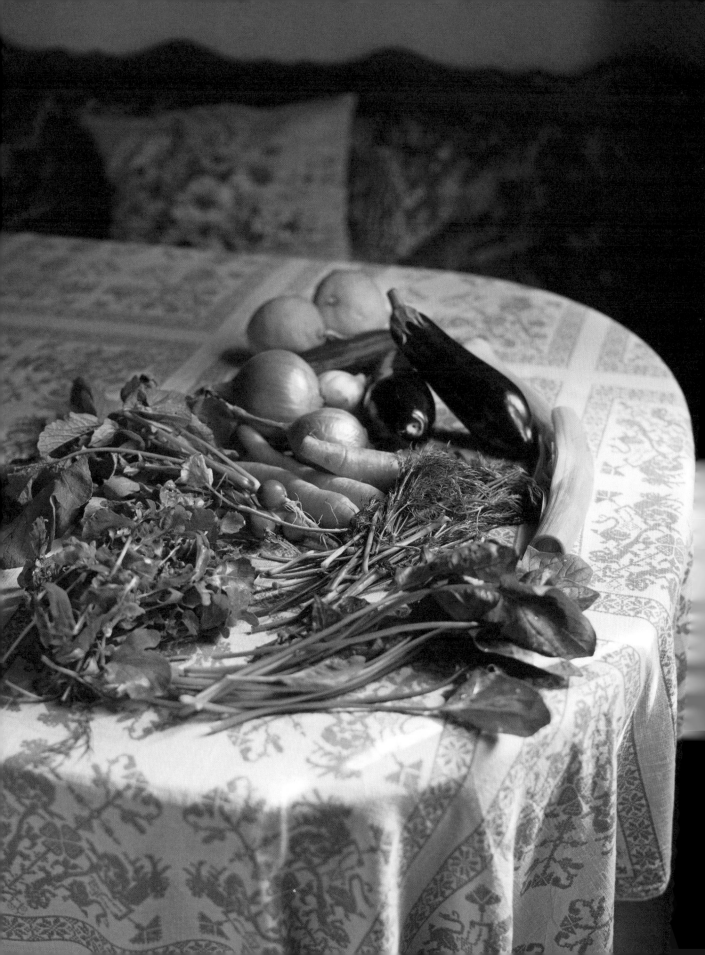

ACKNOWLEDGMENTS

First thanks goes to fellow explorer, photographer David McLain. Fifteen years ago we were wide-eyed, way out over the skies, and with a plum assignment from *National Geographic* when we landed in Sardinia on a mission to find the secret to longevity. We had no idea how big it was. Several articles and four books later, we're back again with this project. He's been a friend and collaborator, and has done more than anyone else to bring the idea of the Blue Zones to life visually. At an age qualifying him as a Blue Zones subject, my dad, Roger Buettner, took to the road to help us track down recipes and loaned us his consummately American palate in deciding whether or not recipes made this book. Because of him, no fermented tofu recipes appear in these pages.

Of the dozens of scientists I've worked with, my first thanks goes to Dr. Gianni Pes, who not only identified Sardinia's blue zone, but nearly two decades later continues to mine insights for the world on living longer and better. For this book, he served as chief scientific consultant as well as a guide in the Sardinian blue zone. He, along with Michel Poulain, founded the concept of Blue Zones with me.

Okinawa's longevity pioneers Drs. Bradley and Craig Willcox, Dr. Makoto Suzuki, and Dr. Hidemi Todoriki provided up-to-date insights on longevity foods. My wonderful fixer, Naomi O'Hara Fujiwara, arranged all the in-home recipe demonstrations along with help from Yukie Miyaguni, Asami Toyokawa, Yoshiki Toyokawa, Sayaka, Mitsuo Nakamoto, Masahiko Tawata, and the Hawaiian wunderkind, Jordon Kondo, who served as a de facto intern on our trip.

Jorge Vindas makes it his business to know every living and emerging centenarian in Nicoya. My fixer since we identified the Nicoya blue zone in 2008, he arranged all the meetings and recipe demonstrations in this book with his affable, can-do attitude, including those with Paulina Villegas, sisters Gioconda and Anabelle Rangel, Xinia Sánchez, and Emilio Briceño Sánchez. Through his Asociación Península de Nicoya Zona Azul foundation, Jorge provides basic necessities to Nicoya's older adults. Stanford's Dr. David Rehkopf provided field insights and did the genetic analysis of the Nicoyan diet. He, along with Luis Rosero Bixby, Dr. Alaro Salas, Dr. Xinia Fenandez Rojas, and the great expert of the Nicoyan diet, Dr. Romano González, all provided scientific input on this book. Dr. Gary Fraser and his work with the Adventist Health Study has informed my work for more than a decade. He's provided new insights for this book.

Thanks to Thea Parikos and Eleni Mazari in Ikaria for always being my home base, guides, and best friends. Also Dr. Christina Chrysohoou for her seminal work on the Ikarian diet. And Athina Mazari, Chrysoula Synagridi, Eleni Karimalis, and Antiopi Koufadaki for sharing their culinary secrets.

Naomi Imatome-Yun, in her quiet fastidiousness, tested all recipes and wrote captions and sidebars; chef Jason Wyrick put expert finishing touches on the recipes. They along with the excellent team at National Geographic including Allyson Johnson, Elisa Gibson, Moira Haney, Melissa Farris, Hilary Black, Moriah Petty, and Judith Klein produced this book. And to Lisa Thomas, my longtime book editor and now National Geographic Books' publisher, congratulations on Blue Zones book #5!

Thanks to my superb team back at Blue Zones headquarters including Amelia Clabots, Aislinn Leonard, Souraya Farhat, and my Right-Hand Man, Sam Skemp. Mostly though, I want to thank my partner, writer Kathy Freston, who helped shape this book, test the recipes, and choose the photos. I look forward to cooking each one of these recipes with you in the years to come.

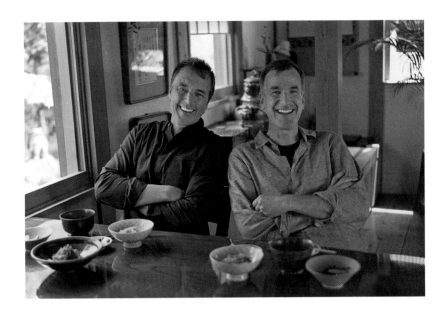

ABOUT THE AUTHOR

DAN BUETTNER is the founder of Blue Zones, an organization that helps Americans live longer, healthier, happier lives. His groundbreaking work on longevity led to his 2005 *National Geographic* cover story, "The Secrets of Long Life," and three national bestsellers: *The Blue Zones, Thrive,* and *The Blue Zones Solution.* He is also the author of *The Blue Zones of Happiness.* He lives in Minneapolis, Minnesota. Visit him on Facebook (facebook.com/BlueZones) and Twitter (@BlueZones), and at bluezones.com.

ABOUT THE PHOTOGRAPHER

DAVID MCLAIN is a Maine-based photographer and filmmaker. Over his career he has shot seven feature-length assignments around the world for *National Geographic;* co-produced and shot *Bounce,* a feature documentary film that premiered at SXSW; and worked around the world for commercial clients including Sony and Apple. McLain has been collaborating with Dan Buettner for the past 20 years and is a founding member of the Sony Artisan program. He lives with his wife and two children in a 220-year-old farmhouse in Maine.

ABOUT THE BLUE ZONES AND BLUE ZONES PROJECT

Blue Zones employs evidence-based ways to help people live longer, better. Beginning in 2004, Dan Buettner teamed with National Geographic and the National Institute on Aging to identify pockets around the world where people lived measurably better, longer lives. After locating the world's blue zones, Buettner took teams of scientists to each location to pinpoint lifestyle characteristics that might explain the unusual longevity. The original research and findings were released in Buettner's best-selling books *The Blue Zones, The Blue Zones Solution,* and *Thrive,* as well as *The Blue Zones of Happiness.*

In 2009, Buettner and Blue Zones worked in partnerships with AARP and the United Health Foundation to apply the Blue Zones principles to Albert Lea, Minnesota. It was a "stunning success," and formed the blueprint for the Blue Zones Project, which has since expanded to 48 communities across the United States, impacting millions of people. This groundbreaking initiative has occasioned double-digit drops in obesity, smoking, and body mass index (BMI).

B̲ͭ̚lue Zones Kitchen

Since 1888, the National Geographic Society has funded more than 13,000 research, exploration, and preservation projects around the world. National Geographic Partners distributes a portion of the funds it receives from your purchase to National Geographic Society to support programs including the conservation of animals and their habitats.

National Geographic Partners
1145 17th Street NW
Washington, DC 20036-4688 USA

Get closer to National Geographic explorers and photographers, and connect with our global community. Join us today at nationalgeographic.com/join

For information about special discounts for bulk purchases, please contact National Geographic Books Special Sales: specialsales@natgeo.com

For rights or permissions inquiries, please contact National Geographic Books Subsidiary Rights: bookrights@natgeo.com

Library of Congress Cataloging-in-Publication Data
Names: Buettner, Dan, author. | McLain, David, (Photographer) photographer.
Title: The Blue Zones kitchen : 100 recipes to live to 100 / Dan Buettner ; photography by David McLain.
Description: Washington, D.C. : National Geographic, 2019.
Identifiers: LCCN 2019012359 (print) | LCCN 2019013534 (ebook) | ISBN 9781426220142 () | ISBN 9781426220135 (trade hardback)
Subjects: LCSH: Cooking. | Blue zones. | LCGFT: Cookbooks.
Classification: LCC TX714 (ebook) | LCC TX714 .B845 2019 (print) | DDC 641.5--dc23
LC record available at https://lccn.loc.gov/2019012359

Printed in China

19/RRDH/1

ILLUSTRATIONS CREDITS

All photos by David McLain unless otherwise noted:

Cover, Oliver Barth; 290 (UP LE), Creativ Studio Heinemann/Getty Images; 290 (UP RT), fcafotodigital/Getty Images; 290 (LO LE), paulista/Shutterstock; 290 (LO RT), Boonchuay1970/Shutterstock; 291 (UP LE), IlonaImagine/Getty Images; 291 (UP RT), Africa Studio/Shutterstock; 291 (CTR LE), Artem Kutsenko/Shutterstock; 291 (CTR RT), Pakorn Kumruen/EyeEm/Getty Images; 291 (LO LE), Kativ/Getty Images; 291 (LO RT), Aleksey Patsyuk/Shutterstock; 292 (UP LE), Akepong Srichaichana/EyeEm/Getty Images; 292 (UP RT), baramee2554/Getty Images; 292 (LO LE), Anastasia Mdivanian/Shutterstock; 292 (LO RT), PicturePartners/Getty Images; 293 (UP LE), Tukaram .Karve/Shutterstock; 293 (UP RT), zevei-wenhui/Getty Images; 293 (CTR LE), Akepong Srichaichana/EyeEm/Getty Images; 293 (CTR RT), Emily Li/Shutterstock; 293 (LO LE), Nipaporn Panyacharoen/Shutterstock; 293 (LO RT), COLOA Studio/Shutterstock; 294 (UP LE), JeniFoto/Shutterstock; 294 (UP RT), onair/Shutterstock; 294 (LO LE), paulista/Shutterstock; 294 (LO RT), Nattawut Lakjit/EyeEm/Getty Images; 295 (UP LE), Alexlukin/Shutterstock; 295 (UP RT), LotusImages16/Getty Images; 295 (CTR LE), anna1311/Getty Images; 295 (CTR), maxsol7/Getty Images; 295 (CTR RT), design56/Getty Images; 295 (LO LE), Boonchuay1970/Shutterstock; 295 (LO RT), Lotus Images/Shutterstock; 296 (UP LE), vaaseenaa/Getty Images; 296 (UP RT), Amy_Lv/Getty Images; 296 (LO LE), Andris Tkachenko/Getty Images; 296 (LO RT), phive/Shutterstock; 297 (UP LE), TS Photography/Getty Images; 297 (UP RT), Noraluca013/Getty Images; 297 (CTR LE), onair/Shutterstock; 297 (CTR RT), xamtiw/Getty Images; 297 (LO LE), sirichai_asawalapsakul/Getty Images; 297 (LO RT), onair/Shutterstock; 298 (UP LE), gowithstock/Shutterstock; 298 (UP RT), Moving Moment/Shutterstock; 298 (LO LE), Pixel-Shot/Shutterstock; 298 (LO RT), Anna Hoychuk/Shutterstock; 299 (UP LE), Soifi/Shutterstock; 299 (UP RT), Etienne Voss/Getty Images; 299 (CTR LE), Kyselova Inna/Shutterstock; 299 (CTR RT), robynmac/Getty Images; 299 (LO LE), Moving Moment/Shutterstock; 299 (LO RT), Rtstudio/Shutterstock; 303, Naomi Fujiwara.